Bugs, Bowels, and Behavior

The Groundbreaking Story of The Gut-Brain Connection

Bugs, Bowels, and Behavior

The Groundbreaking Story of The Gut-Brain Connection

Edited by Teri Arranga,
Claire I. Viadro, MPH, PhD,
and Lauren Underwood, PhD

Foreword by Martha Herbert, PhD, MD

Skyhorse Publishing

Skyhorse Publishing books may be purchased in bulk at
special discounts for sales promotion, corporate gifts,
fundraising, or educational purposes. Special editions
can also be created to specifications. For details, contact
the Special Sales Department, Skyhorse Publishing,
307 West 36th Street, 11th Floor, New York, NY 10018
or info@skyhorsepublishing.com.

Skyhorse® and Skyhorse Publishing® are registered
trademarks of Skyhorse Publishing, Inc.®, a Delaware
corporation.

Visit our website at www.skyhorsepublishing.com

10 9 8 7 6 5 4 3 2 1

Library of Congress Cataloging-in-Publication Data
is available on file.

ISBN: 978-1-61608-736-4

Printed in the United States of America

Chapter 15 is excerpted from *Waging War on the Autistic
Child* by Andrew Wakefield (Skyhorse Publishing, 2012).
Used with permission.

To Ian, whose inspiration has brought forth education to me and to others for the good of children, families, and the public health.

~~ *Teri*

To David, Logan, and Casey, who have taught me so much about love – thank you for patiently tolerating my culinary and health explorations and filling my life with music.

~~ *Claire*

To Rachael, for inspiring me to be the person I am today; for all those who have been there for us along this journey (too many to name – you know who you are); and to Priya, who is always by my side.

~~ *Lauren*

ACKNOWLEDGEMENTS

Thanks are extended to Lauren Underwood, PhD, who kindly performed scientific editing and consulting for this book; Laurette Janak, who reviewed literature; Tony Lyons and Skyhorse Publishing for courage in journalism; the book's excellent designer, Fiona Mayne; AutismOne for support of this work; and all of the courageous clinicians and researchers of integrity who put the health of the public first.

Disclaimer
Information is not provided as medical advice. Patients/caregivers should research all information given. Every person's physiology is unique. All information should be discussed with the patient's personal physician and/or other specialist appropriate to the symptom(s) or body system(s) involved in their individual situation, who provides the patient with regular medical oversight, monitoring, and lab testing, and who keeps up-to-date on the most recent research and interventions. Beginning any significant biomedical or other interventions that may impact physiology or making changes to an established regimen should be discussed with the patient's physician in advance.

CONTENTS

BUGS, BOWELS, BRAINS, BEHAVIOR AND THE EMERGENCE OF BRAIN-BODY-PLANET MEDICINE

By Martha Herbert, PhD, MD

Bugs, bowels, brain, and behavior have been neatly packaged in separate domains of research. Brain and behavior have been linked, but bugs are only recently getting their fair share of attention regarding bowel health. Until not too long ago, linking bugs and bowels with brain and behavior would have been the last thing most behavioral or brain scientists would have imagined. Yet clinical challenges are forcing the issue, and the boundaries between domains are becoming permeable.

The way to build links across these domains is to dive deep under the surface. Our human eyes and other senses perceive human-scale phenomena, but our bodies don't have built-in microscopes or molecular analytics. These beneath-the-surface activities include the underlying levels of biology by which bugs influence the bowels and brain, and they shape how brain creates behavior.

People have often tended to simplify things into a linear stream of events. One of the most common is the idea that genes come first, then they create molecules, and then these molecules cause behaviors. This story about biology assumes that causation occurs in just one direction. It's easy to grasp, and it feels compelling because we hear so much about new genetic discoveries and how genes ostensibly "cause" problems in brain and behavior. But it leaves a lot of steps out of its narrative. Moreover, claims of genetic "causation" are coming apart with overwhelming evidence for greater degrees of complexity; this encourages us to see genes not as uniquely causative but as contributory, and it supports our appreciation of the influence of other types of contributors as well.[1]

Linking bugs, bowels, brain, and behavior is really a problem of multiscale systems biology. This refers to an emerging approach that is the broader scientific movement in which the exploration of bugs, bowels, brain, and behavior resides. The term "multiscale" highlights the many levels at which biological systems operate *simultaneously*. Bug biology, bowel biology, brain biology, and behavior all are in a dance with each other. Control does not come from any one level, but instead there is influence back and forth across many levels in a vastly complex multiscale interconnected web.

A related framework that helps understand the linkages tackled in this rich volume is the "middle-out" approach. Middle-out is neither top-down nor bottom-up. Denis Noble, in his eloquent book *The Music of Life,* uses musical metaphors to show the interplay among genes, multicellular harmonies, organs and systems in the body, and the brain.[2] In his view, genes don't "do" anything, and they don't "determine" things, but rather they set certain parameters that constrain the dance. In this framework, the action is at the physiological level, and behaviors are emergent properties that come out differently depending on the way the physiological dance plays out.

In this multiscale dance extravaganza, one of the critical questions is transduction—how do activities at one level turn into influences at another? A classical example is sensory transduction. We know a fair bit about how light turns into the colors, shapes, and movements we see: light enters the eye, where it triggers a complex computational cascade among a network of highly organized cells in the retina. This generates highly structured nerve impulses that then travel through the brainstem and then into the cerebral cortex through processing stations that make progressively more complex connections, first just with this visual information and then taking account of more and more other information as well. We can tell a similar story about how we hear: vibrations in the air are transduced into what we experience as sound by going through the eardrum into the middle ear, which excites the tiny pitch-sensitive hairs of the cochlea, gets its initial processing in the brainstem, and then gets further sorted out in the primary and associational auditory areas of the cerebral cortex.

In elucidating the links between bugs, bowels, brain, and behavior, we are literally fleshing out the mechanisms by which transduction across the different levels of activity in each of these levels actually occurs. Bugs can exert their influences through myriad mechanisms, such as chemical and immune. These mechanisms directly or indirectly affect the brain—and teasing out just how this influence occurs is at the core of the various chapters in this volume. Bugs in turn have their own behavior, this, in turn, is influenced by the milieu in which they operate—how resilient is the system? What is the nutritional status and how will this bias bug behavior? What are the properties of the foods passing through the gut, and how do they shape gut behavior? What sorts of toxic and electromagnetic modulation may be changing the biochemical, bioenergetic, and resonance properties altering cellular behavior? Are the intestinal villi healthy or worn down? Are the junctions between the cells tight or dysfunctional? How vibrant or vulnerable is the gut wall?

All of these influences on bugs and bowels are, in turn, influenced by brain and behavior (the choice between vegetables and candy has major bug/bowel consequences!)—and by the social, economic, biological, ecological, and physical properties of the world in which the bugs and the host reside. The brain also has myriad vulnerabilities that are impacted by bugs (and many other things as well). These vulnerable tissues and processes include brain blood flow, blood-brain barrier, neurotransmitters, neuron-glial interactions, and neuroinflammation. All of these influence the quality and extent of electrophysiological oscillatory synchrony, which is a fundamental and direct determinant of perception, emotion, cognition, and behavior. Thus, through changing the quality of function at so many levels, bugs and bowels can exert both direct and indirect influence on how the brain thinks and how it modulates our inner bodily regulation and our relations with the world around us. Whether all of these levels operate in harmony and optimal synchronization or whether the organization of their interconnections is disrupted, they are all in this together. This ensemble of harmonies and cacophonies produces our behaviors.

Presently, we are in an evolutionarily unprecedented multiscale planetary crisis. One dimension of this crisis is exposure of organisms to influences outside the boundaries of what their physiological systems are designed to handle. An organism pushed beyond its limits becomes weakened. A weakened organism does a poorer job of protecting its integrity against the very different agendas of bugs—it can't push back, maintain its boundaries, or keep things in balance. When the host is weak, bugs become more invasive, and the balance shifts in favor of their priorities. The cascade of influences creates palpable changes in brain, some of which are elaborated in this volume, and many more of which have not yet received scientific attention.

The process of going beyond a simple linear model to a complex multiscale model is daunting to our minds and belief systems. The world may have seemed more manageable when it was more neatly and discretely compartmentalized. The situation is further complicated by political and economic pressures to leave these connections unexamined since problems might be revealed that would put established institutions into an unfavorable light.

Reassuringly, issues of suffering and survival are trumping the compartmentalized approach. This book is a welcome, courageous, and path-breaking foray into this important bug-bowel-brain-behavior complexity. There is ever so much more to do and to study, and there is more complexity than we may ever fully understand. We may yet be outpaced by the biogeochemical chaos that our socioeconomic systems have unleashed, which we experience not only in our climate crisis and in the destruction of biological and cultural diversity, but also in our own bodies and brains. At this juncture, we need bold brain-body planet medicine. Toward that end, this book offers the kind of unbounded, integrated scientific and practical investigation that gives us hope of survival, reduction of suffering, and a move toward restoring systems integrity.

References

1. Krimsky S and J Gruber, Eds. (2013). *Genetic Explanations: Sense and Nonsense.* Cambridge, MA, Harvard University Press.
2. Noble D. (2006). *The Music of Life: Biology Beyond the Genome.* New York, Oxford University Press.

INTRODUCTION

By Lauren Underwood, PhD

You can ask anyone today whether they know someone with Alzheimer's disease, Parkinson's disease, or autism – conditions that affect various age groups and that result from neurological or immunological sequelae that were secondary to a primary insult – and chances are their answer will be affirmative. Why is this the case? Why is the incidence of chronic illness increasing, and do we know the cause of any of these conditions?

Here are a few dramatic statistics:

The Centers for Disease Control and Prevention (CDC) estimates 1 child in 88 with autism – 1 in 54 boys.[1] Notably, this is an increase from the CDC's 2004 Autism A.L.A.R.M.* A CDC report from the Autism Developmental Disabilities Monitoring Network stated:

> For decades, the best estimate for the prevalence of autism was 4 to 5 per 10,000 children. In 2004, CDC partnered with the American Academy of Pediatrics to issue an Autism A.L.A.R.M. to educate physicians about ASDs. At that time, data from several studies that used the current criteria for diagnosing autism and ASDs such as Asperger's disorder and Pervasive Developmental Disabilities found prevalence rates between 2 and 6 per 1,000 individuals. Put another way—data showed that as many as 1 in 166 children have an ASD. Studies in Europe and Scandinavia have found as many as 12 in 1,000 children with an ASD. Studies done in the United States over the past decade have found rates between 2 to 7 per 1,000 children. [2]

---

*A.L.A.R.M.: Autism is prevalent. Listen to parents. Act early. Refer. Monitor.

In addition to the 1 in 166 children with autism statistic, the A.L.A.R.M. also noted that "1 in 6 children are diagnosed with a developmental disorder and/or behavioral problem."

Therefore, according to the CDC's own numbers, there has been a notable rise in autism prevalence.

But that is not the extent of it.

As per a 2011 report in *Academic Pediatrics*:

> *An estimated 43% of US children (32 million) currently have at least 1 of 20 chronic health conditions assessed, increasing to 54.1% when overweight, obesity, or being at risk for developmental delays are included; 19.2% (14.2 million) have conditions resulting in a special health care need, a 1.6 point increase since 2003.*[3]

A 2011 study in *Pediatrics* concluded:

> *Developmental disabilities are common and were reported in ~ 1 in 6 children in the United States in 2006–2008. The number of children with select developmental disabilities (autism, attention deficit hyperactivity disorder, and other developmental delays) has increased, requiring more health and education services.*[4]

The real question to ask is why are so many people, most notably children, sick.

Do we know the cause of autism, and can this give us clues as to the origins of other conditions with neurological and immunological involvement? Although many spokespersons and media outlets say that the cause is not known, many distinguished researchers and clinicians do have biologically plausible theories concerning factors causal to the epidemic rise in autism. We know more today than we did 70 years ago when the medical condition known as autism was defined by Leo Kanner in his highly referenced paper *Autistic Disturbances of Affective Contact.*[5]

Introduction

In Kanner's paper, autism was described as a psychiatric disorder. This initial description of "infantile autism" became the standard that clinical psychiatrists used and continue to use to diagnose to the syndrome known as autism. What does that mean? It means that autism was defined solely as a mental condition. However, interestingly within the body of that paper, references related to eating and digestion included some of the following:

- *"Eating", the report said, "has always been a problem with him. He has never shown a normal appetite."*

- *He vomited all food from birth throughout the third month.*

- *He vomited a great deal during his first year, and feeding formulas were changed frequently with little success. He ceased vomiting when he was started on solid food.*

- *The father said: "The main thing that worries me is the difficulty in feeding. That is the essential thing, and secondly his slowness in development. During the first days of life he did not take the breast satisfactorily. After fifteen days he was changed from breast to bottle but did not take the bottle satisfactorily. There is a long story of trying to get food down. We have tried everything under the sun. He has been immature all along. At 20 months he first started to walk. He sucks his thumb and grinds his teeth quite frequently and rolls from side to side before sleeping. If we don't do what he wants, he will scream and yell."*

- *John was born September 19, 1937; his birth weight was 7½ pounds. There were frequent hospitalizations because of the feeding problem.*

- *Refusal of food. Donald, Paul ("vomited a great deal during the first year"), Barbara ("had to be tube-fed until 1 year of age"), Herbert, Alfred, and John presented severe feeding difficulty from the beginning of life.*

These references to issues related to both ingestion and digestion were described then, but they were never addressed or related to the original definition of autism. Then 20 years later, Dr. Bernard Rimland's groundbreaking book *Infantile Autism: The Syndrome and its Implications for a Neural Theory of Behavior*[6] suggested that there could be more to autism than simply what had been defined as a psychiatric disorder. This created a movement toward the understanding that autism is a neurological disorder—that is, it is a biological disorder versus being predominantly psychologically based.

To further substantiate, since the publication of Kanner's paper and Rimland's book, numerous studies have been done on autism, and within recent years, many of them identify specific medically based conditions that have been documented that routinely occur among individuals who have been diagnosed with autism. Clinical definitions of autism continue to evolve.

The *Diagnostic and Statistical Manual of Mental Disorders* (currently version DSM-IV-TR)[7] of the American Psychiatric Association, which provides health care professionals with the standard criteria used for the classification of mental disorders, includes autism in a broad category of pervasive developmental disorders. Again, this definition falls into the psychiatric diagnostic category rather than neurological and/or other general medical categories. But, interestingly, the description includes disruptive behavior, communication disorders, social disorders, and intellectual disability in some cases, as well as the display of numerous aberrant behaviors. So, when we acknowledge the real biological conditions underpinning an eventual autism diagnosis, we can see that so-called mental or psychological or behavioral issues can come downstream of physiological events not originating in the brain.

We especially look with interest and hope to the gut. With what scientific and medical research have uncovered in recent years as it relates to autism spectrum disorders and gastrointestinal conditions, there is a dire need to look beyond behavior because – on the most fundamental level – there is a direct relationship between gastrointestinal health, the brain, and behavior.

Consider the following: If you suffer from the stomach flu, food poisoning, or other pathogenic illness related to the gut, how well can you function at work? What interest do you have in talking to others? How well can you even formulate words? Do you feel like you're in a good mood? What do you think about most while your stomach is cramping? The nausea, the gas, the discomfort? Can you think clearly at all with this pain and distress? Practically everyone has had these feelings at some point. How can these visceral descriptions of how illness in the gut can affect an individual go unnoticed? How can it be said that there is not a direct correlation between the state of the bowel and the effect this can have upon behavior? It simply cannot. There IS a direct, definite, and often quite obvious connection.

In addition to the consequential pain from a pathological gut as described above, a gut in this state can correspondingly affect behavior in other ways: pathogenic organisms (aka bugs) and their byproducts can (1) provoke immunological and neurological reactions and (2) instigate a disease state (e.g., to tissue) in the gastrointestinal tract. This disease state can have associated physiological consequences that eventually adversely affect behavior (e.g., when chemical messengers of the immune system are released and result in an inflammatory response in the brain).

This is what *Bugs, Bowels, and Behavior: The Groundbreaking Story of the Gut-Brain Connection* illuminates for the reader: how the interrelationship between the gut and the brain, when disrupted, can lead to chronic illnesses, like autism, and how the results of these disturbances can have a profoundly altering influence upon behavior.

Bugs, bowels, and behavior as studied in the context of autism provide a platform from which similar applications can be related to other chronic illnesses. The evidence that is being compiled reveals the significance of the gut-brain-behavior connection in autism and can be, in some cases, directly correlated to biomedical findings associated with numerous other chronic conditions that have become global health issues.[8] It is known that pathogenic illness can sometimes lead to the expression of autoimmune-type diseases.[9] If there are biological traits that have been observed among individuals with autism who share similar underlying brain mechanisms and pathophysiologies with other chronic illnesses, like those associated with autoimmune diseases, then these other diagnoses may benefit from similar therapeutic categories and treatments. This revelation should be emphasized because, as previously stated, autism is not the only severe chronic illness that has exponentially increased in recent years: the occurrence of Alzheimer's disease, multiple sclerosis, Parkinson's disease, diabetes, schizophrenia, amyotrophic lateral sclerosis, and more – conditions that affect every race, walk of life, and age group – are also escalating. The biomedical similarities shared among autism and these other chronic illnesses cannot be ignored, and by uncovering the underlying mechanisms of their development, which are not yet fully understood, only then will we have the tools necessary to find cures.

References

1. Prevalence of Autism Spectrum Disorders — Autism and Developmental Disabilities Monitoring Network, 14 Sites, United States, 2008. (n.d.). *Centers for Disease Control and Prevention*. Retrieved February 2, 2013, from http://www.cdc.gov/mmwr/preview/mmwrhtml/ss6103a1.htm?s_cid=ss6103a1_w
2. *Centers for Disease Control and Prevention*. (n.d.). Retrieved February 2, 2013, from http://www.cdc.gov/ncbddd/autism/documents/autismcommunityreport.pdf
3. Bethell CD, Kogan MD, Strickland BB, Schor EL, Robertson J, Newacheck PW. (2011). A national and state profile of leading health problems and health care quality for US children: key insurance disparities and across-state variations. *Academic Pediatrics*, 11(3), S22-S33. Retrieved February 2, 2013, from http://www.sciencedirect.com/science/article/pii/S1876285910002500
4. Trends in the Prevalence of Developmental Disabilities in US Children, 1997–2008. (n.d.). *Pediatrics*. Retrieved February 2, 2013, from http://pediatrics.aappublications.org/content/early/2011/05/19/peds.2010-2989.abstract
5. Kanner L. (1943). Autistic disturbances of affective contact. *Nervous child*. 2(3), 217-250.
6. Rimland B. (1965). *Infantile Autism the Syndrome and Its Implications for a Neural Theory of Behaviour*. Taylor & Francis.
7. American Psychiatric Association. (2000). *Diagnostic and statistical manual of mental disorders* (4th ed., text rev.). Washington, DC: Author.
8. Tunstall-Pedoe H. (2006). Preventing Chronic Diseases. A Vital Investment: WHO Global Report. Geneva: World Health Organization, 2005. pp 200. CHF 30.00. ISBN 92 4 1563001. Also published on http://www. who. int/chp/chronic_disease_report/en. *International Journal of Epidemiology*. 35(4),1107.
9. Rose NR. (1998, February). The role of infection in the pathogenesis of autoimmune disease. In *Seminars in immunology* (Vol. 10, No. 1, pp. 5-13). Academic Press.

CHAPTER ONE

THE BIOCHEMICAL CONNECTION BETWEEN THE GUT AND THE BRAIN: HOW FOOD, BUGS, AND THE GUT BARRIER AFFECT HEALTH, BEHAVIOR, AND COGNITION

By Geri Brewster, RD, MPH, CDN

Introduction

The gut is made up of bugs, an informal term that Dictionary.com accurately defines as "any microorganism." Historically, we have for the most part lived in harmony with the bacteria, viruses, and fungal organisms that typically inhabit the gut (called the gastrointestinal microbiota), and these have played a vital role in maintaining human health. The rigors of the modern lifestyle have done much to restructure this once symbiotic relationship, resulting in a significantly disrupted gut environment. This altered environment not only gives us stomach aches but has far-reaching implications for the rest of our body—our brain included.

Comprised of hundreds of trillions of bacterial cells[1-3] and estimates of bacterial species ranging from the hundreds to the tens of thousands,[4-5] the gastrointestinal (GI) microbiota is unique, highly active, and performs numerous beneficial roles. The health of both the gut and the host is a function of the microbiota.[6] However, though the human body is colonized by multiple species of bacteria from mouth to anus,[7] many factors can affect microbial colonization, including birth procedure, diet, environment, health/disease status, medications, anatomy, host defenses, sex, and age.[8] Moreover, failure to acquire and develop a healthy microbiota during infancy may limit the extent to which a balanced,

1

stable microflora can be established later in life. Disruptions in gut flora can be responsible for a host of diseases as a result of overgrowth of pathogenic bacteria.[9] The gut's intricate connection to other areas of the body (through the immune, nervous, and endocrine systems) and its role as a barrier that protects the internal environment from harmful substances originating in the external world mean that an unhealthy gut can lead to health problems in unexpected places in the body.

The gut is also called the enteric nervous system (ENS) or "second brain."[10] The ENS contains about 100 million neurons—far fewer than the brain but many more than the spinal cord or peripheral nervous system—and these neurons exhibit a phenotypic diversity that is unparalleled. All types of central nervous system (CNS) neurotransmitters have been found in the ENS. Neural activity in the gut is triggered by digestion. Although "the brain in the head doesn't need to get its hands dirty with the messy business of digestion,"[10] bidirectional information continually passes between the gut and CNS. This suggests that at least some neurological and gastrointestinal conditions may have both gut and brain components.

It has been observed that while the brain in our head cannot exist without the brain in our gut, the brain in our gut (the ENS) can survive on its own.[10] Interesting, yes? In other words, the gut's independent nature means that the gut can function somewhat autonomously from the brain. Yet because our gut is made up of and substantially governed by bugs, and bugs and their byproducts in turn influence our brains and behavior, paying attention to these interconnected relationships is inherently necessary if we are to keep our entire bodies healthy and well.

Understanding the GI tract

When I think about the gut, I often wonder how many people actually possess an optimal gut environment. Some of the indicators of a properly functioning GI tract include having two bowel movements a day, feeling good after eating, sleeping soundly, having energy throughout the day, and experiencing no extreme mood swings or food cravings. In my experience, these indicators are all too rare. There is hardly a baby born these days who isn't being treated for either severe reflux, necessitating powerful acid blockers, or for constipation, creating an early reliance on laxatives. Even in adults without known gut issues, complaints of pain after eating or afternoon sluggishness are more and more common and increasingly accepted as normal.

The GI tract starts with the mouth and proceeds to the esophagus, stomach, duodenum, small intestine, large intestine (colon), rectum, and, finally, anus. It is the primary barrier between the outside world and the body's internal environment. As the body's gatekeeper, the gut has to constantly analyze everything that goes in to determine what is helpful or harmful. If something is determined to be helpful, the gut absorbs it through the circulatory or lymph systems for the body to use. Gut-associated lymphoid tissue (GALT) is the army responsible for the task of determining what gets absorbed. Conversely, the gut gets rid of anything assessed to be harmful.

GALT interfaces with the small intestine. This interface then affects the entire body via the bloodsteam. From the small intestines, fluids collect in the portal vein and are delivered to the liver. This pathway is the major entry point for water-soluble nutrients such as amino acids, short-chain fatty acids, and water-soluble vitamins. However, because 70 percent of lymph tissue in the body is associated with the gut as GALT, the lymph system provides a secondary route of entry into the body from the intestines. The lymph system is a network that transports chyle (a milky fluid containing products of digestion) and white blood cells throughout the body via the bloodstream.

GALT can be thought of as an immune system in the gut, located beneath the epithelium (cells lining the GI tract) and abundant with lymphocytes and macrophages that fight off the potentially harmful viruses, bacteria, and other microorganisms that constantly plague this area of the body.[11] The populations of immune and inflammatory cells that colonize the enteric immune system are constantly changing in response to luminal conditions and during pathophysiologic states.[12] Through constant vigilance, GALT differentiates commensal (non-harmful) food and bacterial antigens (foreign molecules) from pathogenic antigens. Because GALT is responsible for determining whether or not an antigen that has made it through harsh stomach acid and survived intestinal enzymatic breakdown and microbial defenses will provoke a homeostatic or immune response in the body, GALT development (which is influenced by intestinal microbes) must remain strong. Interestingly, the gut's initial response to a substance is the same whether the substance is healthy or pathogenic; the microbiota, which influences GALT, is what determines whether the final response will be tolerogenic (producing immunological tolerance) or immunogenic (producing an immune response). In short, it is up to the GALT to inhibit the development of allergy or autoimmunity.[13]

To further understand how the gut's immune system functions, it is helpful to be familiar with the term "oral tolerance." Oral tolerance refers to the body's ability to differentiate between pathogens that enter the body through the GI tract and elicit an appropriate immune response versus the diverse group of dietary proteins and compounds that should not normally trigger an immune response. Oral tolerance to dietary antigens is maintained by three different mechanisms: anergy (a state of immune unresponsiveness), cell deletion, and immune suppression. In the presence of a stressor and infection, oral tolerance can break down, allowing GALT to react to the antigens. This, in turn, causes proinflammatory compounds to build up, prompts opening of the tight junctions between the small intestinal cells, allows antigens to enter into circulation, and triggers the subsequent production of IgA, IgG, IgM, and IgE antibodies.[14] Some of the antibodies created in response to this inflammatory cascade get released into the bloodstream and cross the blood-brain barrier, where they can affect brain chemistry and behavior.[15]

Antigens come in many forms. Some oral antigens, like those created from the fluid of lysed (broken down) bacterial cells, furnish one example of how the above process works. These oral antigens, from the lysed cells, can reduce the frequency of diarrhea, mucosal infection, and diverticulitis by increasing IgA and cytokines at the mucosal and luminal levels. While provoking this type of response suggests a mild inflammatory state, it is an appropriate reaction in order to minimize diarrhea and a more aggravated response. In other words, the presence of these antigens and the reaction they provoke will stimulate an immune reaction to prevent a worse response.

Sometimes, food antigens can induce an immunogenic response, especially when presented in the gut with an adjuvant. An adjuvant is an immunological agent that increases the antigenic response. Even chronic infection or inflammation can become adjuvants, perpetuating the cycle of immunogenic responses. This may lead to multiple food allergies or sensitivities.[13]

A heavy metal contained in a pesticide and presenting to the gut with a food antigen can serve as an adjuvant and can stimulate an immune reaction, or if gut inflammation already exists, further inflammation will ensue. Thus, a viscious cycle can begin to occur. In this way, even seemingly benign foods can aggravate the gut.

The GI barrier, gut flora, and inflammatory disease

According to Fasano and Shea-Donohue, the gastrointestinal tract acts as a barrier that finely regulates the trafficking of macromolecules between the external (food, microbes) and internal (systemic, cells, tissues, and so forth) environments.[16] The intestinal mucosal barrier heavily influences the immune response that begins with and results from antigen interaction. If this complex intestinal barrier is broken, foreign molecules can enter, interact with the immune system, and launch an inflammatory response that can lead to a multitude of local intestinal as well as systemic extraintestinal diseases. This concept of a leaky gut or poor barrier function as the initiating trigger for autoimmune disease[17] has gained increasing acceptance.

The functions of normal gut flora are numerous (see Table 1). For this reason, many experts in the field suggest that the gut flora be considered an accessory organ. Perturbations in the gut microbiota can result in a lack of immunoregulation or mucosal tolerance, thereby facilitating the overgrowth of pathogenic microbes and the production of inflammation, particularly in genetically susceptible individuals.[18] Mucosal tolerance is essential to health.[19] When mucosal surfaces such as the GI tract are in a state of balance, they are nonreactive to antigens (whether "self" or "nonself "), and there is no inflammation. This balance involves a complex process of anergy of reactive T cells and induction of regulatory T cells.[20] When there is a loss of mucosal tolerance, the ensuing breakdown in innate immune system functions initiates inflammation. Although inflammation is an essential immune response to an injury or pathogen, ongoing inflammation can contribute to the pathogenesis of a disease condition. The effector T cells of the adaptive immune system potentiate inflammation.[21] Because the gut flora shape intestinal immune responses during both health and

Table 1. Selected functions of healthy gut flora

Functions	Description
Detoxification	Produce cytochrome P450-like enzymes Protect against environmental toxins (e.g., mercury, pesticides, pollution)
Digestion	Break down carbohydrates, sugars, and oxalates Break down dietary fiber Deconjugate primary bile acid Balance intestinal pH
Elimination	Regulate peristalsis and bowel movements Combat diarrhea
Immunity	Modulate immune system and gut-brain connection Promote/support Th1 immunity and immune cells Prevent overgrowth of pathogenic bacteria and yeast Exert antimutagenic and antitumor effects
Inflammation	Produce mucus Modulate leaky gut, thereby reducing inappropriate gut luminal content/immune interactions and reducing immune-mediated inflammation both locally and at a distance
Metabolic effects	Produce short-chain fatty acids Produce and synthesize vitamins (e.g., B vitamins, vitamin K) Assimilate minerals Regulate fat, triglyceride, and cholesterol levels

disease, the bacterial communities in the gut are intimately linked to the proper functioning of the immune system.[6]

The immune responses that arise when the gut flora and mucosal barrier are disturbed are increasingly likely explanations for the high incidence of inflammatory disease in industrialized countries,[9] including perhaps autism spectrum disorders (ASDs). Researchers have identified neuroinflammation in ASD individuals.[22] As shown in Table 2, gut inflammation and a compromised microbiota (referred to as gut dysbiosis) have been associated with a wide variety of GI and systemic health disorders.

Table 2. Some disease conditions associated with gut inflammation

Disease condition
Alcoholic liver disease[23]
Asthma[24]
Atherosclerosis[25]
Chronic fatigue syndrome (CFS)[26]
Eczema[27]
Heart failure[28]
Inflammatory bowel disease (IBD)[29]
Insulin resistance[30] and Type 1 diabetes[31,32]
Irritable bowel syndrome (IBS)[33]
Metabolic syndrome[34]
Obesity[35]
Systemic and localized inflammation[36]

Table 3. Inflammatory conditions of the GI tract

Organ	Inflammatory condition
Mouth	Oral allergy syndrome
Esophagus	Eosinophilic esophagitis, esophagitis
Stomach	Gastritis, ulcers (can be caused by hyperchlorhydria) Gastric polyps (can be caused by hypochlorhydria)
Small intestine	Dysbiosis (microbial imbalance) Small intestinal bacterial overgrowth (SIBO) IBS - pain distention IBD - Crohn's disease Celiac disease
Large intestine	IBS - spastic colon, irritable colon, mucous colitis, spastic colitis IBD - ulcerative colitis

The causes of gut inflammation are complex. Many factors have the potential to create an inflammatory environment in the gut. These include a poor diet, food intolerances or sensitivities, allergies, gut disease, toxins, an unhealthy gut flora, and medications such as antibiotics, proton pump inhibitors (PPIs), and nonsteroidal anti-inflammatory drugs (NSAIDs). Moreover, a number of other inflammatory conditions (listed in Table 3) directly affect the GI tract. Some of the conditions (such as Crohn's disease and celiac disease) are bowel disorders known for causing increased intestinal permeability, a condition in which damaged intestines allow substances to pass through that otherwise shouldn't.

Gut inflammation that is left untreated and worsened by poor diet and external factors previously mentioned can intensify and perpetuate the disease process. Take, for example, some of the more common sequelae of gut inflammation. Gut dysbiosis secondary to antibiotic therapy may lead to gastroesophageal reflux disease (GERD). If not treated, GERD can lead to esophagitis, which can advance to Barrett's esophagus and, ultimately, to esophageal cancer.[37,38] In this example, the inflammation is contained (at least initially) to sequelae within organs of the gut. However, because the gut has a systemic influence on the body in its day-to-day functions, gut inflammation and the intestinal permeability that results have the potential to create inflammation throughout the rest of the body. Systemic diseases associated with increased intestinal permeability include inflammatory joint disease, rheumatoid arthritis, ankylosing spondylitis, Reiter's syndrome, chronic dermatological conditions, schizophrenia, and allergic disorders.[39,40]

Gut, brain, and body
In 1999, the journal *Gut* published an article on neurogastroenterology, described as "a new and advancing subspecialty of clinical gastroenterology and digestive science."[12] Neurogastroenterologists examine the interactions of the CNS, including the brain, with the gastrointestinal tract. Alongside a focus on the neural and endocrine influences on the GI tract, this emerging discipline considers the ENS.

Traditionally, the primary focus of the field of gastroenterology was to describe the genesis of functional gastrointestinal disease.

However, as we have seen, the inflammatory cascade that is ignited in the GI tract by offending substances that trigger an enteric reaction has body-wide implications. Moreover, enteric glial cells and mast cells communicate with the CNS.[41] The enteric glia control gastrointestinal functions and certain neurotransmitter precursors and may serve as a link between the nervous and immune systems of the gut. They synthesize cytokines and appear to be involved in the etiopathogenesis of various pathological processes in the gut, particularly those with neuroinflammatory or neurodegenerative components.[42] In 2005, Pardo and colleagues demonstrated the presence of neuroglial and innate neuroimmune system activation in the brain tissue and cerebrospinal fluid of persons with autism.[43]

The ENS performs a triage role with the flow of information that begins with immune detection and signal transfers from the host of dietary antigens, toxins, bacteria, viruses, and yeast with which it interfaces on a daily basis. This is the basis for the neuroimmunophysiologic communication that exists as enteric neurons are activated. The GI tract, when immunologically challenged, can release various cytokines that can lead to an increase in corticotropin-releasing hormone (CRH), which is involved in the stress response. This, in turn, can affect the CNS, the hypothalamic-pituitary-adrenal (HPA) axis, and the peripheral nervous system. Translocation of bacteria or lipopolysaccharides into a damaged gastrointestinal lining can also alter the HPA axis. This complex system of stressors, antigens, cytokines, and cortisol forms a multifaceted communication network together with the neurological and neuroendocrine systems, all originating in the gut.[44]

The gut-brain connection and gluten
At this point, it may no longer surprise you that the gut is connected to the brain. Have you ever had a "gut feeling" that something was wrong, a slightly unsettled knot in your belly that seems to say that something is amiss? Or had bad dreams after a large dinner? Or experienced brain fog after eating cake? These are just a few well-known examples of the gut-brain connection. Even Charles Dickens was familiar with this topic and, as long ago as the 1800s, used the gut-brain connection as a literary device. Dickens' character Scrooge, when faced with the

ghost of Jacob Marley, did not initially believe in the ghost but blamed the vision on something he had eaten (undigested beef or an underdone potato) that had affected his senses.

To further illustrate the gut-brain relationship, it is worth considering the potential impact of gluten ingestion on the gut, brain autoantibodies, and behavior. In the 1950s and 1960s, doctors found that neurological conditions improved in some psychosis and celiac disease patients when gluten was removed from their diets.[45] Several decades later, in the early 1990s, Reichelt and Knivsberg found abnormal substances that resembled opioid peptides in the urine of autistic people.[46] These peptides were thought to originate from the incomplete breakdown of food, given that their levels exceeded what the CNS could produce on its own. This work resulted in what is now known as the opioid excess theory.[47] This theory states that the incomplete breakdown of gluten and casein produces two different peptides that are known to have opioid activity in the body, namely gluteomorphins (from gluten) and casomorphins (from casein).[46] These peptides are able to escape the gut in the presence of intestinal permeability. The peptides are then able to cross the blood-brain barrier and cause neurological problems.[48]

In a review article in 2002, Knivsberg and colleagues demonstrated that children with autism and urinary peptide abnormalities experienced improvements in social connectedness, willingness to learn, and ability to make transitions after one year on a gluten-free/casein-free diet.[48] Later, Reichelt and Knivsberg wrote a thorough review affirming both the possibility and probability of a gut-brain connection in autism.[49] They conclude that diet affects behavior, which can be correlated to excreted compounds.[49]

One factor that the opioid excess theory fails to recognize is that children with ASD (as well as other individuals) may react to gluten and casein in metabolically different ways. According to a body of work by celiac researcher Dr. Alessio Fasano,[50] there are two distinct categories of individuals who experience difficulty with gluten. The first category includes people with "gluten sensitivity," who experience inflammation from gluten even though they do not initially have visible intestinal damage. People with celiac disease (CD), on the other hand, have an autoimmune reaction to gluten that damages the intestines. The difference between these two conditions stems from how the immune system responds to gluten. Where gluten sensitivity is present, the innate immune system—the body's first line of defense against invaders—responds to gluten ingestion by fighting the gluten directly. This creates inflammation both inside and outside of the digestive system. In those who are gluten-sensitive, gluten has been demonstrated to reduce the tight junctions that serve a barrier function in the gut.[50] Moreover, Fasano's group has shown that the protein zonulin increases intestinal permeability by decreasing tight cellular junctions and that gluten in certain individuals stimulates zonulin production.[51] In the case of celiac disease, both the innate immune system and the adaptive immune system (a more advanced, sophisticated part of the immune system) are involved. However, people with CD and individuals with gluten sensitivity experience near-identical symptoms, including diarrhea, bloating, abdominal pain, joint pain, depression, brain fog, and migraines.[50]

In studying gut permeability and mucosal immune gene expression in individuals with CD and gluten sensitivity, Fasano and colleagues reported that only 57% of those identified as gluten-sensitive carried DQ2 or DQ8 genes, the genes that are tested for when determining gluten metabolism disorders.[50] This finding indicates that those two genes are less involved in gluten sensitivity than they are in celiac disease.[50] On the blood tests, just under half (48%) of those diagnosed as gluten-sensitive had positive antigliadin antibodies (AGA-IgA) or AGA-IgG blood tests, showing that they were making antibodies to the gluten in their diet.[50] AGA-IgA and AGA-IgG are antibodies that the body produces in response to gluten. What is interesting is that little more than half of the gluten-sensitive group carried CD genes, while the rest did not, indicating that the genes are not necessary for the body to produce the AGA. The study also found that none of the participants labeled as gluten-sensitive produced tTG-IgA (tissue transglutaminase antibody) or EMA-IgA (endomysial antibody), which are antibodies very specific to celiac disease that indicate when the body is attacking its own tissue in an autoimmune reaction.

The important take-home message of Fasano's work is the observation that even persons who don't have celiac disease can still be damaged by gluten. As the authors conclude, "In itself, the absence of autoantibodies [the autoimmune antibodies produced in CD but not in gluten sensitivity] and intestinal lesions does not rule out the intrinsic toxicity of gluten, whose intake, even in non-CD individuals, has been associated with damage to other tissues, organs and systems besides the intestine."[50] It's validating to hear a leading expert in celiac disease acknowledge what many of us have witnessed all along: gluten sensitivity or intolerance potentially can wreck your health even if you're not officially diagnosed with CD, and gluten can negatively impact thought, functions, and behaviors. It is not surprising that research over the past several decades has demonstrated that gluten elimination has improved schizophrenia symptoms in some patients.[52] In a recent double-blind, randomized, placebo-controlled rechallenge trial, Biesiekierski and colleagues found that non-CD patients with IBS also claimed considerable improvement in gut symptoms with the institution of a gluten-free diet, further supporting the concept of non-celiac-related gluten sensitivity.[53]

The accumulated evidence indicates that both gluten sensitivity and celiac disease can also exist even in the absence of verified enteropathy and can affect many organs. Studies have identified gluten-related immunological pathogenesis in the joints, bones, heart, thyroid, cerebellum, and in neuronal synapsin I, a protein responsible for synaptogenesis (the formation of synapses) and neurotransmitter release.[54] Gluten ataxia has also been found to be 30 times higher in patients with celiac disease than in the general population.[25] Ultimately, the production of autoantibodies in response to gluten may result in neuroimmune dysregulation and autoimmunity.[54]

Gastrointestinal dysfunction and ASD

Autism is a condition where there is increasingly strong evidence of a gut-brain connection and evidence that healing the gut will help heal the condition. Autism is classified as a behaviorally defined syndrome by the current edition of the *Diagnostic and Statistical Manual of Mental Disorders* (DSM-IV-TR).[55] As discussed below, however, a growing body of evidence suggests that ASD is much more than is covered by the DSM-IV-TR definition. Many knowledgeable researchers and practitioners currently consider ASD to be a systemic disorder that involves immune, neuroimmune, metabolic, gene expression, and gastrointestinal dysfunction.[56]

Nearly every day, my practice and discussions with other practitioners confirm the view of ASD as a systemic disorder. I regularly see children diagnosed with ASD presenting with gut issues, asthma, eczema, food allergies, sleep irregularities, anxiety, and perseverative behaviors. In addition, their parents tell stories about frequent illness and poor dietary histories and a lifetime of exposure to agricultural and other chemicals, biotechnology, medications, and other toxins. In these situations, my goal is to implement dietary strategies that aim toward healing the gut, while enhancing and supporting the body's natural healing and detoxification efforts. Invariably, gastrointestinal dysfunction winds up at the center of my treatment for ASD.

The link between gastrointestinal dysfunction and ASD is not a new concept. Leo Kanner, the psychiatrist and physician whose studies helped form the foundation of modern understandings and approaches to autism, described what seemed to be GI disturbances in many of the subjects profiled in his 1943 paper "Autistic disturbances of affective contact."[57] Eating problems, infant vomiting, large tonsils, and poor nursing are some of the descriptions Kanner used when presenting his case histories. In a 1971 study, Goodwin and coauthors found that six of the fifteen autistic children they studied had bulky, odorous, or loose stools or intermittent diarrhea, and one had celiac disease.[58] In 1999, endoscopic examinations of 36 autistic children with intestinal symptoms showed that over two-thirds of the children had reflux esophagitis (69%) and/or chronic duodenal inflammation (67%), and a sizeable proportion (42%) had chronic gastritis.[59]

In 2006, Valicenti-McDermott evaluated ASD and family autoimmune disease and found that 70% of children with ASD had GI issues compared with 42% of children with a developmental disorder other than ASD.[60] More recently, in a 2010 consensus report, Buie and a group of experts concluded that "gastrointestinal disorders and associated symptoms are commonly reported in individuals with ASD, but key issues such as the prevalence and best treatment of these conditions are incompletely understood."[61] These studies confirm that something more than behavior is going on in children with ASD: some form of gut dysfunction seems to be present.

A 2002 study that examined the GI flora of children with late-onset autism found that ASD children harbored more clostridial species bacteria than control children.[62] When fed a diet of sugar and refined carbohydrates, clostridia produce propionic acid (PPA), a short-chain fatty acid.[63] PPA is also a food preservative found in bread products. Considering the effects of clostridial species overgrowth, a 2008 study demonstrated how PPA produced from clostridia resulted in negative social behaviors in rat models.[63] Specifically, intraventricular infusions of PPA produced reversible repetitive dystonic behaviors, hyperactivity, turning behavior, retropulsion, caudate spiking, and the progressive development of limbic kindled seizures, all of which suggest that this compound has CNS effects. Moreover, this group of researchers noted that PPA produces brain and behavioral abnormalities similar to symptoms observed in human autism.[64] In more recent research, these authors reported that immunohistochemical analysis of brain tissue from PPA rats revealed an innate neuroinflammatory response as a result of the exposure to PPA. This demonstrates a direct influence of a gut compound on behavior.[65] As summarized by the lead researcher involved in this work, Dr. Derrick MacFabe:[66]

> PPA is actively taken up by specific [...] transporters in the gut, cerebral vasculature, and CNS neurons and glia. PPA has a number of interesting neurobiological effects on receptor activation, neurotransmitter release, pH, cholesterol/fatty acid metabolism, mitochondrial function, and immune system activation, making it an ideal compound linking diet, digestive system function, and bacterial infection with ASD.

These studies, which focus on the proliferation of pathogenic bacteria and the organic acids they produce, provide a persuasive framework for beginning to understand the link between the gut flora and behavior as well as cognition.[65] There are several other examples of the relationship between the gut flora and cognition:

- Evidence of a verbal IQ decrement in both IBD and IBS patients when measured against healthy controls as well as the patients' own pre-disease IQ scores, with a particularly pronounced verbal IQ deficit in the IBD patients.[67]

- Presence of psychiatric disorders (especially major depression and anxiety) in up to 94% of IBS patients (and frequent overlap of IBS with fibromyalgia and CFS), with evidence that cognitive-behavioral therapy is effective in IBS sufferers.[68]

- Relief of neurocognitive symptoms, such as short-term memory loss and ability to concentrate, in patients with CFS following reestablishment of gut flora through a probiotic combination containing *Lactobacillus acidophilus* (*L. acidophilus*), *Bifidobacterium infantis* (*B. infantis*), and *Bifidobacterium longum* (*B. longum*).[69]

Healing the gut: probiotics

Could a positive shift in one's microbiota help to reverse some of the conditions described in this chapter? A review of the literature seems to suggest that the answer is yes. According to Fasano and Shea-Donohue, the autoimmune process can be arrested if the interplay between genes and environmental triggers is prevented by re-establishing intestinal barrier function, in part through "novel treatment strategies, such as the use of probiotics."[16]

Probiotics, once considered heretical, are now regarded as mainstream. Over 700 randomized, controlled human studies have been conducted on probiotics and various probiotic strains, yielding strong clinical support for their use in both the prevention and treatment of gastrointestinal disorders and metabolic syndrome.[70] Each strain has demonstrated unique characteristics in improving human immune response, with implications for the nervous and endocrine systems as well. Moreover, probiotic formulations may help both gastrointestinal and systemic conditions. Probiotics can counteract adverse changes in intestinal barrier function, visceral sensitivity, and gut motility. They can also decrease inflammatory cytokines, thereby positively influencing mood in patients whose emotional symptoms and inflammatory immune chemicals are elevated. In one controlled animal study that supported the role of probiotics as a potential antidepressant, *B. infantis* significantly reduced cytokine levels of IFN-gamma, TNF-alpha, and IL-6, and markedly increased plasma concentrations of tryptophan, the precursor to serotonin.[71]

Although most people are aware of probiotics, many assume that purchasing probiotics from the local drugstore or consistently eating yogurt is all it takes to reestablish a balanced flora. Typically, it is not that simple. The intricacy of the gut flora means that just taking a probiotic and "calling it a day" is generally insufficient for the maintenance of intestinal health. Starving out the "bad" bugs through a diet low in simple sugars and flooding the system with "good" bugs is important but may not always get the job done. To truly modify the gut flora, it may be necessary to dig into the communities of microorganisms living in the gut to alter the composition of the existing bacterial population. Many species of microorganisms within the human body are protected within communities called biofilms.[8] If you are curious as to what a biofilm is, just imagine brushing your teeth. Each morning after you brush, your teeth feel squeaky clean; after an hour or so, however, they start to feel a bit slick. This slickness is a polysaccharide film (or biofilm) that the bacteria in your mouth create to protect themselves so that they can stay put. The same thing happens in the gut with the exception that the gut biofilm is not being constantly broken down and rebuilt as with tooth brushing. Biofilms house and shield the gut bacteria (whether good or bad) from invaders, acting as powerful protectors that can be very hard to penetrate. Because gut biofilms can be layers deep and hard to reach, a complex protocol may be needed to promote a more immune-friendly and immune-supportive gut environment.

Effective biofilm protocols involve an individualized set of tools that can take weeks or months to achieve their full effect. I often liken these protocols to the process of gardening. If you picture the terrain of your gut as hard ground, polysaccharide enzymes may first be sent in to turn over the biofilm as a pitchfork turns over soil. Next, antimicrobials are used to clean out the clumps and rocks (the bad bugs). At this stage, prebiotics (food for the good bugs) can be sent in to fertilize the gut, finally allowing probiotics (the good bugs or "seeds") to be planted. Other healthcare practitioners may prefer a different protocol or order of operations, but the important thing is to address biofilms with a qualified, attentive healthcare professional due to the pathogenic nature of many of the bugs present.

Healing the gut: food as medicine
There is no doubt that diet has a major effect on the gut flora. Dietary

factors can shape the gut environment for the proliferation of both beneficial and pathogenic bacteria. For example, fermented foods can provide both prebiotics (nondigestible food ingredients that stimulate the growth and activity of bacteria) and probiotics. Animal products provide nutrients such as essential fatty acids and vitamins A and D, which support innate immunity and are required for the balance of T regulatory and T helper cells. Sugars and refined flour products, on the other hand, feed pathogenic bacteria.

There is much in the literature to support the belief in food as medicine.[72] In my practice, I have used this philosophy of healing to work with children suffering from developmental disorders, including ASDs. Given my experience, I am frequently invited to speak on the topic at health conferences. My lectures on nutritional interventions and ASD often begin with a review of the literature establishing the presence of GI inflammation in many children diagnosed with ASD.[61] This evidence persuasively suggests that GI inflammation may exacerbate ASD symptoms and, conversely, that dietary interventions can ameliorate GI inflammation in at least some children, improving overall outcomes.[61]

As a nutritionist, no one believes more strongly than I that "you are what you eat." I grew up in the 1960s and '70s, when people were becoming alarmingly concerned over environmental pollutants and the adulteration of the food supply. Even as a child, it seemed inherently wrong to me to put synthetic foodstuffs into my body. How would my body use these chemicals? Wouldn't chemicals just pollute my body in the same way that the environment was being polluted? It was clear that the environment was suffering—wouldn't I suffer, too, if I ate chemical foods? My mother shared these concerns. Diagnosed with multiple sclerosis in the late '50s, when medicine had little to offer except muscle relaxants, she began pursuing what was ultimately considered alternative treatment. Dietary, oral, and intramuscular vitamin therapies were the cornerstones of her treatment, followed in the '70s by amalgam removal, chelation, hyperbaric oxygen therapy, chiropractic work, and acupuncture, to name a few. The efficacy of these treatments confirmed my early intuition that, simply stated, what you put in your body directly affects your ultimate health and well-being.

This realization led me to passionately study human nutrition and foods. As my understanding of nutritional biochemistry and disease deepened, it would disturb me when a parent would say, "My doctor said to feed him whatever he'll eat. His diet has no relevance to his condition." Even today, I hear this! I find it tragic that so much potential healing is being turned away simply because many healthcare practitioners equate nutritional health with deficiency diseases of previous centuries. They can't imagine that in this "land of plenty" our diets may be causally related to a child's developmental disabilities, or that nutrition can be used to improve symptoms, prevent the exacerbation or progression of developmental disease and, quite possibly, heal. Medicine seems to have lost sight of its healing mission and has become the practice of symptom suppression. Although this type of practice is valuable in certain situations, I still believe in healing the body and using food as its medicine.

Other dietary influences

Numerous dietary factors can negatively influence inflammatory status. For example, a year after a study reported on food additives and hyperactive behavior in a community sample of 3-year-old and 8- and 9-year-old children,[73] the European Union banned the use of some artificial colors in foodstuffs. Moreover, anyone suffering from a reaction to monosodium glutamate (MSG) can tell you that there is a very definite and immediate connection between the gut and the brain. Glutamates, including MSG, are excitotoxins that overstimulate neurons. Persons with autism have been found to have increased serum glutamate levels.[74] Studies have also found a significant increase in reports of headache and subjectively reported pericranial muscle tenderness after oral administration of MSG.[75] Might some of these reactions be the result of more permeable guts? Possibly.

The increase in world omega-6 consumption over the past century can be considered another very large and uncontrolled dietary experiment that may be contributing to the increased societal burdens of aggression, depression, and cardiovascular mortality.[76] Compensating for the omega-6 to omega-3 imbalance in our diet has yielded favorable results in some studies, such as a small pilot study suggesting that supplementation with high-dose EPA/DHA concentrates may improve behavior in children with attention-deficit/hyperactivity disorder (ADHD).[77] In the study, significant improvements were seen in inattention, hyperactivity, oppositional/defiant behavior, and conduct disorder.

But why are we always playing catch up? At nearly every turn, we find the influence of diet on behavior already amply documented in the literature. In May 2009, an American Academy of Environmental Medicine (AAEM) position paper called for a moratorium on genetically modified (GM) foods,[78] stating that "several animal studies indicate serious health risks associated with GM food," including changes in the gastrointestinal system. The specificity of the association between GM foods and particular disease processes is also supported by animal studies showing significant immune dysregulation, including upregulation of cytokines associated with asthma, allergy, and inflammation.[79,80] GM foods have been shown to cause translocation of gut flora DNA, thereby altering immune response.[81] The evidence is so convincing regarding this particular dietary variable that the AAEM called on physicians "to educate their patients, the medical community, and the public to avoid GM foods when possible and provide educational materials concerning GM foods and health risks." The AAEM also called for long-term independent studies and labeling, concluding that "there is more than a casual association between GM foods and adverse health effects" and that "there is causation" as defined by recognized scientific criteria.

Eliminating common food allergens has also been shown to benefit children's behavior. Interestingly, many common food allergens (such as corn, soy, and wheat) happen to be the most commonly genetically modified foods. Milk is another common food allergen, and conventional milk comes from cows being fed a diet of GM corn and soy. (In marketing language, this constitutes a "vegetarian-fed" cow, which always perplexes me, given that, the last time I checked, cows were herbivores and *should* be eating a "vegetarian" diet.) In a recent study, 64% of children diagnosed with ADHD were actually experiencing a hypersensitivity to food.[82] The study showed that a strictly supervised and restricted elimination diet can be a valuable instrument to assess whether ADHD is induced by food.

Summing up

The deluge of chronic disease being diagnosed in the youngest and most vulnerable members of society demands attention and action. The compelling examples of the gut-bugs-brain connection provided in this chapter also point to the need for ongoing research into the causation of these diseases, including mental health and developmental conditions. However, I believe that enough evidence already exists to suggest we need not wait for the results of this research to begin to initiate change. When diet and microbiota are in concert with the body, the enteric nervous system does not get stimulated into an inflammatory state. It stands to reason, then, that body-wide inflammation such as that occurring in the brain and central nervous system of children with autism can likely be improved through diet. From my perspective, the research adequately demonstrates that the way to build a better brain is through the gut and gut microbiota. It truly may be as simple as changing one side of the equation (what we eat) to affect the other side of the equation (our symptoms).

In the same way that what a mother consumes during gestation is known to influence her baby's neurological development, it appears to me that everything that her baby consumes after birth has to be regarded as important, with the utmost respect given to the gut, in particular. For centuries, the gut was recognized as the least mature organ in a full-term baby, and wet nurses or goat's milk were always at the ready to help soothe a colicky infant. As fragile as the gut is, it is also the most difficult system to repair. Prevention therefore is key, which is why regard for diet and respect for the exquisite complexity of this organ are paramount. The gut is the interface for the health of the entire body, and healing the GI tract can have effects on all body systems. There already exists a great body of knowledge, a very small portion of which I have touched on in this chapter, to suggest that a restoration of respect for the natural order of things needs to be supported, beginning with a less adulterated food supply and support of a healthy gastrointestinal tract.

Evidence supports the promise of a healthier future with a better gut microbiota. It has been a longtime hope of mine that we could give the infants born today a better opportunity to develop an optimum gut microbiota by innoculating their oral cavities with beneficial flora at birth. This would be comparable to the practice of giving infants eye drops (silver nitrate a couple of centuries ago, antibiotic drops now) to prevent potentially blinding eye infections from bacteria contracted during the birth process. While childhood blindness seemed reason enough to begin giving eye prophylaxis at birth, is not the deluge of chronic childhood disease associated with gut-bug-brain inflammation enough to warrant a probiotic boost? I think so.

References

1. Ley RE, Peterson DA, Gordon JI. Ecological and evolutionary forces shaping microbial diversity in the human intestine. *Cell* 124: 837–48, 2006.
2. Savage DC. Microbial ecology of the gastrointestinal tract. *Annu Rev Microbiol* 31: 107–33, 1977.
3. Whitman WB, Coleman DC, Wiebe WJ. Prokaryotes: the unseen majority. *Proc Natl Acad Sci USA* 95: 6578–83, 1998.
4. Xu J, Gordon JI. Inaugural article: honor thy symbionts. *Proc Natl Acad Sci USA* 100: 10452–9, 2003.
5. Frank DN, St Amand AL, Feldman RA, Boedeker EC, Harpaz N, Pace NR. Molecular-phylogenetic characterization of microbial community imbalances in human inflammatory bowel diseases. *Proc Natl Acad Sci USA* 104: 13780–5, 2007.
6. Round JL, Mazmanian SK. The gut microbiota shapes intestinal immune responses during health and disease. *Nat Rev Immunol.* 2009 May;9(5):313-23.
7. Macfarlane S, Furrie E, Macfarlane GT, Dillon JF. Microbial colonization of the upper gastrointestinal tract in patients with Barrett's esophagus. *Clin Infect Dis.* 2007 Jul;45(1):29-38.
8. Macfarlane S, Macfarlane GT. Composition and metabolic activities of bacterial biofilms colonizing food residues in the human gut. *Appl Environ Microbiol.* 2006 Sep;72(9):6204-11.
9. Maslowski KM, Mackay CR. Diet, gut microbiota, and immune responses. *Nat Immunol.* 2011 Jan;12(1):5-9.
10. Gershon M. *The Second Brain: A Groundbreaking New Understanding of Nervous Disorders of the Stomach and Intestine.* New York, NY: HarperCollins Publishers, 1999.
11. Beltina.org Health Encyclopedia. Gut-associated lymphoid tissue (GALT). Available online at: http://www.beltina.org/health-dictionary/gut-associated-lymphoid-tissue-galt.html
12. Wood JD, Alpers DH, Andrews PL. Fundamentals of neurogastroenterology. *Gut.* 1999 Sep;45(Suppl 2):II6-II16.
13. Jones DS (Ed.). *Textbook of Functional Medicine.* Gig Harbor, WA: The Institute for Functional Medicine, 2006.
14. Vojdani A, O'Bryan T, Kellermann GH. The immunology of immediate and delayed hypersensitivity reaction to gluten. *Eur J Inflamm.* 2008;6(1):1-10.
15. Reichelt K. Gluten, milk proteins and autism: dietary intervention effects on behaviour and peptide secretion. *J Appl Nutr.* 1990 Jan;42:1-11.

16. Fasano A, Shea-Donohue T. Mechanisms of disease: the role of intestinal barrier function in the pathogenesis of gastrointestinal autoimmune diseases. *Nat Clin Pract Gastroenterol Hepatol.* 2005 Sep;2(9):416-22.

17. Fasano A. Surprises from celiac disease. *Sci Am.* 2009 Aug;301(2):54-61.

18. Langlands SJ, Hopkins MJ, Coleman N, Cummings JH. Prebiotic carbohydrates modify the mucosa associated microflora of the human large bowel. *Gut.* 2004;53:1610-6.

19. Medzhitov R. Inflammation 2010: new adventures of an old flame. *Cell.* 2010 Mar;140(6):771-6.

20. Dubois B, Joubert G, Gomez de Agüero M, Gouanvic M, Goubier A, Kaiserlian D. Sequential role of plasmacytoid dendritic cells and regulatory T cells in oral tolerance. *Gastoenterology.* 2009 Sep;137(3):1019-28.

21. Maynard CL, Weaver CT. Intestinal effector T cells in health and disease. *Immunity.* 2009 Sep;31(3):389-400.

22. Herbert MR. Large brains in autism: the challenge of pervasive abnormality. *Neuroscientist.* 2005 Oct;11(5):417-40.

23. Banan A, Keshavarzian A, Zhang L, Shaikh M, Forsyth CB, Tang Y, Fields JZ. NF-kB activation as a key mechanism in ethanol-induced disruption of the F-actin cytoskeleton and monolayer barrier integrity in intestinal epithelium. *Alcohol.* 2007 Sep;41(6):447-60.

24. Hijazi Z, Molla AM, Al-Habashi H, Muawad WN, Molla AM, Sharma PN. Intestinal permeability is increased in bronchial asthma. *Arch Dis Child.* 2004 Mar;89(3):227-9.

25. Erridge C, Attina T, Spickett CM, Webb DJ. A high-fat meal induces low-grade endotoxemia: evidence of a novel mechanism of postprandial inflammation. *Am J Clin Nutr.* 2007 Nov;86(5):1286-92.

26. Maes M, Mihaylova I, Leunis JC. Increased serum IgA and IgM against LPS of enterobacteria in chronic fatigue syndrome (CFS): indication for the involvement of gram-negative enterobacteria in the etiology of CFS and for the presence of an increased gut-intestinal permeability. *J Affect Disord.* 2007 Apr;99(1-3):237-40.

27. Majamaa H, Laine S, Miettinen A. Eosinophil protein X and eosinophil cationic protein as indicators of intestinal inflammation in infants with atopic eczema and food allergy. *Clin Exp Allergy.* 1999 Nov;29(11):1502-6.

28. Sandek A, Rauchhaus M, Anker SD, von Haehling S. The emerging role of the gut in chronic heart failure. *Curr Opin Clin Nutri Metab Care.* 2008 Sep;11(5):632-9.

29. Laukoetter MG, Nava P, Nusrat A. Role of the intestinal barrier in inflammatory bowel disease. *World J Gastroenterol.* 2008 Jan;14(3):401-7.

30. Mehta NN, McGillicuddy FC, Anderson PD, Hinkle CC, Shah R, Pruscino L, Tabita-Martinez J, Sellers KF, Rickels MR, Reilly MP. Experimental endotoxemia induces adipose inflammation and insulin resistance in humans. *Diabetes.* 2010 Jan;59(1):172-81.

31. Bosi E, Molteni L, Radaelli MG, Folini L, Fermo I, Bazzigaluppi E, Piemonti L, Pastore MR, Paroni R. Increased intestinal permeability precedes clinical onset of type 1 diabetes. *Diabetologia.* 2006 Dec;49(12):2824-7.

32. Visser J, Rozing J, Sapone A, Lammers K, Fasano A. Tight junctions, intestinal permeability, and autoimmunity: celiac disease and type I diabetes paradigms. *Ann N Y Acad Sci.* 2009 May;1165:195-205.

33. Ohman L, Simrén M. Pathogenesis of IBS: role of inflammation, immunity and neuroimmune interactions. *Nat Rev Gastroenterol Hepatol.* 2010 Mar;7(3):163-73.

34. Vrieze A, Holleman F, Serlie MJ, Ackermans MT, Dallinga-Thie GM, Groen AK, van Nood E, Bartelsman JFW, Oozeer R, Zoetendal E, de Vos WM, Hoekstra JBL, Nieuwdorp M. Metabolic effects of transplanting gut microbiota from lean donors to subjects with metabolic syndrome. Abstract 90. Presented at the Meeting of the European Association for the Study of Diabetes (EASD), Stockholm, September 2010.

35. Bajzer M, Seeley RJ. Physiology: obesity and gut flora. *Nature*. 2006 Dec;444(7122):1009-10.

36. Schwarz B, Salak N, Hofstötter H, et al. [Intestinal ischemic reperfusion syndrome: pathophysiology, clinical significance, therapy]. *Wien Klin Wochenschr*. 1999 Jul;111(14):539-48.

37. Yang L, Lu X, Nossa CW, Francois F, Peek RM, Pei Z. Inflammation and intestinal metaplasia of the distal esophagus are associated with alterations in the microbiome. *Gastroenterology*. 2009 Aug;137(2):588-97.

38. Hoffman M. Esophageal cancer on the rise. *WebMD*. February 01, 2007. Available online at: http://www.webmd.com/cancer/features/esophageal cancer-rise

39. Holden W, Orchard T, Wordsworth P. Enteropathic arthritis. *Rheum Dis Clin North Am*. 2003 Aug;29(3):513-30, viii.

40. Fink MP. Intestinal epithelial hyperpermeability: update on the pathogenesis of gut mucosal barrier dysfunction in critical illness. *Curr Opin Crit Care*. 2003 Apr;9(2):143-51.

41. Grundy D, Al-Chaer ED, Aziz Q, Collins SM, Ke M, Taché Y, Wood JD. Fundamentals of neurogastroenterology: basic science. *Gastroenterology*. 2006 Apr;130(5):1391-411.

42. Rühl A. Glial cells in the gut. *Neurogastroenterol Motil*. 2005;17:777-90.

43. Pardo CA, Vargas DL, Zimmerman AW. Immunity, neuroglia and neuroinflammation in autism. *Int Rev Psychiatry*. 2005 Dec;17(6):485-95.

44. Turnbull LK, Mullin GE, Weinstock LB. Principles of integrative gastroenterology: systemic signs of underlying digestive dysfunction and disease. Chapter 7 in GE Mullin (Ed.), *Integrative Gastroenterology*. New York, NY: Oxford University Press USA, 2011.

45. Kalaydjian AE, Eaton W, Cascella N, Fasano A. The gluten connection: the association between schizophrenia and celiac disease. *Acta Psychiatr Scand*. 2006 Feb;113(2):82-90.

46. Reichelt KL, Knivsberg AM. Can the pathophysiology of autism be explained by the nature of the discovered urine peptides? *Nutr Neurosci*. 2003 Feb;6(1):19-28.

47. Whiteley P, Shattock P. Biochemical aspects in autism spectrum disorders: updating the opioid-excess theory and presenting new opportunities for biomedical intervention. *Expert Opin Ther Tar*. 2002 Apr;6(2):175-83.

48. Knivsberg AM, Reichelt KL, Hoien T, Nodland M. A randomised, controlled study of dietary intervention in autistic syndromes. *Nutr Neurosci*. 2002;5(4):251-61.

49. Reichelt KL, Knivsberg AM. The possibility and probability of a gut-to-brain connection in autism. *Ann Clin Psychiatry*. 2009;21(4):205-11.

50. Sapone A, Lammers KM, Casolaro V, Cammarota M, Giuliano MT, De Rosa M, Stefanile R, Mazzarella G, Tolone C, Russo MI, Esposito P, Ferraraccio F, Cartenì M, Riegler G, de Magistris L, Fasano A. Divergence of gut permeability and mucosal immune gene expression in two gluten-associated conditions: celiac disease and gluten sensitivity. *BMC Med*. 2011 Mar;9(23).

51. Drago S, El Asmar R, Di Pierro M, Grazia Clemente M, Tripathi A, Sapone A, Thakar M, Iacono G, Carroccio A, D'Agate C, Not T, Zampini L, Catassi C, Fasano A. Gliadin, zonulin and gut permeability: effects on celiac and non-celiac intestinal mucosa and intestinal cell lines. *Scand J Gastroenterol.* 2006 Apr:41(4):408-19.

52. Cascella NG, Kryszak D, Bhatti B, Gregory P, Kelly DL, McEvoy JP, Fasano A, Eaton WW. Prevalence of celiac disease and gluten sensitivity in the United States clinical antipsychotic trials of intervention effectiveness study population. *Schizophr Bull.* 2011 Jan;37(1):94-100.

53. Biesiekierski JR, Newnham ED, Irving PM, Barrett JS, Haines M, Doecke JD, Shepherd SJ, Muir JG, Gibson PR. Gluten causes gastrointestinal symptoms in subjects without celiac disease: a double-blind randomized placebo-controlled trial. *Am J Gastroenterol.* 2011 Mar;106(3):508-14.

54. Vojdani A, O'Bryan T, Kellermann GH. The immunology of gluten sensitivity beyond the intestinal tract. *Eur J Inflamm.* 2008;6(2).

55. American Psychiatric Association. *Diagnostic and Statistical Manual of Mental Disorders*, 4th edition, text revision. Washington, DC: American Psychiatric Association, 2000.

56. Herbert MR, Arranga T. Interview with Dr. Martha Herbert—Autism: a brain disorder or a disorder that affects the brain? *Medical Veritas.* 2006;3:1182–94.

57. Kanner L. Autistic disturbances of affective contact. *Nervous Child.* 1943;2:217-50.

58. Goodwin MS, Cowen MA, Goodwin TC. Malabsorption and cerebral dysfunction: a multivariate and comparative study of autistic children. *J Autism Child Schizophr.* 1971 Jan-Mar;1(1):48-62.

59. Horvath K, Papadimitriou JC, Rabsztyn A, Drachenberg C, Tildon JT. Gastrointestinal abnormalities in children with autistic disorder. *J Pediatr.* 1999 Nov;135(5):559-63.

60. Valicenti-McDermott M, McVicar K, Rapin I, Wershil BK, Cohen H, Shinnar S. Frequency of gastrointestinal symptoms in children with autistic spectrum disorders and association with family history of autoimmune disease. *J Dev Behav Pediatr.* 2006 Apr;27(2 Suppl):S128-S136.

61. Buie T, Campbell DB, Fuchs GJ III, Furuta GT, Levy J, VandeWater J, Whitaker AH, Atkins D, Bauman ML, Beaudet AL, Carr EG, Gershon MD, Hyman SL, Jirapinyo P, Jyonouchi H, Kooros K, Kushak R, Levitt P, Levy SE, Lewis JD, Murray KF, Natowicz MR, Sabra A, Wershil BK, Weston SC, Zeltzer L, Winter H. Evaluation, diagnosis, and treatment of gastrointestinal disorders in individuals with ASDs: a consensus report. *Pediatrics.* 2010 Jan;125(Suppl 1):S1-S18.

62. Finegold SM, Molitoris D, Song Y, Liu C, Vaisanen ML, Bolte E, McTeague M, Sandler R, Wexler H, Marlowe EM, Collins MD, Lawson PA, Summanen P, Baysallar M, Tomzynski TJ, Read E, Johnson E, Rolfe R, Nasir P, Shah H, Haake DA, Manning P, Kaul A. Gastrointestinal microflora studies in late-onset autism. *Clin Infect Dis.* 2002;35(Suppl 1):S6-S16.

63. MacFabe DF, Rodriguez-Capote K, Hoffman JE, Franklin AE, Mohammad-Aset Y, Taylor AR, Boon F, Cain DP, Kavaliers M, Possmayer F, Ossenkpp KP. A novel rodent model of autism: intraventricular infusions of propionic acid increase locomotor activity and induce neuroinflammation and oxidative stress in discrete regions of adult rat brain. *Am J Biochem Biotechnol.* 2008;4(2):146-66.

64. Shultz SR, MacFabe DF, Ossenkopp KP, Scratch S, Whelan J, Taylor R, Cain DP. Intracerebroventricular injection of propionic acid, an enteric bacterial metabolic end-product, impairs social behavior in the rat: implications for an animal model of autism. *Neuropharmacology.* 2008 May;54(6):901-11.

65. MacFabe DF, Cain NE, Boon F, Ossenkopp KP, Cain DP. Effects of the enteric bacterial metabolic product propionic acid on object-directed behavior, social behavior, cognition, and neuroinflammation in adolescent rats: relevance to autism spectrum disorder. *Behav Brain Res.* 2010;217:47-54.

66. MacFabe D. The "self-centered bug": can acquired infections influence brain function and behavior in autism and other neurodevelopmental disorders? Presentation at Defeat Autism Now! Spring conference, 2008.

67. Dancey CP, Attree EA, Stuart G, Wilson C, Sonnet A. Words fail me: the verbal IQ deficit in inflammatory bowel disease and irritable bowel syndrome. *Inflamm Bowel Dis.* 2009 Jun;15(6):852-7.

68. Hunt MG, Moshier S, Milonova M. Brief cognitive-behavioral internet therapy for irritable bowel syndrome. *Behav Res Ther.* 2009 Sep;47(9):797-802.

69. Sullivan A, Nord CE, Evengård B. Effect of supplement with lactic-acid producing bacteria on fatigue and physical activity in patients with chronic fatigue syndrome. *Nutr J.* 2009 Jan 26;8:4.

70. Wallace TC, Guarner F, Madsen K, Cabana MD, Gibson G, Hentges E, Sanders ME. Human gut microbiota and its relationship to health and disease. *Nutr Rev.* 2011 Jul;69(7):392-403.

71. Desbonnet L, Garrett L, Clarke G, Bienenstock J, Dinan TG. The probiotic *Bifidobacteria infantis*: an assessment of potential antidepressant properties in the rat. *J Psychiatr Res.* 2008 Dec;43(2):164-74.

72. Srinivasan P. A review of dietary interventions in autism. *Ann Clin Psychiatry.* 2009 Oct-Dec;21(4):237-47.

73. McCann D, Barrett A, Cooper A, Crumpler D, Dalen L, Grimshaw K, Kitchin E, Lok K, Porteous L, Prince E, Sonuga-Barke E, Warner JO, Stevenson J. Food additives and hyperactive behaviour in 3-year-old and 8/9-year-old children in the community: a randomised, double-blinded, placebo-controlled trial. *Lancet.* 2007 Nov; 370(9598):1560-7.

74. Shinohe A, Hashimoto K, Nakamura K, Tsujii M, Iwata Y, Tsuchiya KJ, Sekine Y, Suda S, Suzuki K, Sugihara G, Matsuzaki H, Minabe Y, Sugiyama T, Kawai M, Iyo M, Takei N, Mori N. Increased serum levels of glutamate in adult patients with autism. *Prog Neuropsychopharmacol Biol Psychiatry.* 2006 Dec;30(8):1472-7.

75. Baad-Hansen L, Cairns B, Ernberg M, Svensson P. Effect of systemic monosodium glutamate (MSG) on headache and pericranial muscle sensitivity. *Cephalagia.* 2010 Jan;30(1):68-76.

76. Hibbeln JR, Nieminen LRG, Blasbalg TL, Riggs JA, Lands WEM. Healthy intakes of n-3 and n-6 fatty acids: estimations considering worldwide diversity. *Am J Clin Nutr.* 2006 Jun;83(Suppl 6):S1483-S1493.

77. Sorgi PJ, Hallowell EM, Hutchins HL, Sears B. Effects of an open-label pilot study with high-dose EPA/DHA concentrates on plasma phospholipids and behavior in children with attention deficit hyperactivity disorder. *Nutr J.* 2007 Jul;6:16.

78. Dean A, Armstrong J. Genetically modified foods. Wichita, KS: American Academy of Environmental Medicine, May 8, 2009. Available online at: http://www.aaemonline.org/gmopost.html

79. Kroghsbo S, Madsen C, Poulsen M, Schrøder M, Kvist PH, Taylor M, Gatehouse A, Shu Q, Knudsen I. Immunotoxicological studies of genetically modified rice expressing PHA-E lectin or Bt toxin in Wistar rats. *Toxicology.* 2008 Mar;245(1-2):24-34.

80. Finamore A, Roselli M, Britti S, Monastra G, Ambra R, Turrini A, Mengheri E. Intestinal and peripheral immune response to MON810 maize ingestion in weaning and old mice. *J Agric Food Chem.* 2008 Dec;56(23):11533-9.

81. Smith JM. Seeds of Deception: *Exposing Industry and Government Lies About the Safety of the Genetically Engineered Foods You're Eating.* Portland, ME: Yes! Books, 2003.

82. Pelsser LM, Frankena K, Toorman J, Savelkoul HF, Dubois AE, Pereira RR, Haagen TA, Rommelse NN, Buitelaar JK. Effects of a restricted elimination diet on the behaviour of children with attention-deficit hyperactivity disorder (INCA study): a randomised controlled trial. *Lancet.* 2011 Feb; 377(9764):494-503.

Additional References

Johansson-Lindbom B, Svensson M, Wurbel MA, Malissen B, Márquez G, Agace W. Selective generation of gut tropic T cells in gut-associated lymphoid tissue (GALT): requirement for GALT dendric cells and adjuvant. *J Exp Med.* 2003 Sep;198(6):963-9.

Kunkel EJ, Campbell DJ, Butcher EC. Chemokines in lymphocyte trafficking and intestinal immunity. *Microcirculation.* 2003 Jun;10(3-4):313-23.

Mullin GE, Swift KM. *The Inside Tract: Your Good Gut Guide to Great Digestive Health.* Emmaus, PA: Rodale Books, 2011.

Nagler-Anderson C. Man the barrier! Strategic defences in the intestinal mucosa. *Nat Rev Immunol.* 2001 Oct;1(1):59-67.

Nagler-Anderson C, Shi HN. Peripheral nonresponsiveness to orally administered soluble protein antigens. *Crit Rev Immunol.* 2001;21(1-3):121-31.

Sekirov I, Russell SL, Antunes LCM, Finlay BB. Gut Microbiota in Health and Disease. *Physiol Rev.* 2010 July;90(3):859-904.

Takaishi H, Ohara S, Hotta K, Yajima T, Kanai T, Inoue N, Iwao Y, Watanabe M, Ishii H, Hibi T. Circulating autoantibodies against purified colonic mucin in ulcerative colitis. *J Gastroenterol.* 2000;35(1):20-7.

Watanabe M, Watanabe N, Iwao Y, Ogata H, Kanai T, Ueno Y, Tsuchiya M, Ishii H, Aiso S, Habu S, Hibi T. The serum factor from patients with ulcerative colitis that induces T cell proliferation in the mouse thymus is interleukin-7. *J Clin Immunol.* 1997 Jul;17(4):282-92.

CHAPTER TWO

THEORIES OF GUT-BRAIN AXIS INVOLVEMENT IN CHILDHOOD DEVELOPMENTAL DISORDERS

By Arthur Krigsman, MD

In clinical medicine, the concept of brain function being dependent upon activities occurring in the gastrointestinal (GI) tract is not a novel one. In the setting of gastrointestinal health, this unidirectional gut-brain link is seen upon ingestion of various foods and pharmaceuticals. For example, when one ingests substances containing alcohol, there is rapid absorption of alcohol molecules from the gastrointestinal tract. These molecules are transported within minutes to the brain via the blood. Similarly, when one ingests pharmaceutical substances such as narcotics, there is rapid absorption from the healthy gastrointestinal tract into the bloodstream with transport of the ingested opioid molecules to the brain via the peripheral circulation. Both of these examples serve to illustrate the simple concept of the direct and rapid effect of absorbed intestinal contents on the brain and its function.

From a strictly conceptual standpoint, it is critical to understand that the gastrointestinal tract serves primarily as a biologic interface with the larger environment in which the human organism resides. When speaking of the absorption of "outside molecules," the gastrointestinal tract is by far the single organ most responsible for internalization of substances that are exogenous to the body. Because of the potentially detrimental impact upon the brain of the wide variety of ingested foods (and non-food items), the mammalian body has evolved a variety of protective mechanisms designed to make gastrointestinal absorption as selective a process as possible. This serves to ensure physiologic homeostasis within the body, allowing the body as a whole to function within the very narrow physiological parameters necessary to ensure optimal health. Deviation from these optimal parameters due to inappropriate absorption of gastrointestinal luminal contents usually results in disease.

The digestive process

The highly evolved and selective process of absorption begins immediately after ingestion of foods and is referred to as the process of digestion. In this process, ingested foods are broken down into simpler molecules by the combination of physical chewing activity, salivary enzymes, gastric enzymes, gastric acid, duodenal brush border enzymes, pancreatic enzymes, and bile. Together, these numerous and complex processes serve to transform large ingested molecules into smaller simpler substances that then come in contact with the surface of the small bowel villi responsible for absorption. The actual passage of these simple molecules through the villi is also a highly selective process, the success of which relies heavily upon the intact architectural structure of the villi.

An elaborate transport system exists in which some molecules move across the villous membrane without expenditure of energy (passive transport), whereas other molecules require the expenditure of energy (active transport). Once absorbed, these molecules enter the lymphatic system and are transported to the body's systemic circulation. During their movement through the most superficial layers of the intestinal lining (epithelium), they encounter a highly evolved immunologic defense that is designed to remove molecules that it deems foreign or does not recognize. (In fact, the gastrointestinal tract is the organ that contains the most heavily concentrated system of lymphoid tissue, a fact that further attests to the enormity of the body's exposure to external influences via the gastrointestinal tract and the importance of maintaining its integrity.) When the immunologic defense system is functioning in health, any protein antigens that manage to circumvent the initial degradation phase occurring within the lumen of the bowel are prevented from entering the systemic circulation. Those molecules that somehow succeed in penetrating the immunologic defense system will encounter additional immunologic activity within the circulating portion of the blood to prevent them from causing harm. The focus of this chapter is on the digestive and immunologic activity on the luminal surface of the bowel and within the lining of gastrointestinal tissue that interfaces the GI tract and the lumen—the epithelium. It proposes a mechanism explaining how inflammatory disease of this epithelial lining may be viewed as the initial step in a cascade of gut-brain axis events leading to developmental delay.

Downstream effects of digestive dysfunction

Deficiencies or disease in any of the individual systems of digestion, absorption, and surveillance result in disease states that are thought to have neurologic and immunologic consequences. Examples of this are celiac disease, Crohn's disease, and classic IgE-mediated food allergy. These examples are similar in that damage to the highly evolved system of selective intestinal villous absorption leads to pathological absorption of food and consequent systemic downstream effects, including effects on the central and peripheral nervous systems. In all three examples, the inflammatory disease state has been well characterized on a cellular and molecular level and, to a lesser extent, on a genetic level.

In the case of celiac disease, immunologic destruction of the villous barrier function as a result of dietary exposure to gluten results in inappropriate absorption of a variety of intact food-derived macromolecules, with a consequent increase in systemic elevations of IgG to numerous foodstuffs.[1] Importantly, from a neurologic standpoint, seizure activity and peripheral neuropathy have both been linked to untreated or inadequately treated celiac disease, suggesting that the immunologic activity occurring in the intestinal lining of these patients is having a downstream effect on neurologic function.[2] The precise mechanism of this downstream effect is unclear. Leading theories include immunologic activity directed against the central and peripheral nervous systems and/or the products of inappropriately absorbed gluten molecules or their derivatives acting as neurotoxins.

In the case of Crohn's disease, there is also ample data demonstrating the presence of food-specific IgG in active versus quiescent intestinal inflammation.[3] Interestingly, numerous publications have noted the presence of an altered affect in adult patients with Crohn's disease as compared with other chronic diseases; it is entirely plausible that pathologically absorbed molecules from the gut are acting on the adult brain, negatively impacting affect and personality.[4]

In the third example, that of classic IgE food allergy, an intense immunologic response to pathologically absorbed foodstuffs further contributes to pre-existing immunologic sensitization at the mucosal level, triggering specific immunologic activity involving eosinophils and mast cells. This results in potential multiorgan pathology such as respiratory distress or failure, hives, capillary dilatation and leakage, edema, arthritis/arthralgia, and gastrointestinal bleeding. Neurologic consequences of classic food allergy are not as common as those in celiac disease and Crohn's disease but may include encephalopathy and peripheral neuropathy.[5]

Autism-associated enterocolitis

In the context just described, one can consider the more commonly encountered and unique disease entity of autism-associated enterocolitis and its attendant impact on brain function. However, there is one important distinction to be made between autism-associated enterocolitis and the three examples listed above. Whereas Crohn's disease, celiac disease, and IgE-mediated food allergy have known effects on immunologic and neurologic systemic dysfunction in adults (and less often in children), these diseases do not appear to have *developmental* sequelae. In contrast, because autism-associated enterocolitis presents exclusively in the critical developmental period of infancy or early toddlerhood, existing data relating to its unique inflammatory characteristics provide a scientifically intriguing window onto its impact not only on neurologic function but also on developmental, behavioral, and fundamental cognitive processes.

The focus of the ensuing paragraphs is twofold. First, I synthesize what is known about the mucosal pathology of autism-associated enteritis/enterocolitis (with enteritis defined as inflammation of the small intestine and enterocolitis defined as inflammation of both the small and large intestines), discussing mucosal inflammation, villous destruction, brush border disaccharidase deficiencies, increased intestinal permeability, and elevated antibody production to clostridial floral species. Second, I formulate a mechanistic hypothesis that demonstrates the cumulative role of these processes in the breach of intestinal villous mucosal integrity and the attempts of the gastrointestinal immunologic response to contain this breach. Extension of this hypothesis leads to the question of whether failure to adequately contain the breach could result in more systemic involvement, including that of delays in brain development and function.

1. Mucosal inflammation

The earliest significant description of the cellular infiltrate present in autism-associated inflammatory bowel disease (IBD) was authored by the Inflammatory Bowel Disease Study Group at the Royal Free Hospital in London, England, and was published in the *American Journal of Gastroenterology* in September 2001.[6] The nine authors of this retrospective controlled study demonstrated a number of significant findings:

a. Active ileitis was present in 8% of GI-symptomatic children with autism spectrum disorder (ASD) but not in controls.

b. Chronic colitis was present in 88% of GI-symptomatic ASD children as compared with 4.5% of non-autistic controls. This chronic colitis was patchy in distribution, displaying a pattern distinct from ulcerative colitis but similar to that seen in Crohn's disease.

c. Eosinophilic infiltration of the lamina propria was present significantly more frequently in GI-symptomatic ASD children than in either children with ulcerative colitis or non-autistic controls.

d. Frequency and severity of inflammation was significantly greater in affected ASD children as compared with non-autistic controls but less intense than that seen in ulcerative colitis.

e. Endoscopic features of mucosal inflammation in GI-symptomatic ASD children were less frequent and intense than those seen in ulcerative colitis but significantly more frequent than in non-autistic controls.

Subsequent to this 2001 publication, two additional papers have looked specifically at the frequency and cellular characterization of enterocolitis in GI-symptomatic ASD children. The first, published in 2005 by a group of Venezuelan researchers led by pediatric gastroenterologist Dr. Lenny González, won second prize in the scientific category at the Venezuelan Congress of Pediatrics 2005.[7] In the study, GI-symptomatic ASD children demonstrated duodenal intraepithelial lymphocytosis and colonic lymphoplasmacytosis. Frequent esophagitis, gastritis, duodenitis, and ileocolitis also were noted.

In a second paper, my colleagues and I reviewed histopathologic findings at ileocolonoscopy in 143 consecutive GI-symptomatic ASD children.[8] We found ileitis to be present in more than a third of the children (34.6%) and colitis in more than two-thirds (69.2%). In addition, we noted inflammation of both the ileum and colon together in over one-fourth of GI-symptomatic children (29.1%). When ileitis was present, it was most frequently associated with colitis as opposed to presenting as an isolated small bowel histologic entity. When colitis was present, it tended to be multifocal. Significantly, the presence of histologic ileal and/or colonic lymphoid nodular hyperplasia (LNH) statistically predicted the concurrent presence of histologic ileocolonic inflammation. This strongly suggests that the LNH seen in GI-symptomatic ASD children is part of a larger immunologic-histopathologic process, as opposed to the milder form of LNH frequently encountered by pediatric endoscopists that occurs in the absence of recognizable histologic ileocolonic inflammatory activity. This distinction between LNH accompanied versus unaccompanied by mucosal inflammation is critical and resolves the longstanding misconception that GI mucosal LNH, when encountered, may be immediately dismissed as being of no clinical import. Taken together, our data and the data of Dr. González's group replicate the original observations of Professor John Walker-Smith and his Inflammatory Bowel Disease Study Group team regarding the presence of pathologic mucosal inflammatory cellular infiltrates in conjunction with lymphonodular hyperplasia in GI-symptomatic ASD children.

In 2001, in an effort to further define specific cell populations of colonic lymphocytes in inflamed colonic tissue obtained from GI-symptomatic ASD children, Furlano and colleagues performed immunohistochemical evaluation on colonic biopsies to determine cell lineage and functional markers and histochemical analysis to evaluate the presence of glycosaminoglycans and basement membrane thickness.[9] As compared with normal control subjects, the GI-symptomatic ASD children were found to have:

- significantly more intraepithelial lymphocytes in the surface epithelium
- a significantly higher number of lamina propria eosinophils
- a lymphocyte population with significantly higher proportions of CD3+, CD8+, gamma delta T cells, plasma cells, and proliferating epithelial cells on immunohistochemical analysis of the transverse colon

The gamma delta T cell counts were higher in the GI-symptomatic ASD children than in the children with ulcerative colitis, whereas the ulcerative colitis children had higher proportions of CD3+, CD8+, plasma cells, and proliferating epithelial cells than the GI-symptomatic ASD children.

These immunohistochemical findings correlated well with the histologic findings by these same researchers as described in their 2001 review of the histopathology of the ASD GI disease described above. In addition, the paper noted that basement membrane thickness of GI-symptomatic ASD children was significantly greater than that seen in normal control subjects. Perhaps of even greater interest, the basement membrane thickening in ASD children far exceeds what is seen in Crohn's disease and ulcerative colitis. In addition, glycosaminoglycans were decreased in GI-symptomatic ASD children as compared with normal control subjects but not as much as in children with ulcerative colitis. This again correlates well with the concept of a less intense degree of mucosal destruction in autism-associated colitis as compared with ulcerative colitis. However, the exceedingly thickened basement membrane in ASD as compared with both Crohn's disease and ulcerative colitis suggests a unique attempt at architectural fortification by construction of a physical barrier against epithelial injury "known" by the immune system to be even more systemically harmful to the host than the inflammation seen in ulcerative colitis and Crohn's disease.

After thus defining the inflammatory characteristics of the colon, the Inflammatory Bowel Disease Study Group authors turned their attention in 2002 to those of the small bowel. In the 2002 paper, Torrente and colleagues compared GI-symptomatic ASD children with two control groups consisting of typical children having either celiac disease or no demonstrable bowel pathology (i.e., healthy controls).[10] The research group demonstrated that, in contrast to the relatively mild histopathology seen on routine light microscopy in a series of 25 distal duodenal biopsies obtained from the GI-symptomatic ASD children, there were *marked* abnormalities seen upon immunohistochemistry.

Specifically:
- The density of CD8 intraepithelial lymphocytes was significantly higher in the ASD-GI group as compared with healthy controls but less than in the celiac group.

- Within the lamina propria, excess CD3, CD4, and CD8 were present in the GI-symptomatic ASD children as compared with both control groups, with frequent pericryptal aggregation of the CD3, CD4, and CD8 cells.
- Mean plasma cell density in the GI-symptomatic ASD children was significantly higher than in healthy controls but lower than in children with celiac disease.
- Basement membrane thickening was present both in the GI-symptomatic ASD group and the celiac group; a marked increase in cryptal proliferation in the ASD group was similar to that seen in the celiac group and significantly greater than in the healthy control group.

The most striking finding of this study was the deposition of IgG on the basolateral enterocyte membrane and subepithelial basement membrane in 23 of 25 of the GI-symptomatic ASD children studied, with co-localization of complement C1q on double exposure and confocal microscopy. The significance of this finding is that it confirms the pathological significance of the mucosal lesion and strongly implies an autoimmune origin. Cryptal proliferation was prominent, supporting and extending the findings of others[11] demonstrating Panneth cell hyperplasia in GI-symptomatic ASD small bowel biopsy tissue. Panneth cell hyperplasia is known to occur in situations of excessive cryptal proliferation. The aggregate significance of the small intestinal lesion described in this paper is that it depicts pathology distinct from all known forms of pediatric enteropathies.

In a further effort to demonstrate unique features of the ASD mucosal inflammatory process, my colleague Dr. Stephen Walker and I performed microarray analysis (with qPCR confirmation) on both ileal and colonic biopsies from ASD children and compared them with three non-ASD control groups: healthy children, Crohn's disease, and ulcerative colitis.[12] This study, using the completely objective tool of microarray methodology, provided the first ever description of the *unique molecular features* of inflamed ASD ileal and colonic mucosal tissue and clearly depicted ASD-associated intestinal inflammation as being molecularly distinct from both Crohn's disease and ulcerative colitis. Importantly, it also clearly separates ASD mucosal tissue from normal controls, i.e., the non-specific inflammation seen at light microscopy in GI-symptomatic ASD children is not "normal." Another significant finding of the study was that it provided further insight into the pathologic significance of the oft-seen mucosal LNH. We showed, in methodologically and statistically convincing fashion, that the LNH of GI-symptomatic ASD children shares similar unique molecular features with inflamed ASD mucosal tissue and, therefore, is reflective of GI inflammatory disease – that is, the LNH seen in these children is part of the disease process and may not be dismissed as "normal."

2. Villous destruction

In GI-symptomatic ASD children, we frequently encounter an as-yet-unpublished but readily identifiable endoscopic lesion of the small bowel. The lesion appears visually as a white spot, usually less than 1 mm in diameter, that is superficial to the small bowel mucosa and appears adherent to the mucosal surface. Indeed, this white spot is typically easily displaced from the mucosa upon contact with the tip of the endoscope. Examined at light microscopy with routine H & E (hematoxylin and eosin) staining, the lesion appears to consist of a decapitated single villus (or occasionally two adjacent villi), the internal contents of which are in direct contact with luminal material. Plumes of fibrin (an insoluble protein) rise from within the truncated villus and appear to coat the exposed surface (Figure 1). Significantly, only mild (if any) cellular inflammatory infiltrate is seen within the vicinity of the lesion at light microscopy, a recurring theme first noted by the IBD Study Group at the Royal Free Hospital in the late 1990s. Capsule endoscopy has consistently demonstrated the distal extension of these white spot lesions well into the proximal and mid jejunum, with frequent zones of well-demarcated erosion and/or erythema surrounding many of the lesions. In addition, white spot lesions are often present in the vicinity of scattered small mucosal aphthae (ulcerations). As described, the lesions bear a striking similarity to mucosal changes seen during the early evolution of Crohn's disease as described by Rickert and Carter[13] as well as Sankey and colleagues.[14] This preliminary finding of villous architectural damage is exciting in that it potentially provides a simple anatomic explanation for the increased intestinal permeability found in ASD children (see *Increased intestinal permeability*).

3. Brush border disaccharidase deficiencies

In 1999, Horvath and colleagues demonstrated decreased activity of at least one duodenal brush border disaccharidase or glucoamylase in nearly three-fifths (58%) of GI-symptomatic ASD children and decreased activity of two or more enzymes in approximately one-fourth (24%) of these children.[11] Disaccharidases and glucoamylases are enzymes that help break down larger carbohydrate molecules into simpler carbohydrate molecules. In the Horvath study, lactase (the enzyme involved in the hydrolysis of lactose) was the most frequently deficient brush border enzyme.[11] More recently, Kushak and colleagues found strikingly similar proportions of lactase deficiency (58%) in GI-symptomatic ASD children under 5 years of age.[15] Again, lactase was the most frequently deficient enzyme, followed by sucrase and maltase. Interestingly, light microscopic evidence of cellular mucosal inflammation was absent in the vast majority of children studied (N=199). When present, however, cellular mucosal inflammation was strongly predictive of deficiency of at least one brush border disaccharidase. The frequent presence of disaccharidase deficiency in the absence of light microscopic cellular histopathology is reminiscent of the findings of Torrente[10] described above, in which significant inflammatory activity (and mucosal damage) was present in the absence of cellular infiltrates as seen on conventional light microscopy.

4. Increased intestinal permeability

It is well established within the current body of medical literature that conditions involving mucosal inflammation and diminished intestinal mucosal barrier function often lead to the appearance of inappropriately absorbed intestinal luminal contents within the blood. Although the precise mechanisms by which the pathologically absorbed luminal contents enter the blood may vary from disease to disease, the phenomenon of their presence within the systemic circulation is collectively referred to as increased intestinal permeability. Intestinal permeability has recently been shown to be involved in the pathogenesis of both intestinal and even extraintestinal autoimmune diseases such as Crohn's disease, celiac disease, and type 1 diabetes mellitus.

Formal testing to determine whether increased intestinal permeability from any cause is present in a given patient is most frequently accomplished using a simple test. The procedure involves the simultaneous oral administration of two biologically inert carbohydrates of different molecular sizes and absorption routes and the subsequent measurement of urinary recovery of each molecule. The most commonly used inert carbohydrates are lactulose and mannitol. In situations of intestinal health, neither of these compounds is particularly well absorbed, and those molecules that are absorbed remain structurally intact as they traverse the various organs of the body and are excreted in the urine. The carbohydrates are administered orally after a brief fast, and urine samples are collected over the following 5-6 hours. The inert property of the ingested carbohydrates allows for detection and quantification of the degree of intestinal absorptive dysfunction. Importantly, because lactulose is a relatively large molecule, it is absorbed via a paracellular route. In contrast, mannitol, a relatively small molecule, is absorbed via a transcellular route. Further analysis of the urinary lactulose:mannitol ratio is, therefore, thought to reflect the disease-specific underlying pathophysiologic processes responsible for the abnormal absorption and permeability.

In 1996, D'Eufemia and colleagues evaluated intestinal permeability of lactulose and mannitol in 40 children with ASD.[16] Importantly, the study *excluded*, among other things, clinical (that is, symptomatic) evidence of gastrointestinal disease. Despite the exclusion of children with GI symptoms, a significantly higher proportion ($p=<0.001$) of ASD children demonstrated abnormal intestinal permeability of lactulose (but not mannitol) as compared with a non-autistic control group. None of the children had undergone gastrointestinal endoscopy. Speculating on the significance of abnormal lactulose permeability versus the normal permeability seen with mannitol, the authors concluded that the paracellular pathway may be more affected because of alterations of tight junctions between adjacent cells of the bowel mucosa.

A more recent study by de Magistris and colleagues evaluated intestinal permeability as measured by urinary excretion of lactulose and mannitol in children with ASD and their adult first-degree relatives as compared with non-ASD healthy children and their adult first-degree relatives.[17] As compared with the D'Eufemia study, this study excluded only those patients in whom a gastrointestinal disease had been confirmed but did not exclude patients on the basis of the presence of gastrointestinal symptoms. As a result, the study would be expected to identify a larger proportion of children with abnormal intestinal permeability. The researchers found that more than a third (37%) of ASD children showed abnormal intestinal permeability as compared with zero healthy child controls. Interestingly, one-fifth (21%) of the first-degree adult relatives of ASD children also demonstrated abnormal intestinal permeability as compared with only about 5% of the healthy adult controls. The presence of abnormal intestinal permeability within the ASD group did not predict the presence of GI symptoms as reported by the parents. It would be interesting to perform the reverse analysis to see whether patients with GI symptoms are more likely than those without GI symptoms to have increased intestinal permeability. Regardless, this study confirmed the earlier 1996 report of increased intestinal permeability and is entirely consistent with disruption of mucosal barrier function in children with ASD and their first-degree relatives as compared with non-ASD children and their first-degree relatives.

5. Elevated antibody production to clostridial flora species

It is well established that there are serum antibodies to microbial flora of the intestine in both adult and pediatric patients with Crohn's disease, including antibodies to *Saccharomyces cerevisiae* (*S. cerevisiae*), *Escherichia coli* (*E. coli*), and clostridial species. More recent data has associated the presence of some of these antibodies with a more complicated disease course, including fistulization and perforation.[18] When combined with known Crohn's disease gene associations, the presence of these serologic antibodies may even provide prognostic information as to the statistical risks of developing these potential complications.[19] The association between these antibodies and severity of disease takes into account both the number of different species to which antibodies are being produced and the actual amount of antibody to each individual species. Thus, risk of progression to severe disease may be indicated by low levels of numerous species-specific antibodies or, conversely, by exceedingly high levels of antibody to even a single species. The significance of these findings lies in their statistically predictive value. For example, if one knew that a given patient's serologic status was associated with a statistically higher chance of a more severe disease course, this would support earlier and more aggressive treatment.

No published data exist regarding the frequency of these serologic markers in GI-symptomatic children with ASD. However, in my experience with antibody serologies in over 500 GI-symptomatic children with ASD, a pattern has emerged. The pattern involves marked elevation of the cBir1 antibody early in the course of the bowel disease, with negligible antibody presence against *E. coli* and *S. cerevisiae*. The cBir1 antibody is an antibody to the flagella protein on clostridial bacterial species. In the absence of treatment of bowel inflammation, there is a gradual and much smaller rise in the other antibodies over time, but their absolute values do not approach those seen for cBir1. Importantly, retrospective pooled analysis in our patient group demonstrates that the presence of elevated serum cBir1 antibody is statistically predictive for the presence of histologic ileocolitis as seen upon conventional light microscopy. Of further interest is a pattern of cBir1 antibody normalization in patients who, upon receiving pharmaceutical and dietary interventions for their IBD, achieve GI symptom resolution coupled with evidence of mucosal healing on follow-up biopsies. cBir1 appears to enhance the proinflammatory cytokines IL-6 and IL-1 in peripheral blood monocytes, and studies to determine further cytokine associations are under way.

When discussing the presence of serologic antibodies in the setting of inflammatory bowel disease (both ASD-associated and non-ASD-associated), it is important to understand that current data have not demonstrated that the antibodies' presence stems from infection or overgrowth of the organism to which antibodies are being produced. Therefore, no therapeutic interventions should be based on their presence. It is thought that an immunologic intolerance to *normal* intestinal flora develops as a result of the increased intestinal permeability in IBD. Identifying the presence of serologic antibodies to gut flora is used primarily as a way to distinguish between Crohn's disease and ulcerative colitis and to offer prognostic information as to the likelihood of aggressive disease. The relevance of this information for ASD-associated enterocolitis lies in the clues these antibodies may hold for understanding the immunologic mechanisms at play and how these mechanisms affect both bowel and brain function.

Proposing a conceptual model

By synthesizing the aforementioned mucosal immunohistochemical, histochemical, histopathologic, permeability, and serologic data with the clinical observations seen in countless ASD children over the years by parents and clinicians, it is possible to put forth a conceptual model that links these various processes in ASD as follows (Figure 1):

- At some point within the first year of life, an autoimmune process is triggered, targeting the mucosal lining of the bowel. The autoimmune nature of this inflammatory activity is strongly supported by the specific lymphocyte subpopulations seen with immunohistochemical and histochemical staining in both the small and large bowel.[9,10] Light microscopy severely underestimates the presence of this inflammatory activity. The antigen source is likely both exogenous to the body and strongly antigenic.

- As a direct consequence of this T cell inflammatory activity (and to a lesser extent neutrophilic activity), individual villi are decapitated focally but in cumulatively great numbers. Again, and significantly, light microscopy often fails to identify inflammatory cellular infiltrate, or identifies only mild neutrophilic or lymphocytic invasion, in regions of villous damage and associated superficial mucosal erosion.

- In an effort to maintain barrier function integrity of the now-exposed subepithelial compartment, a fibrinous proteinaceous material is exuded from the truncated villi, covering the exposed surface and forming a white spot lesion, which is the endoscopic hallmark of autism-associated inflammatory bowel disease. Surrounding these white spot lesions is a well-demarcated area of superficial mucosal erosion that is enough to decrease the concentration and activity of the most superficially located disaccharidase (lactase) and, less frequently, other disaccharidases.

- T cells cluster around the crypts, perhaps in a further effort to prevent what the immune system recognizes as potentially devastating pathologic absorption of inadequately processed luminal material.

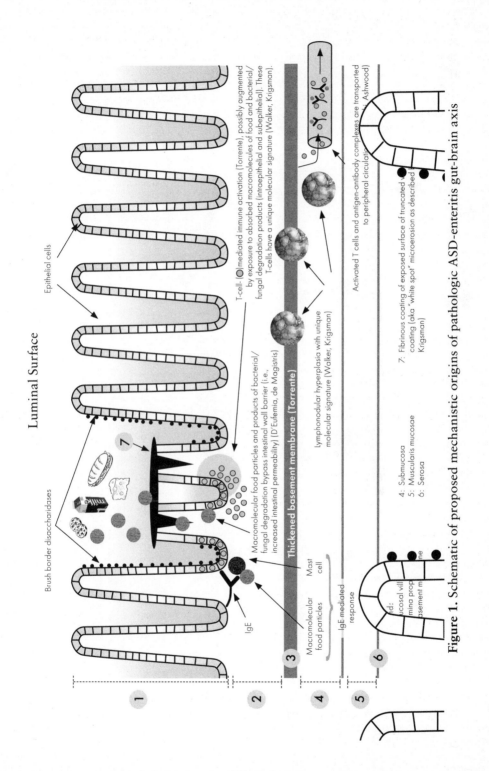

Figure 1. Schematic of proposed mechanistic origins of pathologic ASD-enteritis gut-brain axis

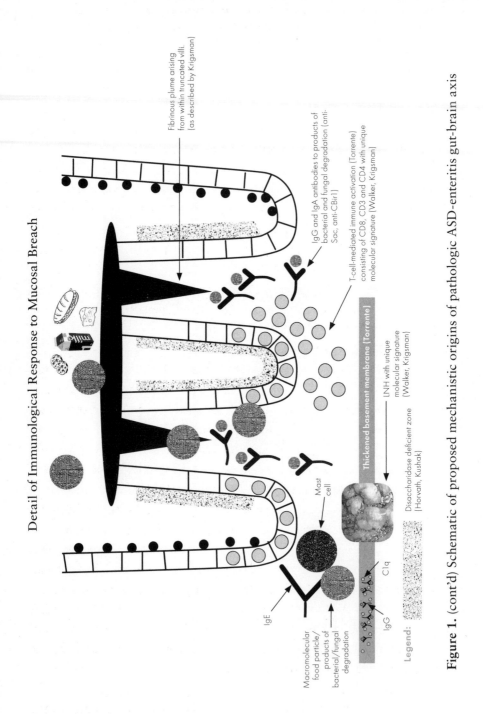

Detail of Immunological Response to Mucosal Breach

Fibrinous plume arising from within truncated villi (as described by Krigsman)

IgG and IgA antibodies to products of bacterial and fungal degradation (anti-Sac, anti-CBir1)

T-cell-mediated immune activation (Torrente) consisting of CD8, CD3 and CD4 with unique molecular signature (Walker, Krigsman)

Thickened basement membrane (Torrente)

LNH with unique molecular signature (Walker, Krigsman)

Disaccharidase deficient zone (Horvath, Kushak)

Mast cell

IgE

Macromolecular food particle/products of bacterial/fungal degradation

Legend: IgG   C1q

Figure 1. (cont'd) Schematic of proposed mechanistic origins of pathologic ASD-enteritis gut-brain axis

42

- Additional architectural protective action undertaken by the immune defenses involves the thickening of the basement membrane with heavy concentration of IgG and complement C1q.

Considering these processes together, it is tempting to view the autistic GI mucosal immunologic response as one that attempts to confine the damage to the epithelium and contain any pathologically absorbed luminal products within the inflamed epithelium. The products of this intense inflammatory activity, including cytokines, remain local to the mucosa but also are transported systemically via the blood. It is entirely conceivable that the proinflammatory molecular products of mucosal cellular-mediated inflammation are transported via the blood to extraintestinal locations such as the brain[20] and the large joints, causing encephalitis and arthritis, respectively.

Further adding to the inflammatory cascade at the luminal surface is the presence of bacterial and fungal flora which, as a result of the loss of intestinal mucosal barrier integrity, are now in direct contact with the high concentration of protective gastrointestinal lymphoid tissue that normally lines the gastrointestinal tract. This exposure triggers production of particularly high levels of serum anticlostridial antibodies (anti cBir1), well above those seen in Crohn's disease and ulcerative colitis. Antibody production against other floral species occurs as well but to a significantly lesser extent. Our data show that the presence of elevated levels of serum anticlostridial antibody is predictive of enterocolonic inflammation, and the cBir1 antibody is associated with production of proinflammatory cytokines. Additional inflammatory cytokine activity occurring in the intestinal mucosa has been documented as well.[21] The contribution, if any, of *abnormal* flora to this ASD-GI mucosal inflammatory process is less well understood.

The ability of luminal contents to bypass selective absorptive pathways is reflected most simplistically in the permeability studies of D'Eufemia and de Magistris.[16,17] The observation that lactulose, rather than mannitol, is the predominant abnormally absorbed analyte is consistent with the concept of disrupted mucosal integrity in the manner described above.

Despite immunologic attempts at repair and containment, the primary autoimmune inflammatory process is ultimately ineffective.

Luminal products, such as incompletely digested food and products of microbial degradation, succeed in reaching the systemic circulation, where further immunologic activation occurs, though at least some of this observed activity may be the result of immune activation occurring at the aforementioned luminal surface. Proinflammatory cytokine activity within the peripheral blood of GI-symptomatic ASD children has been noted in response to specific dietary antigens such as gluten and casein.[22,23] Because of the young age of the child and the critical developmental window during which this process occurs, the successful penetration of luminal bacterial and fungal degradation products, luminal diet-derived products, and the degradation products of the destroyed cells themselves could then potentially serve as catalysts for a variety of mechanisms described elsewhere in this publication, resulting in developmental delay, arrest, or regression.

From the standpoint of clinical gastroenterology, the inflammatory processes described above result in such "conventional" symptoms as diarrhea, constipation, abdominal pain, abdominal distention, and failure to thrive. *The phenomenon of neurodevelopmental dysfunction as the result of gut-brain axis involvement within the setting of gastrointestinal disease allows for the specific neurodevelopmental disease, in this case autism, to be considered no less a GI symptom than diarrhea.*

This mechanistic approach provides a unifying explanation for some intriguing clinical observations frequently made by those who care for ASD patients. Clinical observations point to improvement in cognitive and gastrointestinal function when patients are on one of the following:

- a clear liquid diet (in preparation for colonoscopy)
- a diet that excludes protein (i.e., an exclusively elemental formula)
- a regimen of regular bowel cleanouts
- courses of antibacterial agents
- courses of antifungal agents
- probiotics
- supplemental digestive enzymes
- oral 5-aminosalicylates
- corticosteroids
- immunomodulators

Perhaps the most intriguing observation of all is that improvement in gastrointestinal function frequently correlates with improvement in cognitive and behavioral function. Conversely, worsening of gastrointestinal function is frequently associated with a decline in cognitive and behavioral function.[24,25] Parents often report that when they see the first morning stool, they immediately know what kind of "autism day" lies ahead.

From a treatment standpoint, the presence of chronic gastrointestinal symptoms in the face of demonstrable mucosal pathology warrants treatment for the IBD. In the absence of any data to the contrary, it is clinically reasonable to treat autism-associated IBD in identical fashion to the IBD observed in conventional, non-ASD Crohn's disease. To the extent that this unifying theory of gut-brain axis involvement is correct (i.e., that the neurodevelopmental disorder called "autism" is a gastrointestinal symptom), primary treatment of the IBD holds great promise as a potential treatment for ASD and possibly other neuropsychiatric disorders with known bowel mucosal pathology.

References

1. Husby S, Foged N, Høst A, Svehag SE. Passage of dietary antigens into the blood of children with coeliac disease. Quantification and size distribution of absorbed antigens. *Gut.* 1987 Sep;28(9):1062-72.

2. Bushara KO. Neurologic presentation of celiac disease. *Gastroenterology.* 2005 Apr;128(4 Suppl 1):S92-S97.

3. Lerner A, Rossi TM, Park B, Albini B, Lebenthal E. Serum antibodies to cow's milk proteins in pediatric inflammatory bowel disease. Crohn's disease versus ulcerative colitis. *Acta Paediatr Scand.* 1989 May;78(3):384-9.

4. North CS, Alpers DH. A review of studies of psychiatric factors in Crohn's disease: etiologic implications. *Ann Clin Psychiatry.* 1994 June;6(2):117-24.

5. Kelsay K. Psychological aspects of food allergy. *Curr Allergy Asthma Rep.* 2003 Jan;3(1):41-6.

6. Wakefield AJ, Anthony A, Murch SH, Thomson M, Montgomery SM, Davies S, et al. Enterocolitis in children with developmental disorders. *Am J Gastroenterol.* 2000 Sep;95(9):2285-95.

7. González L, Lopez K, Martinez M, et al. Endoscopic and histological characteristics of the digestive mucosa in autistic children with gastro-intestinal symptoms: preliminary report. *G.E.N. suplemento especial de pediatria.* 2005;1:41-7.

8. Krigsman A, Boris M, Goldblatt A, Stott C. Clinical presentation and histologic findings at ileocolonoscopy in children with autistic spectrum disorder and chronic gastrointestinal symptoms. *Autism Insights.* 2010;2:1-11.

9. Furlano RI, Anthony A, Day R, Brown A, McGarvey L, Thomson MA, et al. Colonic CD8 and gamma delta T-cell infiltration with epithelial damage in children with autism. *J Pediatr.* 2001 Mar;138(3):366-72.

10. Torrente F, Anthony A, Heuschkel RB, Thomson MA, Ashwood P, Murch SH. Focal-enhanced gastritis in regressive autism with features distinct from Crohn's and *Helicobacter pylori* gastritis. *Am J Gastroenterol.* 2004 Apr;99(4):598-605.

11. Horvath K, Papadimitriou JC, Rabsztyn A, Drachenberg C, Tildon JT. Gastrointestinal abnormalities in children with autistic disorder. *J Pediatr.* 1999 Nov;135(5):559-63.

12. Walker SJ, Fortunato J, Gonzalez LG, Krigsman A (2013) Identification of Unique Gene Expression Profile in Children with Regressive Autism Spectrum Disorder (ASD) and Ileocolitis. *PLoS ONE* 8(3); e58058.doi:10.1371/journal.pone.0058058.

13. Rickert RR, Carter HW. The "early" ulcerative lesion of Crohn's disease: correlative light- and scanning electron-microscopic studies. *J Clin Gastroenterol.* 1980 Mar;2(1):11-9.

14. Sankey EA, Dhillon AP, Anthony A, Wakefield AJ, Sim R, More L, et al. Early mucosal changes in Crohn's disease. *Gut.* 1993 Mar;34(3):375-81.

15. Kushak RI, Lauwers GY, Winter HS, Buie TM. Intestinal disaccharidase activity in patients with autism: effect of age, gender, and intestinal inflammation. *Autism.* 2011 May;15(3):285-94.

16. D'Eufemia P, Celli M, Finocchiaro R, Pacifico L, Viozzi L, Zaccagnini M, et al. Abnormal intestinal permeability in children with autism. *Acta Paediatr.* 1996 Sep;85(9):1076-9.

17. de Magistris L, Familiari V, Pascotto A, Sapone A, Frolli A, Iardino P, et al. Alterations of the intestinal barrier in patients with autism spectrum disorders and in their first-degree relatives. *J Pediatr Gastroenterol Nutr.* 2010 Oct;51(4):418-24.

18. Dubinsky MC, Kugathasan S, Mei L, Picornell Y, Nebel J, Wrobel I, et al. Increased immune reactivity predicts aggressive complicating Crohn's disease in children. *Clin Gastroenterol Hepatol.* 2008 Oct;6(10):1105-11.

19. Ippoliti A, Devlin S, Mei L, Yang H, Papadakis KA, Vasiliauskas EA, et al. Combination of innate and adaptive immune alterations increased the likelihood of fibrostenosis in Crohn's disease. *Inflamm Bowel Dis.* 2010 Aug;16(8):1279-85.

20. Vargas DL, Nascimbene C, Krishnan C, Zimmerman AW, Pardo CA. Neuroglial activation and neuroinflammation in the brain of patients with autism. *Ann Neurol.* 2005 Jan;57(1):67-81. *Erratum in Ann Neurol.* 2005 Feb;57(2):304.

21. Ashwood P, Anthony A, Torrente F, Wakefield AJ. Spontaneous mucosal lymphocyte cytokine profiles in children with autism and gastrointestinal symptoms: mucosal immune activation and reduced counter regulatory interleukin-10. *J Clin Immunol.* 2004 Nov;24(6):664-73.

22. Jyonouchi H, Geng L, Ruby A, Zimmerman-Bier B. Dysregulated innate immune responses in young children with autism spectrum disorders: their relationship to gastrointestinal symptoms and dietary intervention. *Neuropsychobiology.* 2005;51(2):77-85.

23. Jyonouchi H, Geng L, Ruby A, Reddy C, Zimmerman-Bier B. Evaluation of an association between gastrointestinal symptoms and cytokine production against common dietary proteins in children with autism spectrum disorders. *J Pediatr.* 2005 May;146(5):605-10.

24. Maenner MJ, Arneson CL, Levy SE, Kirby RS, Nicholas JS, Durkin MS. Brief report: association between behavioral features and gastrointestinal problems among children with autism spectrum disorder. *J Autism Dev Disord.* 2011 Oct 20. DOI 10.1007/s10803-011-1379-6.

25. Adams JB, Johansen LJ, Powell LD, Quig D, Rubin RA. Gastrointestinal flora and gastrointestinal status in children with autism-comparisons to typical children and correlation with autism severity. *BMC Gastroenterol.* 2011 Mar;11:22.

CHAPTER THREE

ROLE OF THE GI TRACT IN NEUROEPIGENETIC REGULATION DURING EARLY DEVELOPMENT AND ITS IMPLICATIONS FOR AUTISM

By Richard C. Deth, PhD[1]; Nathaniel W. Hodgson[1]; Stephen Walker, PhD[2]; Arthur Krigsman, MD[3]; and Malav S. Trivedi[1]

[1]Department of Pharmaceutical Sciences, Northeastern University, Boston, MA 02115
[2] Institute for Regenerative Medicine, Wake Forest University, Winston-Salem, NC 27101
[3] Pediatric Gastroenterology Resources of New York, Far Rockaway, NY 11691

Outline:

1. Redox-dependent epigenetic regulation
2. Brain-specific neuroepigenetic regulation
3. Intestinal absorption of cysteine
4. Prenatal and postnatal epigenetic programming (PrEP and PEP)
5. Casein- and gluten-derived opiate peptides
6. Summary

There is now substantial evidence that autism is a neurodevelopmental disorder caused by a deficiency in antioxidant availability, leading to a state of oxidative stress. The link between the metabolic condition of oxidative stress and neurodevelopmental disorders involves the critical role of DNA methylation and its epigenetic influence over gene expression, which is highly sensitive to oxidative stress. Although the brain is the obvious organ of focus for understanding autism, it is also becoming obvious that dysfunction of the gastrointestinal (GI) tract is a key underlying contributor to autism. This chapter will examine the crucial processes which normally provide adequate antioxidant capacity to support aerobic metabolism, with a particular emphasis on early development.

1. Redox-dependent epigenetic regulation

While the human genome contains about 23,000 genes, only a fraction of them are active in a given cell at a given time. Inactive genes are repressed by being wound into tight complexes with histone proteins, preventing their transcription into messenger RNA, which otherwise would lead to synthesis of the proteins specified by their DNA sequence. Different cell types (neurons, cardiocytes, skin cells, etc.) all contain the same DNA, but they each stably express a unique pattern of genes, with the other genes being stably silenced. The key event for silencing genes is the placement of a single carbon atom, called a methyl group, at specific DNA sites in the gene which interferes with its transcription and promotes its complexation with histones.[1] These methyl groups are called *epigenetic marks* and their influence is called *epigenetic regulation of gene expression.*[2]

The many different roles of epigenetic regulation have only begun to be appreciated in the past several years, but it is already clear that they involve almost every aspect of human physiology. During fetal and infant development, genes are turned on and off by changes in their epigenetic regulation, underlying the progression from pluripotent stem cells to fully differentiated tissues and organs.[3] Tumor cells display an abnormal pattern of DNA methylation, which appears to be responsible for sustaining their uncontrolled rate of growth.[4] In the brain, epigenetic regulation of gene expression is intimately related to memory formation.[5] Abnormal patterns of DNA methylation have been linked to a number of neurodevelopmental,[6] neuropsychiatric,[7] and neurodegenerative disorders,[8] as well as to the effects of drugs of abuse.[9] The importance of epigenetic mechanisms in developmental disorders is exemplified by Rett syndrome, which is commonly caused

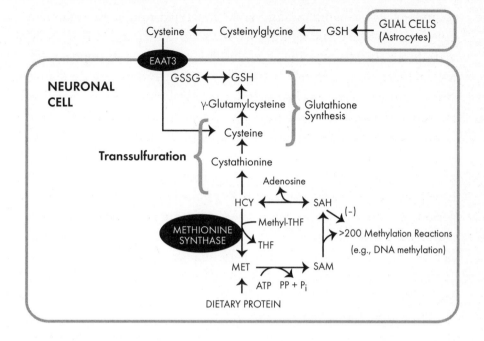

Figure 1. Redox and methylation pathways in neurons. The amino acid cysteine is rate-limiting for glutathione (GSH) synthesis and it is provided either by uptake from astrocyte-derived cysteine or by transsulfuration of homocysteine (HCY). The methionine cycle of methylation (lower right) depends upon both dietary methionine (MET) and remethylation of HCY by methionine synthase. Since formation of HCY from S-adenosylhomocysteine (SAH) is reversible and SAH inhibits methylation, decreased methionine synthase activity (e.g., caused by oxidative stress) both augments GSH synthesis and inhibits methylation reactions. Thus redox status and methylation activity are closely linked.

by mutations in the MECP2 protein, which binds to methylated DNA sites and promotes gene silencing.[10]

Methylation of DNA depends upon adequate levels the methyl donor S-adenosylmethionine (SAM) and is inhibited by the demethylated form of SAM, known as S-adenosylhomocysteine (SAH), as illustrated for a neuron cell in Figure 1. The SAM to SAH ratio, therefore, determines the level of methylation, and this ratio is, in turn, determined by the folate and vitamin B12 enzyme methionine synthase (MS), which converts homocysteine (HCY) to methionine as part of the methionine cycle of methylation. Any decrease in MS activity causes both HCY and SAH to accumulate since conversion of SAH to HCY is reversible, resulting in inhibition of methylation reactions.[11] HCY can alternatively be converted to cystathionine and cysteine via the transsulfuration pathway, increasing synthesis of glutathione (GSH) the primary intracellular antioxidant. Importantly, MS activity is exquisitely sensitive to any increase in oxidative stress, and since one consequence of its inhibition is an increase in transsulfuration and GSH formation, this makes MS inhibition a critical way for cells to maintain their level of antioxidant. However, since decreased MS activity decreases the SAM/SAH ratio, this mode of adapting to oxidative stress will necessarily also result in impaired methylation, including a decrease in DNA methylation, especially if the period of oxidative stress is sustained. This fundamental relationship involving sulfur metabolite pathways means that oxidative stress is a significant threat to normal epigenetic regulation of gene expression, especially during development, thus forming the basis for the "Redox/ Methylation Hypothesis of Autism."[12]

Oxidation, the loss of electrons, is the primary source of energy for cells, and the ongoing production of ATP by mitochondria depends upon conversion of oxygen (O_2) to water (H_2O), accompanied by the inevitable release of a significant portion (1-5%) as highly reactive oxygen species (ROS), which readily oxidize and damage biomolecules.[13] Antioxidants are, therefore, essential to neutralize ROS byproducts by reducing them and to assist in the repair of oxidized biomolecules. When GSH serves this role and gives up its electrons, it is converted to its oxidized GSSG state, which must then be reduced back to GSH. This is accomplished by a fresh supply of electrons provided via a reducing system that starts with electrons from glucose that are transferred through the cofactor NADPH and selenium-containing redox proteins to convert GSSG to GSH.[14] Cells use this system to maintain the correct balance between GSH and GSSG (redox equilibrium), which is usually close to a 100:1 ratio in favor of GSH. Thus, the redox state of cells depends upon both an adequate amount of GSH and the reducing system that keeps the GSH to GSSG ratio high; so, an inadequate supply of antioxidant leads to a condition of oxidative stress. As described below, normal function of the GI tract is essential for maintaining redox status by providing sufficient absorption of cysteine to support adequate levels of GSH. However, autistic children have low levels of GSH and elevated biomarkers of oxidative stress both in blood[15-18] and in brain tissue,[19,20] indicating a systemic deficiency in antioxidant capacity, which can be traced to a GI origin in many cases.

2. Brain-specific neuroepigenetic regulation

While all cells rely upon the same basic antioxidant system, there are significant variations between different organs which, in the case of the brain, allows redox status and cysteine-dependent GSH synthesis to exert even greater epigenetic control. This is accomplished in large part by making GSH a very scarce commodity in neurons so that any change in its level will have a disproportionately greater impact on redox and methylation status. Thus, the level of GSH in neuronal cells is about 0.2 mM, whereas in other cell types, such as liver, its concentration is about 10 mM, a 50-fold difference. This shortage of antioxidant is even more critical since oxygen consumption by the brain is about 10-fold higher than other tissues.[14] Consequently, redox regulation is a particularly powerful mechanism for guiding brain development and for controlling brain function throughout the lifespan.

The low level of GSH in neurons reflects the limited availability of cysteine within the cell, which, in turn, reflects the low concentration outside of the cell in cerebral spinal fluid (CSF). The blood-brain barrier only allows the oxidized form of cysteine (cystine) to enter the CSF, and cystine cannot be taken up by neurons. Instead, cystine is taken up by glial cells such as astrocytes, where it is reduced and converted to GSH. The level of GSH is about 4-fold higher in astrocytes than in neurons.[21] A portion of astrocyte GSH is exported and hydrolyzed to release its cysteine, which is then available for neuronal uptake by the transporter designated EAAT3 (Figure 1). EAAT3 is named for the other members of its protein family that transport excitatory amino acids such as glutamate, but EAAT3 has a strong preference for cysteine and provides > 90% of cellular uptake, making it the single most important controller of neuronal GSH levels and redox status.[22] EAAT3 is prominently expressed in the small intestine, where it appears to also be critical for intestinal absorption of cysteine[23] as well as for cysteine uptake by immune cells, especially regulatory T-cell lymphocytes, which regulate autoimmunity.[24] Interestingly, levels of EAAT3 are higher during growth, indicating the importance of adequate antioxidant for development.[25]

Our laboratory has examined EAAT3-mediated cysteine uptake by human neuronal cells and found that it is regulated by a number of factors that utilize changes in redox status to influence neuronal metabolic activity and modulate gene expression. For example, we found that neurotrophic growth factors (e.g., insulin-like growth factor-1 [IGF-1] and brain-derived growth factor [BDNF]), promote cysteine uptake and increase GSH/GSSG and SAM/SAH in association with an increase in DNA methylation, leading to changes in transcription of a number of genes.[26] The neurotransmitter dopamine increases cysteine uptake and promotes DNA methylation, while alcohol, morphine, enkephalin, and food-derived opiate peptides inhibit cysteine uptake and decrease GSH/GSSG and SAM/SAH, resulting in changes in gene DNA methylation and gene transcription.[27,28] These observations make it clear that EAAT3-mediated redox regulation provides an important opportunity for a wide range of physiological and environmental signals to exert an epigenetic influence on brain development and function.

Another contribution to the low level of GSH in neurons arises from the restricted level of transsulfuration activity in the brain when compared with other tissues. As illustrated in Figure 1, HCY can be converted to cystathionine by cystathionine-beta-synthase (CBS), which is then converted to cysteine by cystathionine-gamma-lyase (CGL). However, this transsulfuration pathway operates at a reduced level in the brain due to lower activity of CGL, limiting the amount of cysteine it provides.[29] As a consequence, EAAT3-mediated cysteine uptake is even more critical as a source of GSH synthesis, increasing the power of factors that regulate its activity. The extent of decrease in transsulfuration shows a remarkable progressive decrease during evolution, evident as an increase in the brain concentration of cystathionine.[30] The level in man is about 2-fold higher than in nonhuman primates, 8-fold higher than in lower mammals, and 40-fold higher than in chickens and ducks. This pattern suggests that utilization of redox-based signaling to control brain function has resulted in positive benefits that favor evolution of species with less and less transsulfuration. It might not, therefore, be surprising that problems that adversely affect redox signaling in the brain might result in a loss of human-specific traits and abilities, such as language and social behavior.

So, how does the brain get by with such low levels of GSH? The answer is selenium. The restricted availability of GSH in the brain is partly compensated for by an increased dependence upon selenoproteins to sustain the flow of antioxidant electrons and to keep GSH in its reduced state. Selenoproteins contain selenium in the form of the amino acid selenocysteine, and they perform a variety of important redox reactions, including the elimination of hydrogen peroxide and the repair of oxidized molecules.[31] To ensure that it has sufficient selenoproteins, the brain (as well as the testes) has evolved a higher capacity to retain precious selenium, and when selenium levels in the plasma are low, other tissues become depleted while brain levels remain high.[32] Unfortunately, selenoproteins are exquisitely sensitive to inhibition by mercury,[33] and any mercury that penetrates the brain will interfere with redox signaling and potentially disrupt normal epigenetic regulation. The very tight, almost irreversible, binding of mercury by selenoproteins contributes to the long-term retention of mercury in the brain and its gradual accumulation across the lifespan. Indeed, it has been proposed that selenoprotein P serves a specific role to protect against mercury toxicity.[34]

3. Intestinal absorption of cysteine

Starting from birth, the systemic availability of cysteine to support GSH synthesis is dependent upon absorption of protein-derived sulfur and selenium-containing amino acids from the GI tract (Figure 2). The epithelial cells that line the intestinal wall express different transporters on their surface, which are critical for uptake of cysteine, methionine, and selenocysteine.[35] These amino acids are then subject to intracellular metabolism within the epithelial cells before being ultimately released to the general circulation on the contralateral surface, either in their free form 'or incorporated into proteins or peptides, including GSH. Availability of transported cysteine or selenium can, therefore, affect the GSH levels and redox status of the epithelial cells themselves, as well as that of the adjacent cells located within the intestinal wall, including immune cells.

EAAT3 was initially cloned from GI epithelial cells,[36] and subsequent studies revealed that it is most prominently expressed in the small intestine, especially in the terminal ileum,[22] a prominent site of

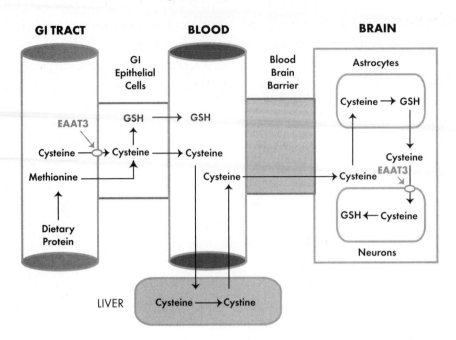

Figure 2. Absorption and systemic distribution of dietary cysteine and methionine. GI epithelial cells take up cysteine and methionine, with EAAT3 being particularly important for cysteine uptake in the distal ileum. A portion of methionine is converted to cysteine via the methionine cycle and transsulfuration of homocysteine. Absorbed cysteine is taken up by the liver, which releases oxidized cystine. Cystine, but not cysteine, is able to traverse the blood-brain barrier and is taken up by astroctyes, which convert it to GSH. Cysteine from astrocyte-derived GSH is available for EAAT3-mediated neuronal uptake, supporting neuronal GSH synthesis.

inflammation in subjects with autism.[37] The highest levels were found in crypt cells and lower villus regions, the locus of multipotent stem cells that sustain the epithelial lining of the gut.[38] EAAT3 shuttles back and forth between the endoplasmic reticulum on the inside of the cell and the surface membrane, and its movement to the cell surface is promoted by growth factors that activate the PI3 kinase signaling pathway, similar to insulin regulation of glucose transporters.[39] In resting cells, about 75% of EAAT3 resides inside the cell where it is inactive, but activation of PI3 kinase increases the proportion of active transporters in the plasma membrane. Once it is positioned in the surface membrane, EAAT3-mediated cysteine uptake is subject to further regulation by opiate and dopamine receptors. Importantly, oxidative stress inhibits

EAAT3 transport activity,[40] and several cysteine residues have been identified as being critical for this mode of regulation,[41] raising the possibility that they might be targets for glutathionylation. Thus, local oxidative stress and inflammation affecting the terminal ileum, such as is observed frequently in autism,[37] can decrease EAAT3-dependent absorption of both cysteine and selenocysteine, resulting in systemic consequences of lower GSH levels and decreased antioxidant capacity.

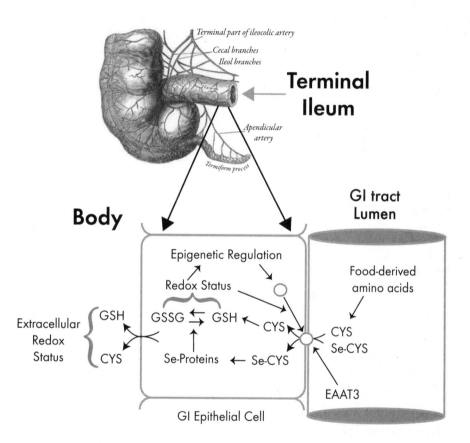

Figure 3. Cysteine and selenocysteine uptake in the terminal ileum. EAAT3 transports diet-derived cysteine (CYS) and selenocysteine (Sel-CYS) into GI epithelial cells in the terminal ileum. Within the cell, cysteine is directed to GSH synthesis and selenocysteine is incorporated into selenoproteins, which maintain GSH in its reduced state. EAAT3 activity is regulated by multiple factors, including intracellular redox status, growth-factor-dependent translocation to the cell surface, epigenetic regulation, and the inhibitory effects of casein- and gluten-derived opiate peptides. Systemic availability of cysteine and GSH depends upon these terminal ileum events.

Notably, the terminal ileum is also an important location for dietary folic acid and vitamin B12 absorption, both of which are essential cofactors for MS activity. Also notably, intestinal microorganisms in the large intestine synthesize folic acid and vitamin B12, representing an additional source. As illustrated in Figure 3, folate uptake into epithelial cells from the intestinal lumen involves the reduced folate carrier (RFC1), while the transport of both folate and vitamin B12 to the body appears to involve the multidrug resistance proteins (MRP). MRP preferentially transports GSH and glutathionylated conjugates of many molecules,[42] possibly including glutathionyl-B12.[43] Thus, under oxidative stress conditions when GSH levels are decreased, the transport of vitamin B12 (and possibly folic acid) to the systemic circulation would be compromised.

It is remarkable that the systemic availability of multiple factors that control redox and methylation status (cysteine, selenocysteine, folate, and vitamin B12) is provided by the same distal segment of the small intestine. Given the importance of methylation-dependent epigenetic regulation for neurodevelopment, it is not surprising that inflammation of the terminal ileum, as first described by Wakefield and colleagues,[37] appears to be an important contributor to autism risk.

4. Prenatal and postnatal epigenetic programming (PrEP and PEP)

Postnatal infant nutrition is most commonly provided by either human breast milk or bovine milk (i.e., formula). Human breast milk is comparatively rich in sulfur-containing amino acids, and colostrum contains 2.5-fold higher levels when compared with mature milk.[44] A comparison of plasma cysteine levels in 12-week-old infants found significantly higher levels for breast-fed versus formula-fed infants.[45] Thus, not surprisingly, breast- feeding appears to provide a superior supply of the essential raw materials for synthesis of the antioxidant GSH. As this source of cysteine is made available, EAAT3 and the factors that modulate its activity serve as critical regulators of the extent to which cysteine may be absorbed.

Breast milk contains a number of different growth factors, including insulin-like growth factor-1, epidermal growth factor, vascular endothelial growth factor, and hepatocyte growth factor, among others.[46,47] These factors activate PI3 kinase, and we found that they stimulate EAAT3-mediated cysteine uptake, accompanied by an increase in GSH levels, an increased SAM/SAH ratio, and increased DNA methylation.[48] Growth factors promote GSH synthesis via both increased cysteine uptake and transcriptional effects, corresponding to short-term and longer-term effects, respectively. These observations imply that breast milk-derived growth factors can stimulate cysteine uptake and increase GSH in the GI epithelium, coincident with the initiation of postnatal digestion. The extent to which antioxidant resources (i.e., cysteine and GSH) are made available to the rest of the body depends upon the efficiency of this process.

Human breast milk is also rich in selenium, and breast-fed infants have higher selenium levels than formula-fed infants.[49] A significant proportion (up to 30%) of breast milk selenium is in the form of glutathione peroxidase (GPx), which is hydrolyzed to selenocysteine

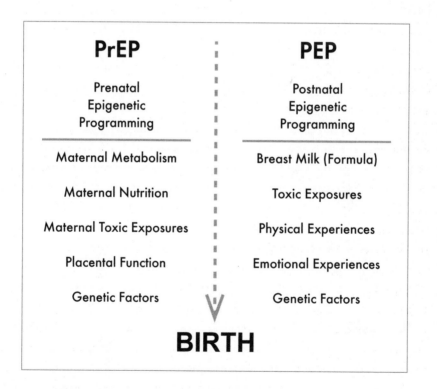

Figure 4. Prenatal and postnatal epigenetic programming. Gene expression is subject to epigenetic regulation via a wide range of factors, many of which impact redox status, thereby affecting DNA and histone methylation. GI tract function plays an important role during postnatal epigenetic programming with lifelong consequences.

during digestion. The importance of GPx activity in breast milk may be to combat oxidation, especially of vulnerable omega-3 fatty acids. However, GPx appears to also represent an important reservoir for delivery of selenium to the developing infant. As a structural analog of cysteine, breast milk-derived selenocysteine can also be transported by EAAT3 and contributes to antioxidant capacity and redox status.[50]

As MS activity and the SAM/SAH ratio are responsive to redox status, it is reasonable to propose that the postnatal transition to independent nutrition is associated with epigenetic responses involving both the GI tract and the body as a whole and that growth factor stimulation of cysteine uptake is a key event in this transition. We call this period of metabolic adaptation *postnatal epigenetic programming* (PEP), as contrasted to *prenatal epigenetic programming* (PrEP), for which maternal nutritional status plays a critical role, and we specifically propose that the GI tract plays a uniquely important role in determining the outcome of PEP.[24] We further suggest that availability of antioxidant resources is the critical determinant of the level of metabolic activity that may be safely achieved without cellular damage. Epigenetic regulation of gene expression provides a molecular mechanism by which the functional state of the GI tract can be matched to the ongoing level of metabolic activity. In other words, the supply of antioxidant must be matched to the demand for antioxidant, and the rate of postnatal growth and development must be restricted so as to not exceed the supply provided by the GI tract. The metabolic consequences of PEP can be profound and can potentially express themselves across the lifespan.

Failure of the GI epithelium to absorb cysteine or selenocysteine increases the availability of these antioxidant resources for utilization by the bacteria that populate the intestine. Indeed, there is a competition between us and the intestinal flora for certain shared nutrients as well as a symbiotic relationship via which we benefit from microbial metabolites including folic acid and vitamin B12. For example, only certain bacteria have the enzymes necessary to synthesize vitamin B12, which we are able to absorb when it is released in our GI tract. Even when we obtain B12 from the consumption of meat, we are only accessing the B12 produced by bacteria residing in the cow, chicken, etc. Cysteine is vital to certain microbes, and when oxidative stress diminishes our uptake of cysteine, cysteine-utilizing microbes flourish and their population expands, shifting the microflora composition toward a state of dysbiosis associated with GI inflammation.[51] Expansion of cysteine-utilizing microbes increases the strength of their competition, which can make it more difficult for GI epithelial cells to take up cysteine, perpetuating the systemic antioxidant deficit. Once established, this vicious cycle can be difficult to interrupt.

Autistic children frequently present with significant GI symptoms, including chronic diarrhea or constipation, foul-smelling stools, and failure to thrive, which can reflect both dysbiosis and inflammation. Endoscopic examination of the bowel can establish a firm diagnosis and set the stage for appropriate treatment strategies. In addition, biopsy samples obtained during endoscopy provide an opportunity for more detailed testing. We carried out a microarray-based analysis of gene expression in biopsy tissue samples from a series of autistic subjects with inflammation of the terminal ileum and compared the results to samples from neurotypical control subjects undergoing endoscopy, who did not exhibit inflammation of the terminal ileum. As illustrated in Table 1, we observed significant differences in the expression of a number of genes that regulate redox and methylation pathways. Expression was lower for all of the enzymes involved in GSH synthesis and transsulfuration, including EAAT3, as well as the D4 dopamine receptor, whose phospholipid methylation activity is dependent upon MS, and NRF2, a transcription factor that controls many oxidative stress-responsive genes. In contrast, expression of the pro-inflammatory cytokine tumor necrosis factor-alpha (TNF-α) was significantly increased, which would be expected in the presence of inflammation. TNF-α levels are elevated in the plasma,[52] cerebral spinal fluid,[53] and brain tissue of autistic subjects,[54] as well as in amniotic fluid during their gestation.[55] Notably, mercury causes a male gender-specific increase of brain TNF-α levels.[56] We found that TNF-α inhibits cysteine uptake[57] and increases transsulfuration,[58] as well as causing a decrease in MS mRNA levels.[57] Taken together, these changes indicate significant alterations of GSH synthesis and methylation pathways in the distal ileum of autistic children, in association with local inflammation, which are likely to contribute to well-documented systemic oxidative stress and impaired methylation.

Table 1. Changes in Redox/Methylation mRNA Levels in Terminal Ileum in Autism

Gene	Name	Fold change	Direction
EAAT3	Excitatory amino acid transporter 3	2.2	Down
GCLC	Gamma glutamylcysteine ligase (catalytic subunit)	1.6	Down
GCLM	Gamma glutamylcysteine ligase (regulatory subunit)	1.7	Down
GSS	Glutathione synthetase	1.5	Down
GSR	Glutathione reductase	1.7	Down
CBS	Cystathionine beta-synthase	2.4	Down
CTH	Cystathionine gamma-lyase	2.6	Down
MTHFR	Methylenetetrahydrofolate reductase	1.6	Down
DRD4	D4 dopamine receptor	2.1	Down
NRF2	Nuclear factor erythroid 2-like 2	3.1	Down
TNFA	Tumor necrosis factor-alpha	1.6	Up

5. Casein- and gluten-derived opiate peptides

Parental and published reports indicating beneficial effects of a gluten-free/casein-free (GF/CF) diet in autism,[59] coupled with evidence of GI inflammation,[37] suggests a possible role for bioactive peptides, which are released from gluten and casein, and have been previously shown to stimulate opiate receptors.[60,61] To investigate this possibility, we examined the redox effects of three peptides that are relatively stable end products of gluten and beta-casein of either human or bovine origin. As illustrated in Figure 5, these peptides share a similar but non-identical amino acid sequence, and their proline residues make them comparatively resistant to further hydrolysis, although they can be hydrolyzed by dipeptidylpeptidase-4 (DPP-IV or CD26).[62] Importantly, studies suggest a role for casein-derived opiate peptides and low DPP-IV activity in sudden infant death syndrome (SIDS).[63-65]

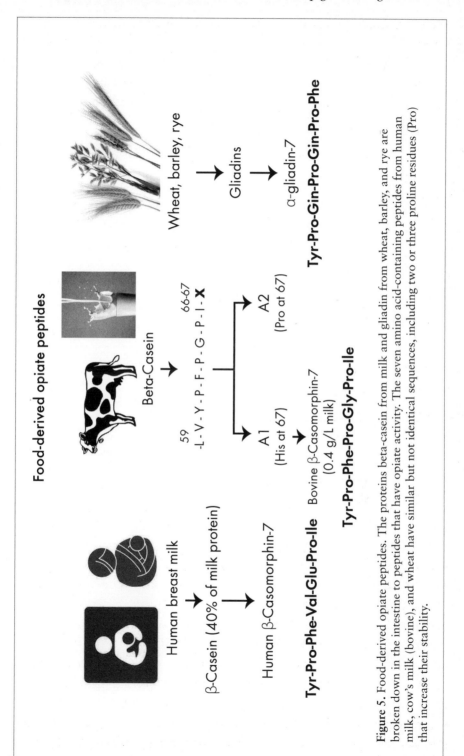

Figure 5. Food-derived opiate peptides. The proteins beta-casein from milk and gliadin from wheat, barley, and rye are broken down in the intestine to peptides that have opiate activity. The seven amino acid-containing peptides from human milk, cow's milk (bovine), and wheat have similar but not identical sequences, including two or three proline residues (Pro) that increase their stability.

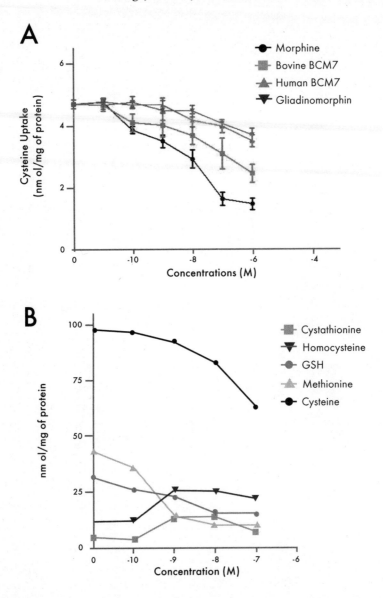

Figure 6. Effects of morphine and opiate peptides on cysteine uptake and thiol metabolite levels. A. Cysteine uptake was measured in cultured human intestinal epithelial cells after 30 min incubation with either morphine, human, or bovine casomorphin-7 (BCM7), or the gliadin-derived peptide gliadinomorphin at the indicated concentrations. Morphine caused the greatest decrease in uptake, followed bovine BCM7, human BCM7 and gliadinomorphin. B. Cellular levels of sulfur metabolites were measured in human neuronal cells following a 4 hr incubation with 1 μM bovine BCM7. Significant decreases in cysteine, GSH, and methionine were observed, while homocysteine and cystathionine increased. This pattern is consistent with decreased cysteine uptake and inhibition of methionine synthase activity.

In cultured cell studies using either human intestinal epithelial cells or human neuroblastoma cells, we found that all three peptides, as well as morphine, inhibited the uptake of cysteine in a dose-dependent manner after a 30-minute period of incubation (Figure 6A). While morphine was clearly the most powerful inhibitor, the bovine (cow's milk) peptide was stronger than the human peptide in both epithelial and neuronal cells. This inhibitory effect was also evident as a decrease in cellular levels of cysteine and GSH (Figure 6B). These peptide effects were completely blocked by naltrexone and naloxone, confirming involvement of opiate receptors. Although cultured cell studies may not fully reflect *in vivo* responses, these results indicate that a GF/CF diet may exert its beneficial effect in autism by facilitating intestinal cysteine uptake, thereby increasing availability of this essential raw material for GSH synthesis. In addition, the greater inhibitory activity of the bovine peptide versus the human peptide supports the generally held belief that breastfeeding offers unique benefits to early development that may reflect the epigenetic consequences of an enhanced antioxidant capacity.

Gluten intolerance is the classic feature of celiac disease. The prevalence of gluten intolerance in the U.S. is increasing, paralleling, to some extent, the increase in autism rates. It is, therefore, tempting to speculate that the population as a whole is experiencing an environmental exposure that causes the uptake and availability of cysteine for antioxidant synthesis to be increasingly critical for a significant number of persons. In this context, autism can be viewed as a neurodevelopmental manifestation of this exposure, with parallels to celiac disease, which has GI tract, immune, and neurological components. As recently reviewed,[66] there are numerous reports of significant improvement in other neurological and neuropsychiatric disorders following institution of a gluten-free diet, accompanied by reports of re-emergence of symptoms upon re-exposure to gluten. Where casein is concerned, cerebral folate deficiency (CFD) is a pertinent example. CFD is associated with autoantibodies to the folate transporter, whose levels decrease on a milk-free diet.[67] Finally, it is worthwhile to note that intestinal uptake of selenocysteine is also critical for normal redox regulation, and levels of selenium are low in autistic children.[68] Since cysteine and selenocysteine are both absorbed from the gut by the same transporter (EAAT3), casein-derived opiate peptides are likely to also inhibit selenocysteine uptake, but this has yet to be directly demonstrated.

6. Summary

Similar to neurodevelopmental disorders of genetic origin, autism appears to result from disruption of epigenetic regulation secondary to impaired DNA methylation, caused by one or more environmental factors. Extensive evidence indicates that oxidative stress and lower levels of GSH are common features of autism, and this will cause impaired methylation. Since the deficit in GSH is systemic, inadequate absorption of cysteine from the GI tract is likely to be an important factor, and this perspective is supported by the presence of GI inflammation in autism and the beneficial effect of a GF/CF diet. Further studies are needed to identify the specific environmental factors that are responsible for decreased absorption of cysteine, but recognition of these causative elements provides a rationale for treatment regimens that address oxidative stress and methylation deficits.

References

1. Dietz SC, Carroll JS. Interrogating the genome to understand oestrogen-receptor-mediated transcription. *Expert Rev Mol Med*. 2008;10:e10.
2. Feinberg AP. Epigenetics at the epicenter of modern medicine. *JAMA*. 2008;299(11):1345-1350.
3. Watanabe A, Yamada Y, Yamanaka S. Epigenetic regulation in pluripotent stem cells: a key to breaking the epigenetic barrier. *Philos Trans R Soc Lond B Biol Sci*. 2013;368(1609):20120292.
4. Vincent A, Van Seuningen I.On the epigenetic origin of cancer stem cells. *Biochim Biophys Acta*. 2012;1826(1):83-8.
5. Hudson AJ. Consciousness and cell memory: a dynamic epigenetic interrelationship. *Can J Neurol Sci*. 2011;38(5):681-8.
6. Gonzales ML, LaSalle JM. The role of MeCP2 in brain development and neurodevelopmental disorders. *Curr Psychiatry Rep*. 2010;12(2):127-134.
7. Nishioka M, Bundo M, Kasai K, Iwamoto K. DNA methylation in schizophrenia: progress and challenges of epigenetic studies. *Genome Med*. 2012;4(12):96.
8. Gapp K, Woldemichael BT, Bohacek J, Mansuy IM. Epigenetic regulation in neurodevelopment and neurodegenerative diseases. *Neuroscience*. 2012. doi:pii: S0306-4522(12)01151-7.
9. Robison AJ, Nestler EJ. Transcriptional and epigenetic mechanisms of addiction. *Nat Rev Neurosci*. 2011;12(11):623-37.
10. Lasalle JM, Yasui DH. Evolving role of MeCP2 in Rett syndrome and autism. *Epigenomics*. 2009;1(1):119-130.

11. Finkelstein JD. Metabolic regulatory properties of S-adenosylmethionine and S-adenosylhomocysteine. *Clin Chem Lab Med.* 2007;45(12):1694-9.

12. Deth R, Muratore C, Benzecry J, Power-Charnitsky VA, Waly M. How environmental and genetic factors combine to cause autism: A redox/methylation hypothesis. *Neurotoxicology.* 2008;29(1):190-201.

13. de Oliveira DM, Ferreira Lima RM, El-Bachá RS. Brain rust: recent discoveries on the role of oxidative stress in neurodegenerative diseases. *Nutr Neurosci.* 2012;15(3):94-102.

14. Schafer FQ, Buettner GR. Redox environment of the cell as viewed through the redox state of the glutathione disulfide/glutathione couple. *Free Radic Biol Med.* 2001;30(11):1191-212.

15. James SJ, Cutler P, Melnyk S, *et al.* Metabolic biomarkers of increased oxidative stress and impaired methylation capacity in children with autism. *Am. J. Clin. Nutr.* 2004;80(6):1611-1617.

16. James SJ, Melnyk S, Fuchs G, *et al.* Efficacy of methylcobalamin and folinic acid treatment on glutathione redox status in children with autism. *Am. J. Clin. Nutr.* 2009;89(1):425-430.

17. Paşca SP, Dronca E, Kaucsár T, *et al.* One carbon metabolism disturbances and the C677T MTHFR gene polymorphism in children with autism spectrum disorders. *J. Cell. Mol. Med.* 2009;13(10):4229-4238.

18. Al-Gadani Y, El-Ansary A, Attas O, Al-Ayadhi L. Metabolic biomarkers related to oxidative stress and antioxidant status in Saudi autistic children. *Clin. Biochem.* 2009;42(10-11):1032-1040.

19. Chauhan A, Audhya T, Chauhan V. Brain region-specific glutathione redox imbalance in autism. *Neurochem Res.* 2012;37(8):1681-9.

20. Rose S, Melnyk S, Pavliv O, Bai S, Nick TG, Frye RE, James SJ. Evidence of oxidative damage and inflammation associated with low glutathione redox status in the autism brain. *Transl Psychiatry.* 2012;2:e134.

21. Sun X, Shih AY, Johannssen HC, *et al.* Two-photon imaging of glutathione levels in intact brain indicates enhanced redox buffering in developing neurons and cells at the cerebrospinal fluid and blood-brain interface. *J. Biol. Chem.* 2006;281(25):17420-17431.

22. Erickson RH, Gum JR Jr, Lindstrom MM, McKean D, Kim YS. Regional expression and dietary regulation of rat small intestinal peptide and amino acid transporter mRNAs. *Biochem Biophys Res Commun.* 1995;216(1):249-57.

24. Waly MI, Hornig M, Trivedi M, Hodgson N, Kini R, Ohta A, Deth R. Prenatal and Postnatal Epigenetic Programming: Implications for GI, Immune, and Neuronal Function in Autism. *Autism Res Treat.* 2012;2012:190930. doi: 10.1155/2012/190930.

25. Howell JA, Matthews AD, Welbourne TC, Matthews JC. Content of ileal EAAC1 and hepatic GLT-1 high-affinity glutamate transporters is increased in growing vs. nongrowing lambs, paralleling increased tissue D- and L-glutamate, plasma glutamine, and alanine concentrations. *J Anim Sci.* 2003;81(4):1030-9.

26. Hodgson N, Trivedi M, Deth RC. Soluble Oligomers of Amyloid β Cause Changes in Redox State, DNA Methylation and Gene Transcription by Inhibiting EAAT3 Mediated Cysteine Uptake. *J Alz Dis* (Under Review).

27. Waly M, Olteanu H, Banerjee R, *et al.* Activation of methionine synthase by insulin-like growth factor-1 and dopamine: a target for neurodevelopmental toxins and thimerosal. *Mol. Psychiatry.* 2004;9(4):358-370.

28. Trivedi M, Hodgson N, Al-Muhairy S, Walker S, Krigsman A, Deth R. Inhibition of cysteine uptake by morphine and casein and gluten-derived opiate

peptides is associated with changes in DNA methylation and gene expression. (Manuscript in preparation)

29. Vitvitsky V, Thomas M, Ghorpade A, Gendelman HE, Banerjee R. A functional transsulfuration pathway in the brain links to glutathione homeostasis. *J Biol Chem.* 2006;281(47):35785-93.

30. Tallan HH, Moore S, Stein WH. L-cystathionine in human brain. *J. Biol. Chem.* 1958;230(2):707-716.

31. Whanger PD. Selenium and the brain: a review. *Nutr Neurosci.* 2001;4(2):81-97.

32. Köhrle J, Jakob F, Contempré B, Dumont JE. Selenium, the thyroid, and the endocrine system. *Endocr Rev.* 2005;26(7):944-84.

33. Ralston NVC, Ralston CR, Blackwell JL 3rd, Raymond LJ. Dietary and tissue selenium in relation to methylmercury toxicity. *Neurotoxicology.* 2008;29(5):802-811.

34. Suzuki KT, Sasakura C, Yoneda S. Binding sites for the (Hg-Se) complex on selenoprotein P. *Biochim. Biophys. Acta.* 1998;1429(1):102-112.

35. Zerangue N, Kavanaugh MP. Interaction of L-cysteine with a human excitatory amino acid transporter. *J Physiol.* 1996;493 (Pt 2):419-23.

36. Kanai Y, Hediger MA. Primary structure and functional characterization of a high-affinity glutamate transporter. *Nature.* 1992;60(6403):467-71.

37. Wakefield AJ, Murch SH, Anthony A, *et al.* Ileal-lymphoid-nodular hyperplasia, non-specific colitis, and pervasive developmental disorder in children. *Lancet.* 1998;351(9103):637-641.

38. Rome S, Barbot L, Windsor E, Kapel N, Tricottet V, Huneau JF, Reynes M, Gobert JG, Tomé D. The regionalization of PepT1, NBAT and EAAC1 transporters in the small intestine of rats are unchanged from birth to adulthood. *J Nutr.* 2002;132(5):1009-11.

39. Sims KD, Straff DJ, Robinson MB.Platelet-derived growth factor rapidly increases activity and cell surface expression of the EAAC1 subtype of glutamate transporter through activation of phosphatidylinositol 3-kinase. *J Biol Chem.* 2000;275(7):5228-37.

40. Trotti D, Danbolt NC, Volterra A. Glutamate transporters are oxidant-vulnerable: a molecular link between oxidative and excitotoxic neurodegeneration? *Trends Pharmacol Sci.* 1998;19(8):328-34.

41. Trotti D, Nussberger S, Volterra A, Hediger MA. Differential modulation of the uptake currents by redox interconversion of cysteine residues in the human neuronal glutamate transporter EAAC1. *Eur J Neurosci.* 1997;9(10):2207-12.

42. Peng KC, Cluzeaud F, Bens M, Duong Van Huyen JP, Wioland MA, Lacave R, Vandewalle A. Tissue and cell distribution of the multidrug resistance-associated protein (MRP) in mouse intestine and kidney. *J Histochem Cytochem.* 1999;47(6):757-68.

43. Jeong J, Ha TS, Kim J. Protection of aquo/hydroxocobalamin from reduced glutathione by a B12 trafficking chaperone. *BMB Rep.* 2011;44(3):170-5.

44. McNally ME, Atkinson SA, Cole DE. Contribution of sulfate and sulfoesters to total sulfur intake in infants fed human milk. *J Nutr.* 1991; 121:1250-4.

45. Minet JC, Bissé E, Aebischer CP, Beil A, Wieland H, Lütschg J. Assessment of vitamin B-12, folate, and vitamin B-6 status and relation to sulfur amino acid metabolism in neonates. *Am J Clin Nutr.* 2000; 72:751-7.

46. Ozgurtas T, Aydin I, Turan O, Koc E, Hirfanoglu IM, Acikel CH, Akyol M, Erbil MK. Vascular endothelial growth factor, basic fibroblast growth factor, insulin-like growth factor-I and platelet-derived growth factor levels in human milk of mothers with term and preterm neonates. *Cytokine* 2010; 50:192-4.

47. Murphy MS. Growth factors and the gastrointestinal tract. *Nutrition.* 1998; 14:771-4.

48. Hodgson N, Waly M, Deth RC. EAAT3-mediated cysteine uptake in human neuroblastoma cells is PI3 kinase-dependent. Society for Neuroscience Meeting Abstracts, Nov. 2008.

49. Dorea JG. Selenium and breast-feeding. *Br J Nutr.* 2002; 88:443-61.

50. Watts SD, Torres-Salazar, D, Divito CB, Amara SG. EAAT3 cysteine transport: Potential mechanism of cysteine binding and translocation. Society for Neuroscience Meeting Abstracts, Nov. 2009.

51. Isaacs PE, Kim YS. The contaminated small bowel syndrome. *Am J Med.* 1979;67(6):1049-57.

52. El-Ansary AK, Ben Bacha AG, Al-Ayadhi LY. Proinflammatory and proapoptotic markers in relation to mono and di-cations in plasma of autistic patients from Saudi Arabia. *J Neuroinflammation.* 2011;8:142.

53. Chez MG, Dowling T, Patel PB, Khanna P, Kominsky M. Elevation of tumor necrosis factor-alpha in cerebrospinal fluid of autistic children. *Pediatr Neurol.* 2007;36(6):361-5.

54. Li X, Chauhan A, Sheikh AM, Patil S, Chauhan V, Li XM, Ji L, Brown T, Malik M. Elevated immune response in the brain of autistic patients. *J Neuroimmunol.* 2009;207(1-2):111-6.

55. Abdallah MW, Larsen N, Grove J, Nørgaard-Pedersen B, Thorsen P, Mortensen EL, Hougaard DM. Amniotic fluid inflammatory cytokines: Potential markers of immunologic dysfunction in autism spectrum disorders. *World J Biol Psychiatry.* 2011 Dec 19. [Epub ahead of print]

56. Thomas Curtis J, Chen Y, Buck DJ, Davis RL. Chronic inorganic mercury exposure induces sex-specific changes in central TNFα expression: importance in autism? *Neurosci Lett.* 2011;504(1):40-4.

57. Muratore CR, Hodgson NW, Trivedi MS, Abdolmaleky HM, Persico AM, Lintas C, De La Monte S, Deth RC. Age-dependent decrease and alternative splicing of methionine synthase mRNA in human cerebral cortex and an accelerated decrease in autism. *PLoS One* (In press).

58. Zou CG, Banerjee R. Tumor necrosis factor-alpha-induced targeted proteolysis of cystathionine beta-synthase modulates redox homeostasis. *J Biol Chem.* 2003;278(19):16802-8.

59. Whiteley P, Haracopos D, Knivsberg A-M, *et al.* The ScanBrit randomised, controlled, single-blind study of a gluten- and casein-free dietary intervention for children with autism spectrum disorders. *Nutr Neurosci.* 2010;13(2):87-100.

60. Huebner FR, Lieberman KW, Rubino RP, Wall JS. Demonstration of high opioid-like activity in isolated peptides from wheat gluten hydrolysates. *Peptides.* 1984;5(6):1139-47.

61. Brantl V, Teschemacher H, Henschen A, Lottspeich F. Novel opioid peptides derived from casein (beta-casomorphins). I. Isolation from bovine casein peptone. *Hoppe Seylers Z Physiol Chem.* 1979;360(9):1211-6.

62. Kikuchi M, Fukuyama K, Epstein WL. Soluble dipeptidyl peptidase IV from terminal differentiated rat epidermal cells: purification and its activity on synthetic and natural peptides. *Arch Biochem Biophys.* 1988;266(2):369-76.63.

63. Sun Z, Zhang Z, Wang X, Cade R, Elmir Z, Fregly M. Relation of beta-casomorphin to apnea in sudden infant death syndrome. *Peptides.* 2003;24(6):937-43.

64. Wasilewska J, Sienkiewicz-Szłapka E, Kuźbida E, Jarmołowska B, Kaczmarski M, Kostyra E. The exogenous opioid peptides and DPPIV serum activity in infants with apnoea expressed as apparent life threatening events (ALTE). *Neuropeptides.* 2011;45(3):189-95.

65. Wasilewska J, Kaczmarski M, Kostyra E, Iwan M. Cow's-milk-induced infant apnoea with increased serum content of bovine β-casomorphin-5. *J Pediatr Gastroenterol Nutr.* 2011;52(6):772-5.

66. Jackson JR, Eaton WW, Cascella NG, Fasano A, Kelly DL. Neurologic and Psychiatric Manifestations of Celiac Disease and Gluten Sensitivity. *The Psychiatric Quarterly.* 2011. Available at: http://www.ncbi.nlm.nih.gov/pubmed/21877216. Accessed September 30, 2011.

67. Ramaekers VT, Sequeira JM, Blau N, Quadros EV. A milk-free diet downregulates folate receptor autoimmunity in cerebral folate deficiency syndrome. *Dev Med Child Neurol.* 2008;50(5):346-352.

68. Jory J, McGinnis W. Red-Cell Trace Minerals in Children with Autism. *American Journal of Biochemistry and Biotechnology.* 2008;4:104-8.

CHAPTER FOUR

BIOFILM: A CAUSE OF CHRONIC GASTROINTESTINAL ISSUES IN ASD

By John H. Hicks III, MD

> Biofilm is the term given to a community of microorganisms living together under or within a self-produced polymer matrix.

Introduction

Community existence is an instinctive and natural way for species to flourish and survive, even under the most difficult climates and conditions. It is an amazing evolutionary response that sustains life and propagates the group. By forming what are called biofilms, groups of cooperative microscopic entities survive and thrive in environments that would typically destroy a single species. Specifically, biofilm is the term given to a community of microorganisms living together under or within a self-produced polymer matrix. These communities may consist of one species of microbe, or a variety of different organisms including bacteria, viruses, yeast, fungi, protozoa, and single-cell microorganisms that live in extreme environments (often referred to as extremophiles).[1] The polymer matrix, which provides rigidity and structure for the microorganisms, is primarily made up of polysaccharides. It adheres firmly to a given surface, providing strong protection to the resident organisms while allowing them to thrive and prosper.

Ubiquitous in nature, biofilms occur in rivers, streams, ponds, and hot acid pools. They are even to be found in the harsh glacial habitats of Antarctica.[2] Biofilms in the natural environment offer constructive potential benefits such as self-purification of streams and rivers, a benefit that could be extended to the treatment of waste water and pollution. Microbes that naturally break down carbon can provide invaluable assistance in breaking down oil particles resulting from accidental oil spills. Using specific bacteria in a controlled manner could conceivably return to a natural state an environment that has been unnaturally polluted and compromised. Additionally, biofilms can be helpful to the mining industry in preventing acid runoff. Biofilms also benefit growing vegetation in the natural environment. Microbes that form a biofilm in the area between the soil and roots of plants can provide increased access to nutrients for themselves and the plant that would otherwise not be available.

Biofilms are not contained exclusively within the external environment of nature, however, nor are their consequences always benign or beneficial. It is now known that biofilm communities are responsible for sundry contamination occurrences. An example is found in clogged and corroded pipes, which often lead to sanitation issues. According to the Center for Biofilm Engineering at Montana State University, biofilm organisms can attach to each other or to any moist, aqueous environment, which provides a highly diverse spectrum of unlimited potential attachments, including soil particles and animal and human tissues.[1-3] Biofilms can also attach securely to the metals and plastics used in implanted medical devices such as joint replacements, heart valves, and indwelling catheters, resulting in many new, invasive, and destructive infections; due to biofilms, joint replacements have had to be removed and replaced. Biofilms can be created from bacteria and other organisms within the human body and survive from food that is consumed. Finally, biofilms are capable of adapting to human environments as varied as plaque on teeth, sinuses, tonsils, eustachian tubes in the middle ear, and the intestines, where they are creating some of the biggest issues for patients with autism spectrum disorders (ASDs).

How biofilms work

Initially, the organisms structure weak, reversible bonds which, over time, mature and become uncompromisingly firm and secure. Strong protein adhesion molecules hold these more permanent attachments together. At this point, biofilms are far more difficult to control and eliminate. The biofilms secrete extracellular signal molecules within the matrix that act as auto-inducers (chemical signaling molecules) to start up detailed genetic programs. At a particular level of auto-inducer concentration, planktonic microorganisms attract and attach themselves to the cell adhesion areas. The extracellular polymeric matrix provides a proficient pathway for cellular communication between the assorted organisms. When the chemical messages gain sufficient strength, the group begins to function as a unit.

As a symbiotic group, biofilm organisms take on various unique characteristics. One example is the ability to synchronize genetic information through a process called quorum sensing.[4-6] Quorum sensing may take place between a single species or a diverse group of microbes. In addition, quorum sensing helps the organisms communicate more efficiently with each other and further assist in the formation and survival of the biofilm community. As different species of microbes share information back and forth, the individual strains and the group as a whole coordinate gene information, replication, and accept extracellular DNA, which they then incorporate into their own genome. This process allows the organisms living within the biofilm to become more virulent and resistant to antimicrobial agents.[1,4,6,7]

An example of this process is when specific fungi pass resistance against antibiotics onto bacteria sharing the same biofilm. The receiving bacteria cooperate and accept the new cellular information and likewise donate their DNA intelligence. This, in turn, allows the fungi to become more resistant to antifungals. Hence, biofilm organisms create an exchange and division of labor that enables them to develop powerful resistance to antibiotics and antifungal agents by preventing penetration of the antimicrobials and their metabolism or breakdown. This ability to exchange genetic information also allows organisms to more effectively evade the natural immune system defenses of the host.[1] Current research suggests that *E. Coli* bacteria have the ability to form a biofilm in 24 hours and can become virtually immune to antibiotics due to a low level of metabolic activity.[8] Other studies estimate that biofilm organisms are 1000 times more resistant to antibiotics than planktonic or free-living bacteria.[6,9-11]

In short, large varieties of microbes living within a biofilm community hold the potential for diverse genetic information exchange, along with new forms of activity from previously known microbe species.[12] This is one of the most critical issues with biofilms and ASD individuals. In individuals with ASD, cell-mediated immunity is often compromised and their system is producing excess antibodies (see *The body's response to biofilms*). However, this is precisely the system (cytotoxic T cells and natural killer cells) that is needed to protect an individual from the formation of biofilms. The biofilms therefore form quickly and strip nutrients from the host, producing toxins and releasing stronger organisms that, in turn, create more gut overgrowth and further issues with detoxification and neurologic function.

Biofilm adaptation

When free-floating bacteria sense stress in a human host, they will often begin to form a biofilm. The bacteria starting the biofilm will look for a location that has sufficient iron, which is necessary for their survival. At the same time, however, the organisms in a biofilm modulate their virulence because they depend on their host. Generally, biofilms are slow to create overt and debilitating symptoms, though this is dependent on the type and species of organisms and the toxins they produce.[1] The formation of a biofilm enables microorganisms to change their growth rate and metabolic rate and, over time, become more resistant to substances designed to exterminate them. Because of their ability to hide from the host's natural immune defenses, biofilm organisms therefore cannot be eradicated without external help and assistance.

Because biofilm organisms are not actively invading the human body but are instead attached to tissues or medical implants (and are protected by their immune-fighting, extracellular matrix), they can easily seed and repopulate new areas. When biofilms naturally mature, they release free-living organisms into central fluid portions of the matrix. The released organisms then seed or swim away in clumps to establish new biofilms elsewhere in the host. As the biofilms persist, they become the source of recurrent fevers and persistent inflammation in the body. In time, through continual overgrowth, some organisms produce toxins that negatively affect the systems of the host.[2,8] In this way, biofilm microorganisms can be responsible for illnesses ranging from mild respiratory infections to pneumonia, and from septic shock to necrotizing fasciitis, or flesh-wasting disease.[7,13]

Another common example is found when persistent otitis media bacteria create biofilms in the ear that escape through the eustachian tube to settle in the warm, moist tissues of the gastrointestinal tract. Many ASD children have a significant history of recurrent ear infections that can be a mechanism for the establishment of biofilms in the gastrointestinal tract. As planktonic bacteria, fungi, and parasites are attracted and attach to new adhesion sites, the biofilm grows and changes from its original form. The newly fashioned mix of respiratory and intestinal organisms shares DNA information and different resistance and survival strategies, and may become invasive. This, in turn, can lead to recurrent seeding and chronic relapsing infections.[3]

Along with the sharing of DNA, biofilms involve intracellular communication from chemical messengers that signal biofilm formation or resolution (dismantling of the biofilm) and indicate when to produce toxins. For some species, auto-inducers dictate when to produce a biofilm and when to release planktonic bacteria to search out another host.[4] Different varieties of biofilm use many different ways to communicate with the varied organisms in their cluster. In cholera, for example, the main messenger is a compound called CAI-1. Low levels of this compound in the Vibrio cholerae produce biofilms, but as the level of CAI-1 increases, pathogenic toxins are released to indicate that it is time to leave the body.[4] Other species collaborate and use other types of molecules for auto-induction communication. Gram-positive bacteria use small peptides, N-acyl homoserine lactones and furanosyl borate diester.[6] *Pseudomonas aeruginosa* (*P. aeruginosa*), often found in the lungs of people with cystic fibrosis, produces two signaling molecules: one that is long, and one is that short.[5] The practical implications of these communication differences are that biofilms are not all the same as regards the organisms that are involved and the matrix that is formed. Therefore, their resistance mechanisms will vary, meaning that there is no single protocol or way to treat all biofilms.

The body's response to biofilms

As previously mentioned, the body uses cell-mediated immunity, a specific response dictated by the immune system, to attempt to attack, control, and eliminate biofilms. Cell-mediated immunity activates macrophage cells, natural killer cells, cytotoxic T cells, and antigen-specific T-lymphocytes which destroy pathogens and stimulate the production of cytokines. Although cytokines recruit more immune assistance, they also increase inflammation. When the immune system is compromised and shifted out of balance (in what is termed a Th2 immune shift), the antibody response side of the immune system is highly overactive, and the opposing/balancing cell-mediated Th1 side is recurrently and persistently suppressed. In this situation, the immune system is unable to activate the necessary response. Contributors to immune system imbalances of this type are numerous and include genetic predisposition, toxic substances, vaccination residuals, and heavy metals.

Biofilms (along with other types of organisms such as cell wall deficient species, L forms, stealth organisms, viruses, and certain spirochetes) have the ability to exploit Th2 immune shifts and debilitate immune system function. Another factor contributing to immune dysfunction is bacterial-induced vitamin D receptor dysfunction. Biofilms and certain other intracellular organisms produce compounds that bind and inhibit vitamin D receptor function. As a result, microbial pathogens increase and cause persistent infection and inflammation, with suppression of the needed cell-mediated immune response. This can cause a wide variety of chronic diseases, increased susceptibility to other infections, and a decline in innate immunity.[14]

Biofilms and autism spectrum disorders

With the increasing incidence of autoimmune diseases, recurrent infections, and chronic illnesses, it has become clear that existing treatment information and protocols are incomplete and that some components of disease are being insufficiently or inadequately addressed. With ASDs, in particular, certain pieces of this mismatched puzzle have been evident for a number of years. Immune dysfunction, heavy metal toxicity, an inability to detoxify waste and toxins, along with the resultant dysbiosis of the gastrointestinal system are well known to be persistent and recalcitrant to modification by current and accepted means of treatment.

Clearly, the role that biofilms play as one of the sources of chronic or recurrent infections that are highly resistant to biocides and antibiotics is an important part of the ASD story.[3,15] The Centers for

Disease Control and Prevention and the National Institutes of Health currently report that 65% of all infections are quite possibly caused by biofilms.[1,8,9] Some of the more common organisms related to chronic infections are *Helicobacter pylori, Clostridium* species, *Streptococcus* species, *Bacillus* species, *Pseudomonas* species, *Klebsiella* species, *Proteus* species, *Candida* species, *Enterococcus* species, and *Serratia* species, to name a few. Biofilms are implicated in many diverse, unrelenting, and debilitating infections, some of which overlap with ASD, such as Lyme disease, arthritis, sarcoidosis, Crohn's disease, irritable bowel syndrome, recurrent strep infections, cystic fibrosis, chronic ear infections, chronic sinusitis, periodontal disease, and many others.[1-3,5,8,16] Further examples of biofilm infections include but are not limited to urinary tract infections, osteomyelitis, chronic prostatitis, gingivitis from plaque, relapsing fevers, chronic sinusitis, toxic shock syndrome, kidney stones, and endocarditis.[2,9,11,16]

Because biofilms produce toxins, an extensive and wide variety of cell and tissue abnormalities can result. With toxins traveling freely in the bloodstream, the extent of their penetration is limited only by the protective nature of the blood-brain barrier. However, heavy metal toxicity such as is found in many individuals with ASD (specifically aluminum) renders the blood-brain barrier more permeable and vulnerable to penetration and biofilm influence. In ASD, the consequences of biofilm toxicity can include cognitive impairment, processing abnormalities, and memory problems. In addition, the pathogenic toxins generated by biofilms are highly permeable and can ultimately access all parts of the body to affect any gland, organ, or system.[17,18] It is therefore reasonable to conclude that biofilm toxins affect and influence multiple body systems. In several studies on ASD individuals with gastrointestinal issues, it was found that disordered gut flora contributed to a vast increase of the *Clostridium* and *Ruminococcus* species of bacteria. This particular bacterial overgrowth leads to changes in pH balance, which affects digestion and greatly impairs the proper absorption of minerals and cofactors necessary for cell energy and neurotransmitter production.[19]

Streptococcus also has the ability to form biofilms, and it is evident that biofilms can be a source of persistent and recurrent streptococcal infections in ASD. There are many different species of *Streptococcus,* and they live in a wide variety of environments. By living in biofilms, streptococci can make adaptive changes and survive in a greater variance of pH, thereby tolerating greater levels of cellular acidity than is typical. Studies also show that streptococci living in a biofilm have the ability to incorporate foreign DNA, moderate their metabolism and replication rate, and be highly resistant to antibiotics. *Streptococcus* bacteria have the potential to form biofilms that seed and produce toxins in all areas of the body. As testing techniques continue to improve, it appears likely that a relationship between bacterial biofilms and pediatric autoimmune neuropsychiatric disorders associated with streptococcal infections (PANDAS) will be established. Like heavy metal toxicity, the *Streptococcus* bacterium also appears able to change the permeability of the blood-brain barrier, thereby changing the permeability of the central nervous system. This could lead to the neuropsychological symptoms seen with PANDAS. A 2005 study has shown that *Clostridium histolyticum* can also cause neuropsychiatric symptoms, which can be temporarily eased by the use of the prescription antibiotic vancomycin.[19]

Disrupting and eradicating biofilms

The knowledge base regarding biofilms and awareness of their medical implications have increased rather slowly, in part because microbiology was and is based on the study of pure cultures of planktonic bacteria rather than complex mixed microbial communities. Fortunately, methods of identifying, culturing, and testing microbes are now improving.[1,3] This will open the door to much-needed information and insights about how to control and eliminate biofilm-related chronic diseases.

In the early formation phase of a biofilm, disruption is relatively straightforward, as the biofilm is more easily detached. However, as the rigid protein matrix structure matures, biofilms become increasingly more difficult to destroy. One solution is to render the matrix softer and more penetrable. Laboratory studies and experiments are being carried out to manipulate the quorum sensing communication process as a way to modify the matrix and eradicate biofilms. Most of this work has not yet reached human trials, however, and many of the compounds under consideration are toxic to humans.[7] Moreover, it is wise to be cautious and prudent, as we do not know the full implications of manipulating quorum sensing. For example, when the entire genome of *P. aeruginosa* was screened, it was discovered that quorum sensing controlled at least thirty-nine genes,[5] showing that intricate and complex interactions occur within different species and may create unanticipated reactions. In some species, manipulation of the quorum sensing molecules will automatically increase their virulence and some species will activate invasion of the tissues.

In looking for a way to treat biofilms, it is obvious that traditional antibiotic therapy is not sufficient, even at atypical high doses. Current antibiotics are proving to be ineffective against these potent communities of microbes. Moreover, antibiotics may negatively contribute to the internal environment by increasing microbial resistance and virulence in certain species.[6,9] Many infections reoccur more powerfully after multiple rounds of different antibiotics, each time with increasingly destructive signs and symptoms.

Beneficial microorganisms living in the gut provide a natural protection against disease-causing microbes, help to develop the immune system, and aid in the digestion and assimilation of food and nutrients. Some types of gastrointestinal biofilms are normal, and use of antibiotics can result in the destruction of our natural beneficial probiotic biofilm. Without this protection, pathogenic bacteria can flourish, destroying gut tissue integrity and increasing gut permeability. Leaky gut tissue then allows movement into the bloodstream of compounds and substances that will create inflammation, generate food and environmental sensitivities, and negatively impact and alter immune function. Additionally, a leaky gut will create a persistent Th2 shift and increase susceptibility to other dangerous pathogens. Weakening of gut motility and function leads to decreased toxin clearance and increased proinflammatory cytokines. This, in turn, can result in diminished absorption of essential nutrients, even in the presence of daily supplementation. With these issues in mind, it is clearly imperative to rid the intestines of pathogenic biofilms to allow for complete healing of the digestive, immune, and all other affected body systems.

The first line of defensive therapy is an effective and potent probiotic, which allows healthy, beneficial, and protective bacteria to repopulate the internal gut environment and prevent the attachment and replication of pathogens that are released as the biofilm regresses. Whenever possible, it is beneficial to identify the specific organisms involved in the biofilm. This can be done through specialized stool testing and culturing, as well as antigen and DNA processing. The type of organism determines whether the cell's surface charge is Gram-positive or Gram-negative. Gram-positive bacteria are more sensitive to the destructive effects of antibiotics and the natural defenses of the immune system, whereas Gram-negative bacteria are more resistant. Furthermore, the positivity or negativity determines what ions or elements are attracted or bound to the cell. These ions may be minerals (such as calcium, magnesium, chloride, or potassium) or heavy metals (such as mercury, aluminum, cadmium, and lead). The nature of the bond between cells and ions (or elements), which provide cross bridging, can greatly enhance the complexity of a biofilm matrix.

Secondly, it is necessary to penetrate the matrix of the biofilm to weaken its protective shield and thereby permanently eradicate the resident microorganisms. One of the most effective and beneficial ways to do this is with enzymatic therapy, using enzymes that specifically break apart protein and carbohydrate molecular bonds. There are several brands of enzymes that contain multiple strains and proprietary blends to facilitate biofilm deactivation and penetration. Enzymes have also been shown capable of preventing biofilm formation. Unfortunately, in some biofilms the process of matrix disruption has the effect of making certain species even more virulent and invasive.[20] In such cases the organisms move to different locations, increasing the level of infection throughout the body. As the biofilm spreads and matures, different species attach and detach, contributing to and increasing genetic modification through an exchange of extracellular DNA.[21] The choice to use or not use enzymes will depend on the types of organisms that each person has within their biofilm. It cannot be assumed that enzymes alone will completely destroy a biofilm once the matrix has matured and is more resistant to degradation.[7]

In cases where enzymatic therapy is inadequate, chelating agents may be needed to remove iron, which is necessary for microbes' survival and the creation of biofilms. For this process, the use of lactoferrin and ethylenediaminetetraacetic acid (EDTA) compounds that remove iron, minerals, and heavy metals are recommended. These compounds may be the most effective additional therapy to prevent biofilms from forming and to remove them once firmly established.[22] (However, attempting to remove heavy metals at the same time as treating the biofilm may increase activity of some yeast components. This is another reason to proceed cautiously with an experienced practitioner who will monitor the situation - organisms, order of operations, and individualization/ timing of each treatment - on a regular basis.) Biofilm studies also show that subinhibitory levels of antibiotics, when combined with enzymatic therapy, can assist in reducing the biofilm burden.[23] These are given in low intermittent doses to avoid the increasing resistance typically induced by high doses of antibiotics.[9,10,24,25] Antibiotics that target the cell cycle will not be as effective, given that biofilms often modify cell metabolism and replication.

Thirdly, the innate immune system needs to be balanced and reactivated. In this way, the immune system can most efficiently regulate a defense against pathogenic biofilms and destroy existing biofilms. Because many of the organisms that make up a biofilm become planktonic and move to different locations, it is critical that the overall immune system be addressed to function optimally. Any Th2 shift must be corrected to stimulate and balance the Th1 side of the immune system to clear pathogens. This can be accomplished with specific immune-boosting supplements called transfer factors. Transfer factors, both general and specific, significantly aid in shifting the immune system back to neutral, increasing the activity of the immune system's natural killer cells. Transfer factors also tag or mark cells that harbor pathogenic organisms, thereby boosting the T-lymphocyte cells' ability to remove the pathogens.[26]

It is imperative to make sure that vitamin D levels are normal and that the receptors are functioning properly. Genetic predisposition to polymorphism or gene variance can influence the activity of the vitamin D receptors that are essential to the uptake of vitamin D. Vitamin D plays an essential role in calcium and bone metabolism, induction of cell differentiation, inhibition of cell growth, and modulation of the immune and hormone systems.[14,27] If the vitamin D receptors are shown to be impaired, an agonist that stimulates the receptors to function properly may be used. Some medications given for high blood pressure have the side effect of being a vitamin D agonist.

In devising a therapeutic protocol, it is needful to prepare for the expulsion of free radicals. Some form of cell protection is critical. The level of protection will be dictated by the length of time the biofilm has been present in the body and the organisms involved. Essential fatty acids (such as black currant oil) provide optimal cell membrane protection along with cell-protective antioxidants like glutathione and antioxidants from berries (including blueberries, blackberries, raspberries, and strawberries).

Other biofilm treatment options to be considered include homeopathic and vibrational remedies. These substances offer assistance in both removing and preventing biofilms. Furthermore, the impact that diet has on the various organisms must be recognized and addressed. Sugar, vinegar, simple carbohydrates, and corn act as food for microbes; therefore, intake of these should be limited and their complete digestion should be sought.

It is important to address all of the pathogens residing within a biofilm. Fungi such as *Candida* will not respond to standard antifungal substances when protected in a biofilm. A different approach is needed. The use of natural products such as cellulase enzymes that dissolve yeast, and other remedies such as olive leaf extract, uva ursi, cranberry with berberine, or Indian Fire Tree Bark tea can be effective. These substances also provide strong antibacterial protection for the immune system.

As a cautionary note, quickly killing a multitude of organisms all at once may release large quantities of toxins, overwhelming an already compromised detoxification system. This can elicit a Herxheimer reaction, which is typically referred to as "die off." A reaction of this type stems from the release of toxins into the bloodstream, which stimulates the production of inflammatory cytokines and generates temporary hormonal imbalances. It can also prompt diarrhea or nausea as the body strives to clean up and clean out. Activated charcoal can reduce the toxin load on the body and help to eliminate the additional toxic burden, thereby reducing the incidence of Herxheimer reactions.

Conclusion

Attention to biofilms is expanding and gaining momentum. Biofilms have constructive, beneficial potential and yet are also associated with chronic diseases and illnesses that are recurrent and persistent. Nature has gifted biofilms with impressive survival abilities, including group communication and genetic adaptability. These varied communities of organisms are highly resistant to current treatments and protocols, including antibiotics and antifungal substances. Therefore, understanding the role that biofilms play in the human body is critical. Combined therapies are warranted, including probiotics, enzymes, natural immune stimulants, and detoxifying supplements. All of these can lend assistance to the immune system to clear and eradicate these potent and powerful microbes.

References

1. Proal A. Understanding biofilms. *Bacteriality: Exploring Chronic Disease.* May 26, 2008. Available online at: http://bacteriality.com/2008/05/26/biofilm/
2. Parsek MR, Singh PK. Bacterial biofilms: an emerging link to disease pathogenesis. *Annu Rev Microbiol.* 2003;57:677-701.
3. Costerton JW, Stewart PS, Greenberg EP. Bacterial biofilms: a common cause of persistent infections. *Science.* 1999 May 21;284(5418):1318-22.
4. Higgins DA, Pomianek ME, Kraml CM, Taylor RK, Semmelhack MF, Bassler BL. The major *Vibrio cholerae* autoinducer and its role in virulence factor production. *Nature.* 2007 Dec 6;450(7171):883-6.
5. Singh PK, Schaefer AL, Parsek MR, Moninger TO, Welsh MJ, Greenberg EP. Quorum sensing signals indicate that cystic fibrosis lungs are infected with bacterial biofilms. *Nature.* 2000 Oct 12;407(6805):762-4.
6. Estrela AB, Wolf-Rainer A. Combining biofilm-controlling compounds and antibiotics as a promising new way to control biofilm infections. *Pharmaceuticals.* 2010;3(5):1374-93.
7. Cvitkovitch DG, Li YH, Ellen RP. Quorum sensing and biofilm formation in Streptococcal infections. *J Clin Invest.* 2003 Dec;112(11):1626-32.
8. Cho H, Jönsson H, Campbell K, Melke P, Williams JW, Jedynak B, *et al.* Self-organization in high-density bacterial colonies: efficient crowd control. *PLoS Biol.* 2007 Oct 30;5(11):e302.
9. Lewis K. Riddle of biofilm resistance. *Antimicrob Agents Chemother.* 2001 Apr;45(4):999-1007.
10. Stoodley P, Purevdorj-Gage B, Costerton JW. Clinical significance of seeding dispersal in biofilms: a response (Comment). *Microbiology.* 2005 Nov;151(11):3453.
11. Brockhurst MA, Hochberg ME, Bell T, Buckling A. Character displacement promotes cooperation in bacterial biofilms. *Curr Biol.* 2006 Oct 24;16(20):2030-4.
12. Jefferson KK. What drives bacteria to produce a biofilm? *FEMS Microbiol Letter.* 2004;236:163-73.
13. Waite RD, Struthers JK, Dowson CG. Spontaneous sequence duplication within an open reading frame of the pneumococcal type 3 capsule locus causes high-frequency variation. *Mol Microbiol.* 2001 Dec;42(5):1223-32.
14. Waterhouse JC, Perez TH, Albert PJ. Reversing bacteria-induced vitamin D receptor dysfunction is key to autoimmune disease. *Ann N Y Acad Sci.* 2009 Sep;1173:757-65.

15. Marphetia T. Chronic middle ear infections linked to resistant biofilm bacteria. Press release, Medical College of Wisconsin, July 11, 2006. Available online at: http://cmbi.bjmu.edu.cn/news/0607/41.htm

16. Hall-Stoodley L, Costerton JW, Stoodley P. Bacterial biofilms: from the natural environment to infectious disease. *Nat Rev Microbiol.* 2004;2(2):95-108.

17. Morrison HI, Ellison LF, Taylor GW. Periodontal disease and risk of fatal coronary heart and cerebrovascular diseases. *J Cardiovasc Risk.* 1999 Feb;6(1):7-11.

18. Stewart R, Hirani V. Dental health and cognitive impairment in an English national survey population. *J Am Geriatr Soc.* 2007 Sep;55(9):1410-4.

19. Parracho HM, Bingham MO, Gibson GR, McCartney AL. Differences between the gut microflora of children with autistic spectrum disorders and that of healthy children. *J Med Microbiol.* 2005 Oct;54(10):987-91.

20. Ceri H, Olson ME, Stremick C, Read RR, Morck D, Buret A. The Calgary Biofilm Device: new technology for rapid determination of antibiotic susceptibilities of bacterial biofilms. *J Clin Microbiol.* 1999 Jun;37(6):1771-6.

21. Li YH, Lau PC, Lee JH, Ellen RP, Cvitkovitch DG. Natural genetic transformation of *Streptococcus mutans* growing in biofilms. *J Bacteriol.* 2001 Feb;183(3):897-908.

22. Singh PK, Parsek MR, Greenberg EP, Welsh MJ. A component of innate immunity prevents bacterial biofilm development. *Nature.* 2002 May 30;417(6888):552-5.

23. Starner TD, Shrout JD, Parsek MR, Appelbaum PC, Kim G. Subinhibitory concentrations of azithromycin decrease nontypeable *Haemophilus influenzae* biofilm formation and diminish established biofilms. *Antimicrob Agents Chemother.* 2008 Jan;52(1):137-45.

24. Marshall TG, Marshall FE. Sarcoidosis succumbs to antibiotics—implications for autoimmune disease. *Autoimmun Rev.* 2004 Jun;3(4):295-300.

25. Cogan NG, Cortez R, Fauci L. Modeling physiological resistance in bacterial biofilms. *Bull Math Biol.* 2005 Jul;67(4):831-53.

26. White A. *A Guide to Transfer Factors and Immune System Health*, 2nd ed. North Charleston: BookSurge Publishing, 2009.

27. Dusso AS, Brown AJ, Slatopolsky E. Vitamin D. *AJP-Renal Physiol.* 2005 Jul;289(1):F8-F28.

CHAPTER FIVE

OLD FRIENDS, NEW TREATMENT: HELMINTHI THERAPY IN AUTISM

By Judith Chinitz, MS, MS

Introduction

My son, Alex, was diagnosed with autism in 1996, three weeks after his second birthday. Our pediatrician at the time dismissed his perpetual diarrhea and vomiting (present since the antibiotics he was given 36 hours after his birth) as symptoms of his autism. "He's sick because he's autistic," she said. "He's autistic because he's sick," I responded. Seventeen years later, it still amazes me how right I was, before I even knew the first thing about autism spectrum disorders (ASDs).

When I was getting my graduate degree in special education, I was taught that autism was a rare condition, present from birth. It could be recognized early, I was told, because the infants would stiffen when picked up, not wanting to be held. How could I, then, recognize it in my own son, when he wouldn't be put down and wanted to be held every minute of every day? At first, the only symptoms of his impending autism were gastrointestinal: projectile vomiting, chronic diarrhea, lack of appetite. It was after a major stomach virus that the first true autistic symptom appeared–Alex stopped responding to his name. Even then, what stood out the most were not the "mental" symptoms but the physical ones.

I met Dr. Sidney Baker, cofounder of the network formerly known as Defeat Autism Now! (DAN!), on March 8th, 1997, almost exactly a year after Alex was diagnosed with autism. Sid eventually became both my friend and mentor. It was at that very first meeting that Sid explained to me the holistic nature of the human body, describing how our various body systems work together in a harmonious whole. He pointed to an artificial spider web he had hung up in the corner of his

of this intertwining. He then explained the
that what is happening in autism involves
m triangle.

ay from Dr. Baker holds as true now as
illness involving many systems of the
bnormalities in the digestive system
une system) and our children's abnormal
coming clearer. The study of the gut biome, an
unto itself, and its relationship to health and disease
ploding area of research. The traditional systems approach
dicine–wherein doctors specialize in the immune system, *or* the
gastrointestinal system, *or* the central nervous system (CNS)–has
done us a disservice. We forget that these systems are not entities unto
themselves but work together as a whole. Disturbance of one system
leads to disturbance of all systems.

As an example, in his brilliant book *The Second Brain*,[12] Dr.
Michael Gershon gives a thorough explanation of how serotonin, which
so many people associate with "brain illnesses" such as depression, is a
major player in the gut and immune system. (Recalling that 70% of our
immune system IS the gut, it should not be surprising that about 60-
70% of the serotonin in our bodies is to be found there.) Dr. Candace
Pert's book, *Molecules of Emotion*,[13] also explores the concept that
our mind and body are connected. She explains, in fascinating detail,
how the same chemical that causes you to feel nervous about speaking
in front of an audience can cause the diarrhea that you experience after
making your public speech.

Importance of the gut flora
As I look back over my many years in the autism biomedical field, a
few moments stand out as being truly formative events in my learning
and thinking process. That first meeting with Sid Baker was one such
moment. Another formative experience occurred at the spring 2010
DAN! conference when I attended Dr. Jeremy Nicholson's lecture on
abnormal bacterial metabolites in the urine of children with autism.[1]
In a published paper, Dr. Nicholson and colleagues had demonstrated
via analysis of urinary organic acids that children with autism have
abnormal gut bacteria when compared with controls. Although the

concept of bacterial dysbiosis had been around since before Alex's autism diagnosis and was old news to me, it was encouraging to hear that empirical confirmation of the concept had been published by an eminent researcher in a major journal. What enthralled me even more that day were Dr. Nicholson's closing words, which were to the effect that every abnormality we see in autism–in the immune and digestive systems and CNS–can be mostly explained by disruption of the development of normal gut flora early in life.

What did he mean by "normal gut flora"? Dr. Nicholson was specifically referring to the hundreds of trillions of bacteria that inhabit the human digestive system. These bacteria are responsible for normal digestion, the production of vitamins, protection from invading pathogens, and more. However, bacteria are not the only inhabitants of the human gut. For example, none of us–even the healthiest person– are free of yeast. There is even a growing understanding in the scientific world that some parasites are also a *normal* part of human microflora and fauna.

In 2010, Heijtz and colleagues published a paper in the *Proceedings of the National Academy of Science* titled "Normal gut microbiota modulates brain development and behavior."[2] The paper makes it clear that the microorganic residents of our bodies (which actually outnumber our own cells by a factor of 10) are crucial to normal brain development. In the researchers' words:

> *Microbial colonization of mammals is an evolution-driven process that modulates host physiology, many of which are associated with immunity and nutrient intake. Here, we report that colonization by gut microbiota impacts mammalian brain development and subsequent adult behavior. [...] Our results suggest that the microbial colonization process initiates signaling mechanisms that affect neuronal circuits involved in motor control and anxiety behavior.*

A theory first known as the *hygiene hypothesis* – and now also called the *old friends hypothesis* or the *biome depletion theory* – states that as human beings evolved, we were inhabited by microorganisms that evolved with us (bacteria, yeast, and parasites). That is, microorganisms were a normal part of the human organism, and our bodies developed in such a way as to accommodate their continued presence. We formed a symbiotic relationship with the inevitable microbes that inhabit us and help develop normal immunity. In short, our immune systems developed around the microbes' omnipresence, and our resident flora were as much a part of us as our liver or heart. This theory is now supported by a growing body of medical research, and, in fact, our intestinal biome is now considered to be a renewable organ. Without these "old friends," moreover, things go terribly wrong with our immune systems. In our current evolutionary-unfriendly germ-free world, chronic inflammatory illnesses are becoming the norm.

When I gave a talk on the topic of the hygiene hypothesis and its relationship to autism at an AutismOne conference in 2007, I received a follow-up email from Dr. Kevin Becker (a researcher at the National Institutes of Health [NIH]) within days of arriving home. Dr. Becker sent me his recently published paper titled "Autism, asthma, inflammation and the hygiene hypothesis."[3] I was thrilled to know someone at the NIH was paying attention! Dr. Becker's paper concludes:

> ...*Similarities between autism, asthma, and inflammatory disorders raise the possibilities of shared mechanisms between these disease types. These include altered immune function in both types of disorders.... [...] Altered patterns of infant immune stimulation may hypersensitize the early immune system not toward allergic sensitivity and bronchial hypersensitivity but to inflammatory or cytokine responses affecting brain structure and function leading to autism. It is well documented that immune cytokines play an important role in normal brain development as well as pathological injury in early brain development.* **It is hypothesized that immune pathways altered by hygiene practices in western society may effect [sic] brain structure or function contributing to the development of autism** (emphasis added).[3]

Helminths and inflammation

I first read about the hygiene hypothesis in a 1999 *New York Times* article about a researcher (then at the University of Iowa, now at Tufts

University) named Dr. Joel Weinstock.[4] The report described Dr. Weinstock's trial using the eggs of a nonpathogenic parasite to treat individuals with inflammatory bowel disease (IBD). Parasitic worms, known as helminths, include whipworms, hookworms, tapeworms, pinworms, and others. Up until 100 years ago or so, we all hosted a variety of these parasitic organisms, which required our bodies as homes. We acquired these organisms shortly after birth, along with a host of other natural flora including bacteria and yeasts. Parasites are easily acquired through soil or water, and, even now, most human beings still have them. Without the early acquisition of parasites and the subsequent immunological reaction they stimulate during the time when our immune systems are learning to differentiate good from bad and self from non-self (mainly in the first two years of life), it is thought that the immune system cannot develop properly.

Dr. Weinstock's trial used the eggs of *Trichuris suis*, whipworms native to the intestines of pigs. In humans, porcine whipworms cannot colonize and instead die in a few weeks. Helminth therapy involves drinking the invisible whipworm eggs in an ounce or two of saline solution. The eggs or ova then make their way to the large intestine where they hatch. In Dr. Weinstock's small-scale study, *Trichuris suis* ova (TSO) were given to six patients with diseases such as Crohn's disease and ulcerative colitis. Five of the six went into remission and the sixth improved dramatically.[4] Dr. Weinstock later explained how the immune systems of these patients had previously been tipped into chronic autoimmunity; by stimulating a certain part of the immune system with TSO therapy, he believed he could tip the scales back, resulting in remission of symptoms.[5] Since 1999, Dr. Weinstock has published additional papers[6-9] exploring the safety and efficacy of TSO for IBD.

A 2012 paper by Dr. Weinstock and his colleague, Dr. David Elliott, reviews the ways that helminths may benefit the immune system, discussing both the "protective effects of helminths" and "the immune pathways altered by helminths that may afford protection."[11] The two authors observe:

> *Exposure to commensal and pathogenic organisms strongly influences our immune system. Exposure to helminths was frequent before humans constructed their current highly hygienic*

environment. Today, in highly industrialized countries, contact between humans and helminths is rare. Congruent with the decline in helminth infections is an increase in the prevalence of autoimmune and inflammatory disease.

Dr. Graham Rook (one of the foremost researchers into the therapeutic possibilities of helminths) and his colleague Dr. Lowry shared similar observations about the rise in inflammatory diseases of the brain as well as gut and immune system in a 2008 paper:

The hygiene hypothesis proposes that several chronic inflammatory disorders (allergies, autoimmunity, inflammatory bowel disease) are increasing in prevalence in developed countries because a changing microbial environment has perturbed immunoregulatory circuits which normally terminate inflammatory responses. [...] Therefore, some psychiatric disorders in developed countries might be attributable to failure of immunoregulatory circuits to terminate ongoing inflammatory responses.[22]

To understand how helminth therapy may mediate abnormal inflammation, it is important to understand the role of cytokines in the immune system. A cytokine is the name for the immune system's chemical messengers, just as neurotransmitters are the chemical messengers of the CNS. In the immune system, cytokines are classified into groups. Two of the best known groups are Type 1 T helper cells (Th1, a family of chemicals associated with autoimmune illnesses) and Type 2 T helper cells (Th2, a family of chemicals associated with allergy and asthma). Th2 was created, in an evolutionary sense, to help our bodies handle parasites. That is, humans developed living in dirt. Until 100 years ago, when we developed indoor plumbing and began to wear shoes, all humans – from shortly after birth – had a native helminth population (acquired from constant exposure to feces in the dirt (both animal and human) and unpurified water. The Th2 family of cytokines developed to keep helminth populations in reasonable check. When the immune system does not develop properly (in part through lack of exposure to stimuli such as helminths), Th2, through mechanisms that are not yet fully understood, begins to react to normally non-harmful environmental stimuli such as pollen and cat dander or begins to attack our own bodies–or both. More than that, the regulatory system (the "off switch" to the proinflammatory Th1/Th2 systems) does not develop, and our bodies are unable to stop the inflammatory cascade.

At this point in time, no one knows exactly how parasites reduce inflammatory cytokines and boost the regulatory system, but there is no doubt that this is their effect. We do know that helminths suppress our immune systems in order to survive and keep our bodies from killing them off. When parasites are used in small, therapeutic doses, it appears that the immune suppression that they bring about can turn off out-of-control inflammation.

Immune abnormalities in autism

Recalling that the cytokines of the immune system are known as neurotransmitters when we're talking about the CNS, it should be fairly obvious that dysregulation of these chemicals in the immune system means they are also dysregulated in the CNS and in the gut, and vice versa. Keeping this in mind, what do we know about immune abnormalities in autism? Two decades ago in 1986, Warren and colleagues explored this question in 31 patients with autism and found several immune-system abnormalities, including "decreased numbers of T lymphocytes; and an altered ratio of helper to suppressor T cells."[14] That is, they found higher levels of proinflammatory cytokines in relation to suppressor (regulatory) ones. Similarly, in 2001, Jyonouchi and colleagues observed "excessive innate immune responses"[15] in children with ASD, while Croonenberghs and colleagues agreed the following year that "There is now some evidence that autism may be accompanied by abnormalities in the inflammatory response system."[16] These same authors hypothesized that "increased production of proinflammatory cytokines could play a role in the pathophysiology of autism."[16]

One of the more important papers on this subject came out in 2005.[17] Describing how the immune system of the brain (the glial cells) is abnormally activated in ASD, possibly causing and maintaining the symptoms of autism, Drs. Pardo, Vargas, and Zimmerman wrote the following:

We recently demonstrated the presence of neuroglial and innate neuroimmune system activation in brain tissue and cerebrospinal fluid of patients with autism, findings that support the view that neuroimmune abnormalities occur in the brain of autistic patients and may contribute to the diversity of the autistic phenotypes. The role of neuroglial activation and neuroinflammation are still uncertain but could be critical in maintaining, if not also in initiating, some of the CNS abnormalities present in autism.[17]

There are many other papers along these lines. In 2008, an interesting article reported researchers' efforts to cause inflammation in the intestines of rats to see what would happen in the CNS.[18] The authors proved their hypothesis that causing inflammation in one part of the body would subsequently be manifested in the CNS as well, observing that the treated rats "exhibited a marked, *reversible* (emphasis added) inflammatory response within the hippocampus, characterized by microglial activation and increases in tumor necrosis factor-alpha (TNF-alpha) levels."[18] (TNF-alpha is a proinflammatory cytokine.) That same year, some of the researchers continued their investigations, this time injecting rats very early in life with toxins from bad bacteria (lipopolysaccharides or LPS).[19] These rats showed significantly greater susceptibility to seizures as adults as well as greatly increased release of inflammatory cytokines after the seizures.[19] Although rodent studies are not equivalent to studies in humans, these results are obviously very significant and certainly establish that, as Dr. Baker always says, "Inflammation is inflammation." The human body is a whole, and every tendril in the web is attached to every other.

Future directions
Abnormal immune activation in the body and brains of children with autism is well established at this point. How or whether this immune activation is the cause of the autistic symptoms or whether it's a symptom of something else is not known. But as Dr. Nicholson said, alterations in the gut flora early in life could certainly lead to altered immunity and altered development. The puzzle may not yet be complete, but a picture is certainly starting to emerge.

Almost daily, the idea that our current overly-hygienic lifestyle has destroyed our natural digestive biome and that changes to our native microflora are connected to a host of chronic diseases appears in the medical literature. The concept that the brain and the gut influence each other is also prevalent in the literature. In an intriguing paper in *Gastroenterology* in 2010, Bercik and colleagues[20] studied the relationship of chronic gastrointestinal inflammation on behavior in rats, after having shown in a prior paper that mice who were experimentally made to be depressed or anxious were more susceptible to gut inflammation.[21] In the second study, the researchers showed the opposite also to be true: animals who were experimentally made to have gut inflammation were more prone to anxiety and depressive behaviors.[20] The investigators concluded that their study "provides support for a bidirectional relationship between behavior and gut inflammation; depression increases vulnerability to gut inflammation, which, in turn, induces depression/anxiety-like behavior."[20]

Returning to autism, Dr. William Parker of Duke University traces the gut-brain connection in his comments on the biome depletion theory:

> *...The immune system and our biome did not evolve in isolation. Other organs, including our brain, were evolving at the same time, and are intertwined with our immune system in ways that are only beginning to be understood. The implications are potentially far reaching. For example, the association of autism with inflammation and the epidemic nature of this disease in post-industrial societies point toward The Biome Depletion Theory. The identification of viral "triggers" which may be involved in autism is consistent with* **the idea that epidemics of autism...are a result of biome depletion** (emphasis added).[23]

The treatment implications of these ideas are significant. In treating inflammation, we can affect both gut and brain health. While there is still much that we don't know about how our "old friends" work (including our once-native populations of helminths), we do already know a great deal. Research into the therapeutic possibilities of helminths is increasing worldwide, with various studies exploring their use in multiple sclerosis, allergy (including peanut allergy), asthma,

IBD, and, soon, autism. There are no clinical studies completed as of yet on the effects of these old friends on autism (although the Albert Einstein College of Medicine, under the direction of Dr. Eric Hollander, has begun one on affected adults), but the anecdotal data are truly compelling. For the past 6 or 7 years, intrepid parents of ASD children have been using therapeutic doses of helminths to attempt to modulate their children's immune systems. By introducing small doses of whipworms and/or hookworms, they are trying to reverse the upregulation of the Th1 and Th2 systems. These parents report global improvements: reduction of gut symptoms, allergies, and anxiety; improved socialization and language; and reduction of aggressive and self-injurious behaviors.

Thus far, small therapeutic doses of helminths have a superb safety record and low incidence of side effects. While helminth treatment is not yet FDA-approved for any condition, Coronado Biosciences, the company that has licensed TSO therapy in the United States, has completed its Phase 1 clinical trial and begun its Phase 2, the next step toward getting FDA approval, for Crohn's disease first. The Phase 1 trial, a safety study, showed that TSO was safe and well-tolerated.[10]

In a talk several years ago, Dr. Martha Herbert (assistant professor of neurology at Harvard Medical School and a pediatric neurologist at Massachusetts General Hospital in Boston) concluded her talk by saying, "When faced with prolonged uncertainty, use your best judgment." That statement has become one of my mantras. I often point out to clients that expressions such as "gut reaction," having a "gut feeling," "butterflies in your stomach," and not being able to "stomach" something are not arbitrary. On the contrary, our digestive system's tie-in to our brain is something we're all (probably too) familiar with. If you'll forgive the intentional pun, my gut tells me that in the not-very-distant future, helminthic therapy (and other approaches to restore our relationship with our old friends) will become standard medical treatment. As one team of researchers elegantly concludes after discussing helminths and inflammatory diseases, "In some not too distant futurity, there may come a day when we all take 'helminth supplements' along with our Omega 3 fatty acids, vitamins, and whatever else goes to make up a modern balanced diet."[24]

References

1. Yap IK, Angley M, Veselkov KA, Holmes E, Lindon JC, Nicholson JK. Urinary metabolic phenotyping differentiates children with autism from their unaffected siblings and age-matched controls. *J Proteome Res*. 2010 Jun 4;9(6):2996-3004.
2. Heijtz R, Wang S, Anuar F, Qian Y, Björkholm B, Samuelsson A, Hibberd ML, Forssberg H, Pettersson S. Normal gut microbiota modulates brain development and behavior. *Proc Natl Acad Sci U S A*. 2011 Feb 15;108(7):3047-52. Epub 2011 Jan 31.
3. Becker KG. Autism, asthma, inflammation, and the hygiene hypothesis. *Med Hypotheses*. 2007;69(4):731-40. Epub 2007 Apr 6.
4. Newman A. In pursuit of autoimmune worm cure. *The New York Times*, August 31, 1999. Retrieved March, 25, 2008 from http://query.nytimes.com/gst/fullpage.html?res=9A0DE6DB113BF932A0575BC0A96F958260&scp=1&sq=in%20pursuit%20of%20an%20autoimmune%20cure&st=cse
5. Weinstock JV, Elliott DE. Helminths and the IBD hygiene hypothesis. *Inflamm Bowel Dis*. 2009 Jan;15(1):128-33.
6. Elliott DE, Summers RW, Weinstock JV. Helminths as governors of immune-mediated inflammation. *Int J Parasitol*. 2007 Apr;37(5):457-64. Epub 2006 Dec 28.
7. Summers RW, Elliott DE, Qadir K, Urban JF Jr, Thompson R, Weinstock JV. *Trichuris suis* seems to be safe and possibly effective in the treatment of inflammatory bowel disease. *Am J Gastroenterol*. 2003 Sep;98(9):2034-41.
8. Summers RW, Elliott DE, Urban JF Jr, Thompson R, Weinstock JV. *Trichuris suis* therapy in Crohn's disease. *Gut*. 2005 Jan;54(1):87-90.
9. Walk ST, Blum AM, Ewing SA, Weinstock JV, Young VB. Alterations of the murine gut microbiota during infection with the parasitic helminth *Heligmosomoides polygyrus*. *Inflamm Bowel Dis*. 2010 Nov;16(11):1841-9.
10. Coronado Biosciences. Coronado Biosciences announces Phase 1 clinical trial results for TSO in Crohn's disease. Burlington, MA: Coronado Biosciences, February 28, 2012. http://ir.coronadobiosciences.com/Cache/1001164055.PDF?D=&O=PDF&IID=4308955&Y=&T=&FID=1001164055
11. Elliott DE, Weinstock JV. Helminth-host immunological interactions: prevention and control of immune-mediated diseases. *Ann N Y Acad Sci*. 2012 Jan;1247:83-96. Epub 2012 Jan 12.
12. Gershon MD. *The Second Brain: The Scientific Basis of Gut Instinct and a Groundbreaking New Understanding of Nervous Disorders and the Intestine*. New York: Harper Collins, 1998.
13. Pert CB. *Molecules of Emotion: The Science Behind Mind-Body Medicine*. New York: Touchstone, 1997.
14. Warren RP, Margaretten NC, Pace NC, Foster A. Immune abnormalities in patients with autism. *J Autism Dev Disord*. 1986 Jun;16(2):189-97.
15. Jyonouchi H, Sun S, Le H. Proinflammatory and regulatory cytokine production associated with innate and adaptive immune responses in children with autism spectrum disorders and developmental regression. *J Neuroimmunol*. 2001 Nov;120(1-2):170-9.
16. Croonenberghs J, Bosmans E, Deboutte D, Kenis G, Maes M. Activation of the inflammatory response system in autism. *Neuropsychobiology*. 2002;45(1):1-6.
17. Pardo CA, Vargas DL, Zimmerman AW. Immunity, neuroglia and neuroinflammation in autism. *Int Rev Psychiatry*. 2005 Dec;17(6):485-95.

18. Riazi K, Galic MA, Kuzmiski JB, Ho W, Sharkey KA, Pittman QJ. Microglial activation and TNF alpha production mediate altered CNS excitability following peripheral inflammation. *Proc Natl Acad Sci U S A*. 2008 Nov 4;105(44):17151-6. Epub 2008 Oct 27.

19. Galic MA, Riazi K, Heida JG, Mouihate A, Fournier NM, Spencer SJ, Kalynchuk LE, Teskey GC, Pittman QJ. Postnatal inflammation increases seizure susceptibility in adult rats. *J Neurosci*. 2008 Jul 2;28(27):6904-13.

20. Bercik P, Verdu EF, Foster JA, Macri J, Potter M, Huang X, Malinowski P, Jackson W, Blennerhassett P, Neufeld KA, Lu J, Khan WI, Corthesy-Theulaz I, Cherbut C, Bergonzelli GE, Collins SM. Chronic gastrointestinal inflammation induces anxiety-like behavior and alters central nervous system biochemistry in mice. *Gastroenterology*. 2010 Dec;139(6):2102-12.e1. Epub 2010 Jun 27.

21. Varghese AK, Verdu EF, Bercik P, Khan WI, Blennerhassett PA, Szechtman H, Collins SM. Antidepressants attenuate increased susceptibility to colitis in a murine model of depression. *Gastroenterology*. 2006 May;130(6):1743-53.

22. Rook G, Lowry CA. The hygiene hypothesis and psychiatric disorders. *Trends Immunol*. 2008 Apr;29(4):150-8. Epub 2008 Mar 6.

23. Parker W. Reconstituting the depleted biome to prevent immune disorders. *The Evolution & Medicine Review*, October 13, 2010. Retrieved October 13, 2010 from http://evmedreview.com/?p=457

24. Zaccone P, Fehervari Z, Phillips JM, Dunne DW, Cooke A. Parasitic worms and inflammatory diseases. *Parasite Immunol*. 2006 Oct;28(10):515-23.

Other articles of interest

Careaga M, Van de Water J, Ashwood P. Immune dysfunction in autism: a pathway to treatment. *Neurotherapeutics*. 2010 Jul;7(3):283-92.

Feillet H, Bach JF. Increased incidence of inflammatory bowel disease: the price of the decline of infectious burden? *Curr Opin Gastroenterol*. 2004 Nov;20(6):560-4.

Fumagalli M, Pozzoli U, Cagliani R, Comi GP, Riva S, Clerici M, Bresolin N, Sironi M. Parasites represent a major selective force for interleukin genes and shape the genetic predisposition to autoimmune conditions. *J Exp Med*. 2009 Jun;206(6): 1395-1408.

Gupta S, Aggarwal S, Rashanravan B, Lee T. Th1- and Th2-like cytokines in CD4+ and CD8+ T cells in autism. *J Neuroimmunol*. 1998 May;85(1):106-9.

Hamilton G. Why we need germs. *The Ecologist Report*. June 1, 2008. Retrieved August 4, 2008. http://www.mindfully.org/Health/We-Need-Germs.htm

Hayes KS, Bancroft AJ, Goldrick M, Portsmouth C, Roberts IS, Grencis RK. Exploitation of the intestinal microflora by the parasitic nematode *Trichuris muris*. *Science*. 2010 Jun 11;328(5984):1391-4.

Li X, Chauhan A, Sheikh AM, Patil S, Chauhan V, Li XM, Ji L, Brown T, Malik M. Elevated immune response in the brain of autistic patients. *J Neuroimmunol*. 2009 Feb;207(1-2):111-6. Epub 2009 Jan 20.

Maizels RM, Yazdanbakhsh M. Immune regulation by helminth parasites: cellular and molecular mechanisms. *Nat Rev Immunol*. 2003 Sep;3(9):733-44.

Mangan NE, Fallon RE, Smith P, van Rooijen N, McKenzie AN, Fallon PG. Helminth infection protects mice from anaphylaxis via IL-10-producing B cells. *J Immunol.* 2004 Nov;173(10):6346-56.

Molloy CA, Morrow AL, Meinzen-Derr J, Schleifer K, Dienger K, Manning-Courtney P, Altaye M, Wills-Karp M. Elevated cytokine levels in children with autism spectrum disorders. *J Neuroimmunol.* 2006 Mar;172(1-2):198-205. Epub 2005 Dec 19.

Reddy A, Fried B. The use of *Trichuris suis* and other helminth therapies to treat Crohn's disease. *Parasitol Res.* 2007 Apr;100(5):921-7. Epub 2007 Jan 6.

Rook G. The hygiene hypothesis and the increasing prevalence of chronic inflammatory disorders. *Trans R Soc Trop Med Hyg.* 2007 Nov;101(11):1072-4.

Schnoeller C, Rausch S, Pillai S, Avagyan A, Wittig BM, Loddenkemper C, Hamann A, Hamelmann E, Lucius R, Hartmann S. A helminth immunomodulator reduces allergic and inflammatory responses by induction of IL-10-producing macrophages. *J Immunol.* 2008 Mar;180(6):4265-72.

Turner JD, Jackson JA, Faulkner H, Behnke J, Else KJ, Kamgno J, Boussinesq M, Bradley JE. Intensity of intestinal infection with multiple worm species is related to regulatory cytokine output and immune hyporesponsiveness. *J Infect Dis.* 2008 Apr;197(8):1204-12.

CHAPTER SIX

THE NOT SO SMALL WORLD OF GUT MICROBES: HOW THEY INFLUENCE BEHAVIOR AND THE BRAIN IN BIG WAYS

By James Jeffrey Bradstreet, MD, MD(H), FAAFP

When I approach a child, he inspires in me two sentiments: tenderness for what he is, and respect for what he may become.
–Louis Pasteur

Autism and the gastrointestinal tract

Autism spectrum disorders (ASDs) are complex developmental abnormalities defined on the basis of the severity of symptoms in three domains: language, socialization, and stereotypical behaviors. Although it is recognized that various chromosomal, mitochondrial, and metabolic disorders can present with autistic features, the biological aspects of ASD are not generally considered in the evaluation and diagnosis of the condition. However, as odd as it may seem to some readers, the microbial world of the gastrointestinal tract has been increasingly recognized as a potential source of neuropsychiatric symptoms.[1]

While it is somewhat easy to understand how brain inflammation could lead to autistic features, it is more challenging to comprehend the role of the gut ecosystem (microbiome) in both creating and maintaining an ongoing central nervous system (CNS) inflammatory response. However, Professor Jeremy Nicholson and his colleagues

97

have reminded us that approximately 50% of the metabolic output of the body actually comes from the biochemistry of the bacteria living in the gut.[2] Nicholson's group was able to distinguish a distinct pattern of metabolites in children with autism that differed from both healthy controls and their unaffected siblings. Importantly, this metabolic view of the microbiome does not require that gastrointestinal symptoms such as diarrhea or pain be present to generate the biochemical changes that could be triggering autism symptoms. This is a critical turning point in our understanding of the role of the gut ecosystem in shaping neuropsychiatric consequences. In this perspective of autism, the biochemical output of the gut ecosystem alters brain development and chemistry. Is that enough to generate the symptom complex we label as autism? Perhaps, although I suspect autism represents a perfect storm caused by the interaction of the microbiome with an altered immune response both in the gut and in the brain.

Immune dysregulation and autism

Although there is much more to discuss with regard to the microbiome, let's first move our discussion of the gut-brain connection over to the brain and immune system. During the last three decades, we have seen accumulating evidence of immune dysregulation in ASD. Although the nature of the immune aberrations is somewhat elusive and inconsistent, the general pattern indicates an imbalance resulting in proinflammatory and autoimmune conditions.[3,4] These effects are present in the gut and the brain of a significant subset of ASD-affected individuals.[5] As early as 1982, Weizman and colleagues found abnormal cell-mediated immune responses to brain proteins in 13 of 17 ASD children tested.[6] More recently, Chez and colleagues noted extremely high cerebrospinal fluid (CSF) to plasma ratios of TNF-alpha (a powerful inflammatory mediator), even in immunologically treated cases of ASD.[7] The potential role of TNF-alpha in autism is incompletely understood. To better grasp its importance, it is useful to consider the research of Professor Edward Tobinick from the University of California in Los Angeles, who has been studying the effect of TNF-alpha reduction on a variety of CNS disorders. In his model of CNS dysfunction, TNF-alpha serves as a powerful inhibitor of synaptic (nerve-to-nerve) communication. Dr. Tobinick has pioneered the use of entanercept (a drug that acts as a false receptor to TNF-alpha and, therefore, removes it from the brain and circulation) in disorders such as traumatic brain injuries and stroke.[8] He also found dramatic and rapid improvement in primary progressive aphasia,[9] wherein reduction of TNF-alpha through use of entanercept resulted in nearly immediate return of speech.

A team headed by Persico in Italy pursued genome-wide evaluations of postmortem autism brains to assess the transcriptional messages from DNA and determine what pattern, if any, was present in autism.[10] They compared the observations of genomic expression in autism to those of Rett syndrome and Down syndrome. To their surprise, a common central mechanism of developmental abnormalities appeared in these three very distinct disorders. In their own words, "Our results surprisingly converge upon immune, and not neurodevelopmental genes, as the most consistently shared abnormality in genome-wide expression patterns. A dysregulated immune response, accompanied by enhanced oxidative stress and abnormal mitochondrial metabolism seemingly represents the common molecular underpinning of these neurodevelopmental disorders."[10] Researchers at Johns Hopkins University also found persistent neuroinflammatory changes in autistic brains at time of autopsy, even into the fourth decade of life.[11] These findings were reinforced by research from the New York State Institute for Basic Research in Developmental Disabilities, which found significant differences in the innate and adaptive immune responses in the brains of individuals with autism when compared with controls.[5]

The potential role of viruses

Collating these various observations, it seems clear that the brain's immune system is responding to immunological cuing in a persistent proinflammatory way. It also seems clear that some incompletely understood vector or force must be driving the ongoing central inflammatory response in ASD. It is tempting to speculate that a persistent neurotropic pathogen (such as a virus or atypical bacteria) is present in the CNS of autistic individuals, but after several decades, none has been identified with any consistency. However, in 2004, I worked with molecular virologists at Coombe Women's Hospital in Dublin, Ireland, and we reported the first three cases of measles virus

(MV) F gene in the CSF of ASD children with concurrent gastrointestinal inflammation.[12] This group of molecular virologists had previously reported a significant association of MV present in the intestinal biopsies of children with autism and a new variant of enterocolitis.[13] In that previous report, they stated:

Seventy-five of 91 patients [82.4%] with a histologically confirmed diagnosis of ileal lymphonodular hyperplasia and enterocolitis were positive for measles virus in their intestinal tissue compared with five of 70 control patients [7.1%]. Measles virus was identified within the follicular dendritic cells and some lymphocytes in foci of reactive follicular hyperplasia.[13]

In 2004, these investigators also reported the presence of MV F gene in the CSF from 19 of 28 (68%) autism cases but in only 1 of 37 (3%) controls (p<0.00001).[14] Because the three original CSF cases[12] were part of this cohort, only 19 cases in all have been positively identified and reported to date.

Even with the detection of the MV gene in the CSF and intestinal biopsies of children affected with autism, the actual cause-and-effect relationship between the MV genome and autistic symptoms is hotly debated.[15] Recently, Persico's Italian team looked at postmortem brain samples of autistic individuals using sophisticated gene amplification techniques.[16] In that investigation, they attempted to isolate DNA presence from 8 DNA viruses (viruses that have DNA as their genetic material and replicate using a DNA-dependent DNA polymerase): cytomegalovirus (CMV), Epstein-Barr virus (EBV), herpes simplex virus type 1 (HSV-1), herpes simplex virus type 2 (HSV-2), humanherpes virus 6 (HHV-6), BK virus (BKV), JC virus (JCV), and simian virus 40 (SV-40). Only the latter three, all members of the polyoma subgroup of papovaviruses, showed a statistically significant association. Although the research team did not look for the genetic presence of any other viruses, even this limited evaluation showed that the autism group carried a more substantial viral burden.

Importantly, viruses are well known to cohabitate with humans in the absence of apparent disease. We have been programmed to think that germs (viruses and bacteria) cause disease, an understanding fostered by Koch and Loeffler in the late 1800s. Although these German physicians were partially correct, even in the worst epidemics, not all exposed individuals develop symptoms of illness. Ultimately, it is the body's defenses that either do or do not prevent a germ from creating disease. Those defenses are far more complicated than mere antibodies or programmed immunity. To prevent disease, viruses must first be excluded from the body by healthy barrier defenses and then must be kept from replicating their DNA or RNA. For DNA viruses, our bodies must spend a lifetime keeping the viral DNA inhibited, or, as is the case with chickenpox and its later reoccurrence as shingles, the virus will continue to cause symptoms. Our systems contain many viruses without actually eliminating them. In the case of the SV-40, BK, and JC viruses noted by Persico's team, it is not so much the presence of the DNA (which was significantly more common in ASD) that is noteworthy as the unknown of how active or inhibited the viruses are.

Returning to the intestinal microbiome

How the gut's complex ecosystem, the intestinal microbiome, influences total body defenses (including brain immune systems) is not fully understood, but it is clear that with 70% of the immune system residing in the gut, the microbiome is an important variable that must be considered. In the absence of consensus on CNS pathogens, some researchers also have focused on the intestinal microbiome as a potential source for immune activation and toxins capable of influencing the brain's development. This is an appealing theory that fits at least some of the clinical and laboratory observations, including those previously mentioned from Nicholson's group at Imperial College in London. In 2000, Sandler and colleagues observed that 8 of 10 children with ASD, regardless of intestinal symptoms, significantly improved after treatment with vancomycin (an antibiotic with activity against anaerobic bacteria).[17] The researchers did not attempt to identify the specific organisms that may have been responding to the vancomycin but speculated that the response might be related to colonization, overgrowth, or infection by anaerobic clostridia in the children's intestinal tract. More recently, Finegold (who took part in the vancomycin study) and colleagues applied highly specific and

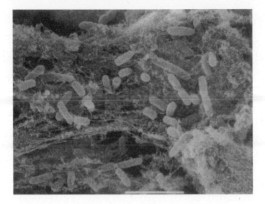

A rare scanning electron micrograph (a useful image though not related to autism) of biofilm with infective E. coli taken from intestinal sections obtained at surgery. (Courtesy of Andrade et al.[20])

sensitive pyrosequencing DNA detection techniques to evaluate the bacteria present in the feces of children with ASD.[18] Their results support the potential reasons why vancomycin could have been effective but, at the same time, point us away from clostridial species to other anaerobic bacteria. One of the predominant organisms vastly overrepresented in the ASD group (as well as in their siblings) was the *Desulfovibrio* species.

Commercial and hospital laboratories are not yet able to reliably measure the gut ecosystem through culturing techniques. Even the advanced research tool of pyrosequencing can only assess the fecal flora and will not give us a full picture of the mucosal-related biofilm-embedded flora. In 2010, Sproule-Willoughby and colleagues stated that "The human gastrointestinal tract hosts a complex community of microorganisms that grow as biofilms on the intestinal mucosa."[19] The biofilm is the adherent mucus with its community of microbes. This system provides a protective bacterial and immunological defensive barrier for the gut. Sproule-Willoughby and colleagues also observe that, as bacterial communities, biofilms "are not well characterized, although they are known to play an important role in human health."[19] There is little research to guide clinicians seeking to treat or change the biofilm-related microbial environment, which is a challenging task that will be discussed later.

Cysteine and glutathione

The finding that the *Desulfovibrio* species is overrepresented in individuals with autism is intriguing because of its potential relationship to observations of cysteine deficiency in ASD. Because *Desulfovibrio* will compete with the host organism (a child with autism) for cysteine, this provides at least one potential mechanism for the observed deficiency of cysteine in ASD.[21] From the late 1990s, I began observing cysteine deficiency on amino acid testing of children with ASD. The availability of cysteine is considered to be the rate-limiting step in the body's ability to manufacture intracellular glutathione.

It would hard to overemphasize the role of glutathione in human health. It is the main intracellular antioxidant, and for decades it has been known to protect neurons from oxidative stress.[22] In addition to more recent observations in autism, glutathione deficiency has long been associated with a variety of disorders that include Parkinsonism,[23] schizophrenia,[24] attention-deficit/hyperactivity disorder (ADHD),[25] HIV,[26] inflammatory bowel disease,[27] and premature aging.[28] While working on research with Professor S. Jill James from the University of Arkansas, I observed dramatically lower cysteine and glutathione as well as corresponding increases in oxidative markers in the ASD population.[29] In that study, we also found increased frequencies of genetic vulnerabilities to oxidation and glutathione metabolism.

Within a healthy biofilm resides a variety of commensal bacteria which are, in part, regulated by cysteine-dependent peptide proteins called defensins. Defensins, which are critical to host immune function and protection,[30] represent another important feature of the intestinal-immune puzzle. Defensins are produced by Paneth cells along the intestinal surface and by dendritic immune cells in lymphoid tissue. Defensins are an inducible yet nonspecific antimicrobial defense mechanism that regulates the gut microbiome.[31] As such, defensins might be considered the extracellular (or cell surface, as with dendritic cells) counterpart of glutathione. It's likely, although at this time still speculative, that the type and magnitude of cysteine deficiency observed in ASD creates a relative defensin deficiency, just as it creates a glutathione deficiency. This would be especially relevant to the local intestinal mucosal environment where *Desulfovibrio*, as a dominant organism, would be locally competing for cysteine resources. In inflammatory bowel disease, as a related example, we see sulfur-dependent bacteria implicated in causation[32] at the same time that we see deficiencies in the Paneth production of defensins.[33]

Thus far, we have touched on overlapping observations involving the following:

- CNS inflammation and brain oxidative stress (cysteine-glutathione deficiency)
- An abnormally skewed microbiome capable of competing with the body for valuable cysteine resources
- Low cysteine in the blood of ASD children
- Evidence of oxidative stress
- Potential responses to antibiotics capable of reducing anaerobic bacteria including *Desulfovibrio*
- Suspected defensin deficiency

Is this enough to explain the catastrophic developmental changes that we label as autism? Maybe, and we are certainly getting closer, but there is more to this story.

Biome depletion

Over the past several decades, both children and their mothers have been exposed to increasingly powerful broad-spectrum antibiotics. This is an unprecedented factor in human development since there is growing acceptance that humans coevolved mutually with their microbiome.[34] This antibiotic assault has radically altered the gut microbiome in a way that predisposes to inflammatory bowel disease.[35] At the same time, cultural changes as humans left farms and gathered in cities have resulted in what is referred to by William Parker of Duke University as "biome depletion."[36] Simply stated, human biome depletion recognizes the regulatory role of helminth species (worms). Rather than being the yucky and presumed-to-be-evil bloodsuckers envisioned by most of us, there is abundant evidence that certain helminths are mutualistic symbionts. In an excellent review on this subject, McKay states:

There is unequivocal evidence that parasites influence the immune activity of their hosts, and many of the classical examples of this are drawn from assessment of helminth infections of their mammalian hosts. Thus, helminth infections can impact on the induction or course of other diseases that the host might be subjected to. Epidemiological studies demonstrate that world regions with high rates of helminth infections consistently have reduced incidences of autoimmune and other allergic/inflammatory-type conditions.[37]

Elliott and colleagues at the University of Iowa also discuss our dependent relationship with worms at some length:

Immune-mediated diseases (e.g., inflammatory bowel disease, asthma, multiple sclerosis, and autoimmune diabetes) are increasing in prevalence and emerge as populations adopt meticulously hygienic lifestyles. This change in lifestyles precludes exposure to helminths (parasitic worms). Loss of natural helminth exposure removes a previously universal Th2 and regulatory immune biasing imparted by these organisms. Helminths protect animals from developing immune-mediated diseases (colitis, reactive airway disease, encephalitis, and diabetes). Clinical trials show that exposure to helminths can reduce disease activity in patients with ulcerative colitis or Crohn's disease.[38]

Mount Sinai School of Medicine has an ongoing trial of helminthic therapy for autism, but no results are available at the time of this writing. The study is investigating *Trichuris suis* ova (TSO), also called pig whipworm eggs. As with any monotherapy for a complex disorder such as autism, it is doubtful that TSO will produce dramatic results in language and stereotypical symptoms over a short course of treatment. TSO does show impressive results in refractory inflammatory bowel disease,[39] but there we are not dealing with complex CNS and developmental abnormalities. When applied to existing respiratory allergies, TSO had no measurable benefit on nasal allergy symptoms in a recent controlled study.[40] It has been observed that there is a mutually exclusive relationship between *Schistosoma* infection and multiple sclerosis, implying a protective effect of helminthic colonization.[41] Although helminths have been shown to have a protective effect by preventing the induction of experimental encephalomyelitis,[42] it is not known whether they can reverse the course of established brain inflammation as observed in ASD.

It is reasonable–even likely–that the immune regulatory role of both the human biome and the microbiome needs to be established in the maternal environment prior to pregnancy.[43,44] Data point to very early immune programming of the brain's future developmental response and also establish a link between maternal immune dysregulation and ASD. It may be that the same microbiome and biome effects that disrupt the maternal immune system are passed along environmentally to a woman's offspring. As will be described in detail later, the ecosystem of the gut is set very early in life.

Changing the intestinal ecosystem

This brings up the issue of artificially changing the intestinal ecosystem. It seems logical that if the nature of the gut flora is the problem, one might attempt to change the flora with different and presumably healthier bacteria (probiotics). This has been discussed briefly by Garvey,[45] but no systematic investigation has been published with regard to ASD. Nonetheless, numerous clinicians and parents undertake the use of bacteria supplementation in an effort to induce a "better" gut ecosystem.[46] My personal experience provides a mixture of results from the use of probiotic supplements. Some children immediately benefit from probiotics, demonstrating improved bowel function, decreased hyperactivity, increased eye contact, and better attention. However, the dose and type of probiotic tolerated seems highly variable. Some children do well only with small doses (in bacterial terms, this is 1-10 billion bacteria per day). Other children are helped only by massive doses (upwards of 450 billion/day). There is support in the pediatric literature for high-dose *Lactobacillus* in ulcerative colitis (UC).[47,48] VSL#3® has been tested in adults and has proven efficacy for UC in this older population as well.[49] However, evidence is lacking for VSL#3® efficacy in Crohn's disease, a different type of inflammatory bowel disease.[50]

The nature of inflammatory bowel disease in autism is immunologically distinct from both UC and Crohn's disease.[51] This creates the need for specific testing for the ASD population of any proposed probiotic. At this point, any large-scale, scientifically rigorous study of probiotics in ASD is unlikely to be financially feasible. Despite this research obstacle, clinicians can reasonably try probiotics in their patient population using an N of 1 study model. In essence, each child's baseline can serve as their own control point for observations. The probiotic can be initiated, starting at low doses, and subsequently increased to tolerance. It is especially helpful to use biomarkers of gut inflammation, where possible. (For a review of these biomarkers and their clinical application to autism interventions, please see Bradstreet et al.[52])

There is growing evidence that the immune system programs itself to accept a specific microbiome very early in life.[53] Within days of birth, the gut of all infants is colonized by the child's mother, the environment (such as hospital or home), and the diet (breast milk or formula). Other influences on the composition of the child's gut microbiome are the method of delivery (vaginal versus surgical) and combinations of different environmental and feeding variables.[54] Once established, the microbiome drives nutrient digestion and absorption, which further determine the composition of the intestinal ecosystem.[55] There is evidence that this ecosystem becomes stable by one year of life; even after exposure to antibiotics, it tends to return to the immunologically programmed microbiome within a few months (HS Winter, MD, personal communication, January 2011).

When and how the microbiome becomes disrupted in autism is poorly understood, but we would expect it to be altered in undesirable ways very early in development. As mentioned earlier, vancomycin resulted in temporary improvement of autistic symptoms. After a few months, however, the children relapsed, implying a return to the old microbiome. Microbiome disruption caused by antibiotics can be potentially life-threatening, as with *Clostridium difficile* colitis, which, in some cases, is refractory to treatment with antibiotics. In these cases, the new harmful microbiome becomes established, and the host lacks the ability to revert to the earlier ecosystem. Contributors to this situation include the facts that the chronic form of colitis is debilitating and creates nutritional deficiencies, the inflammatory response alters local bacterial regulatory factors, and the clostridia biochemically defend their ecological niche.

In these entrenched, chronic cases of colitis in adults, doctors have resorted successfully to fecal bacteriotherapy (FB), also known as fecal transfer or transplantation.[56] This has been successful in pediatric cases as well.[57] Recently, fecal transfer or transplantation also has been proposed as a microbiome modification strategy for autism.[18] However, this potential therapy presents some daunting challenges, including the likelihood of significant consumer resistance. I have had the pleasure of discussing the early use of fecal bacteriotherapy with Professor Emeritus Tore Midtvedt, MD, PhD, from the Karolinska Institute in Sweden. In the early 1950s, Dr. Midtvedt was asked to help a Norwegian community plagued with chronic infectious diarrhea, which had resisted all eradication efforts by local physicians. With a great deal of effort, Dr. Midtvedt's team identified an ideal donor and was able to infuse the feces into infected individuals using enemas, which completely resolved the diarrhea in all the treated patients. However, even in the 1950s this experience was complicated by the challenges of finding a suitable donor. The difficulties of donor screening and identification have only escalated in the era of widespread antibiotic use and occult viruses such as HIV. Despite these challenges, FB research continues at several institutions.

Fecal bacteriotherapy can be accomplished in a variety of ways.[58] The simplest technique would involve swallowing oral time-delayed capsules. This is envisioned but, to my knowledge, is not available to consumers at this time. Recent high-end research has used colonoscopy to deliver the fecal transplant to the cecum (first portion of the large bowel). Both nasogastric tubes and retention enemas have also been used to deliver the new microbiome. Most FB protocols involve pretreating the gut with an antibiotic (for example, vancomycin) or antibiotic combinations, but this risks further disruptions to the ecosystem. Since there have been few clinical trials published, the best methods are not yet established. Moreover, no one as yet has published the application of this therapy to treat the microbiome of ASD. Given the link between bowel flora and at least some of the behaviors observed in autism as well as potential benefits for the immune dysregulation observed in ASD, I suspect we will see more discussions and possible clinical trials with FB and ASD.

Putting the pieces together

Linking our observations into a logical disease model that can guide diagnostic evaluations and therapeutic efforts poses challenges. Nonetheless, the data indicate that the following chain of events could likely lead to and maintain the autistic state.

1. Disruption occurs to the maternal ecosystem both before and during pregnancy.
2. The altered microbiome produces flora that disrupt the immune balance of the mother and her offspring, including (in some cases) production of antibodies directed against the fetal brain.
3. Further complications are induced by biome (helminthic) depletion, such that the pregnant woman is unable to counter the autoimmune and proinflammatory influences of her microbiome disruption.
4. This results in early-life establishment of an undesirable microbiome for the offspring.
5. Cysteine depletion is created at least in part by overgrowth of sulfur-dependent intestinal bacteria.
6. Cysteine-dependent defensin deficiency presumably also occurs, altering the microbiome and permitting greater numbers of potentially pathogenic organisms.
7. Glutathione deficiency and increased intracellular oxidative stress result in all organs. The brain is especially sensitive to glutathione deficiency.
8. Alterations in the blood-brain barrier ensue, which can introduce toxins and viruses to the brain.
9. Glutathione deficiency alters TNF-alpha responses in the brain in undesirable ways.
10. TNF-alpha mediates synaptic plasticity and interferes with neuronal communication in ways described for other neurological disorders.

This potential model allows a combination of antecedents to open the door to brain inflammation and altered development (perhaps from as early as intrauterine development). It is conceivable that these antecedents also allow viral persistence and/or replication to take place where it would otherwise be inhibited. Intervening in the process, therefore, should start early in life and ideally prior to conception to allow proper conditioning of the maternal biome and microbiome. Early intervention of this type represents no small challenge, however, given the resistance to change noted in the gut ecosystem. For existing cases of autism, early and appropriate restoration of the gut flora could offer significant benefits. In clinical observations, we have seen efforts to benefit the microbiome prove successful, even if only temporarily. Improved diagnostic methods of detecting microbiome disruption (such as pyrosequencing) soon may become clinically available to guide clinicians in therapeutic interventions. However, as discussed earlier, methods to assess the biofilm ecosystem are still in their infancy. Despite these challenges, progress is being made in our efforts to alter the intestinal ecosystem in ways that reduce gut pathology and improve the microbiome.

Dietary changes may offer significant advantages in combination with these other therapeutic efforts. Anecdotal observations support interventions ranging from gluten and casein elimination to even more restrictive and challenging diets such as the Specific Carbohydrate Diet™. All of these dietary changes would be expected to modify the immune and microbiome responses of the child. The elimination of carbohydrates clearly would alter the microbiome in anyone, but in ASD it may have a more dramatic effect based on recent observations of specific enzyme deficiencies in ASD involving enzymes called disaccharidases. A team of researchers recently observed deficiencies in these carbohydrate enzymes as well as sugar transport mechanisms in ASD, with the expected alterations in bacterial colonization.[59]

The final stage in digestion of carbohydrates can take place only when double sugars (disaccharides) are adequately broken down into single sugars at the surface of intestinal cells. In the presence of enzyme deficiencies, this implies that oral enzyme supplementation with exogenous enzymes (particularly those with carbohydrate and disaccharidase activity) might be helpful. In clinical cases, the benefits of enzyme supplementation are clear, but a recent study that evaluated this strategy came up short. The researchers found no statistical differences in autism or gastrointestinal symptoms after 6 months of enzyme therapy.[60] Given the complexity of the gut ecosystem, it isn't that surprising to see failure in a single intervention such as enzyme supplementation. It will likely take multiple complex strategies to create a healthy gut-brain relationship.

Fortunately, the research continues. Novel microbiome therapies such as fecal bacteriotherapy loom as potentially viable future treatments, even as biome therapy with TSO is being investigated. Probiotics are readily available already, although dosing and strain selection are still incompletely understood. Methods to address brain inflammation are being discussed and some have proposed anti-inflammatories derived from nature to address this need.[61] Overall, it seems clear that the complex interactions of maternal and child immune and intestinal environments play a major role in the development of ASD and, therefore, are important targets for therapeutic interventions.

References

1. Gonzalez A, Stombaugh J, Lozupone C, Turnbaugh PJ, Gordon JI, Knight R. The mind-body-microbial continuum. *Dialogues Clin Neurosci.* 2011;13(1):55-62.

2. Yap IK, Angley M, Veselkov KA, Holmes E, Lindon JC, Nicholson JK. Urinary metabolic phenotyping differentiates children with autism from their unaffected siblings and age-matched controls. *J Proteome Res.* 2010 Jun 4;9(6):2996-3004.

3. Careaga M, Van de Water J, Ashwood P. Immune dysfunction in autism: a pathway to treatment. *Neurotherapeutics.* 2010 Jul;7(3):283-92.

4. Gupta S, Samra D, Agrawal S. Adaptive and innate immune responses in autism: rationale for therapeutic use of intravenous immunoglobulin. J *Clin Immunol.* 2010 May;30(Suppl 1):90-6. Epub 2010 Apr 1.

5. Li X, Chauhan A, Sheikh AM, Patil S, Chauhan V, Li XM, Ji L, Brown T, Malik M. Elevated immune response in the brain of autistic patients. *J Neuroimmunol.* 2009 Feb 15;207(1-2):111-6. Epub 2009 Jan 20.

6. Weizman A, Weizman R, Szekely GA, Wijsenbeek H, Livni E. Abnormal immune response to brain tissue antigen in the syndrome of autism. *Am J Psychiatry.* 1982 Nov;139(11):1462-5.

7. Chez MG, Dowling T, Patel PB, Khanna P, Kominsky M. Elevation of tumor necrosis factor-alpha in cerebrospinal fluid of autistic children. *Pediatr Neurol.* 2007 Jun;36(6):361-5.

8. Tobinick E Perispinal etanercept for neuroinflammatory disorders. *Drug Discov Today.* 2009 Feb;14(3-4):168-77. Epub 2008 Dec 6.

9. Tobinick E. Perispinal etanercept produces rapid improvement in primary progressive aphasia: identification of a novel, rapidly reversible TNF-mediated pathophysiologic mechanism. *Medscape J Med.* 2008 Jun 10;10(6):135.

10. Lintas C, Sacco R, Persico AM. Genome-wide expression studies in Autism spectrum disorder, Rett syndrome, and Down syndrome. *Neurobiol Dis.* 2012 Jan;45(1):57-68. Epub 2010 Dec 2.

11. Vargas DL, Nascimbene C, Krishnan C, Zimmerman AW, Pardo CA. Neuroglial activation and neuroinflammation in the brain of patients with autism. *Ann Neurol.* 2005 Jan;57(1):67-81. Erratum in: *Ann Neurol.* 2005 Feb;57(2):304.

12. Bradstreet JJ, El Dahr J, Anthony A, Kartzinel JJ, Wakefield AJ. Detection of measles virus genomic RNA in cerebrospinal fluid of children with regressive autism: a report of three cases. *Journal of American Physicians and Surgeons.* 2004 Summer;9(2):38-45.

13. Uhlmann V, Martin CM, Sheils O, Pilkington L, Silva I, Killalea A, Murch SB, Walker-Smith J, Thomson M, Wakefield AJ, O'Leary JJ. Potential viral pathogenic mechanism for new variant inflammatory bowel disease. *Mol Pathol.* 2002 Apr;55(2):84-90.

14. Bradstreet JJ, El Dahr J, Montgomery SM, Wakefield AJ. TaqMan RT-PCR detection of measles virus genomic RNA in cerebrospinal fluid in children with regressive autism. Presented at the 2004 International Meeting for Autism Research (IMFAR).

15. Dubik M, Offit PA. Measles virus RNA and autism revisited. *AAP Grand Rounds.* 2004;12(5):56-7.

16. Lintas C, Altieri L, Lombardi F, Sacco R, Persico AM. Association of autism with polyomavirus infection in postmortem brains. *J Neurovirol.* 2010 Mar;16(2):141-9.

17. Sandler RH, Finegold SM, Bolte ER, Buchanan CP, Maxwell AP, Väisänen ML, Nelson MN, Wexler HM. Short-term benefit from oral vancomycin treatment of regressive-onset autism. *J Child Neurol.* 2000 Jul;15(7):429-35.

18. Finegold SM, Dowd SE, Gontcharova V, Liu C, Henley KE, Wolcott RD, Youn E, Summanen PH, Granpeesheh D, Dixon D, Liu M, Molitoris DR, Green JA 3rd. Pyrosequencing study of fecal microflora of autistic and control children. *Anaerobe.* 2010 Aug;16(4):444-53. Epub 2010 Jul 9.

19. Sproule-Willoughby KM, Stanton MM, Rioux KP, McKay DM, Buret AG, Ceri H. In vitro anaerobic biofilms of human colonic microbiota. *J Microbiol Methods.* 2010 Dec;83(3):296-301. Epub 2010 Oct 12.

20. Andrade JA, Freymüller E, Fagundes-Neto U. Adherence of enteroaggregative *Escherichia coli* to the ileal and colonic mucosa: an in vitro study utilizing the scanning electron microscopy. *Arq Gastroenterol.* 2011 Sep;48(3):199-204.

21. James SJ, Cutler P, Melnyk S, Jernigan S, Janak L, Gaylor DW, Neubrander JA. Metabolic biomarkers of increased oxidative stress and impaired methylation capacity in children with autism. *Am J Clin Nutr.* 2004 Dec;80(6):1611-7.

22. Siesjö BK, Rehncrona S, Smith D. Neuronal cell damage in the brain: possible involvement of oxidative mechanisms. *Acta Physiol Scand Suppl.* 1980;492:121-8.

23. Jenner P. Altered mitochondrial function, iron metabolism and glutathione levels in Parkinson's disease. *Acta Neurol Scand Suppl.* 1993;146:6-13.

24. Do KQ, Trabesinger AH, Kirsten-Krüger M, Lauer CJ, Dydak U, Hell D, Holsboer F, Boesiger P, Cuénod M. Schizophrenia: glutathione deficit in cerebrospinal fluid and prefrontal cortex in vivo. *Eur J Neurosci.* 2000 Oct;12(10):3721-8.

25. Dvoráková M, Sivonová M, Trebatická J, Skodácek I, Waczuliková I, Muchová J, Duracková Z. The effect of polyphenolic extract from pine bark, Pycnogenol on the level of glutathione in children suffering from attention deficit hyperactivity disorder (ADHD). *Redox Rep.* 2006;11(4):163-72.

26. Kalebic T, Kinter A, Poli G, Anderson ME, Meister A, Fauci AS. Suppression of human immunodeficiency virus expression in chronically infected monocytic cells by glutathione, glutathione ester, and N-acetylcysteine. *Proc Natl Acad Sci USA.* 1991 Feb 1;88(3):986-90.

27. Iantomasi T, Marraccini P, Favilli F, Vincenzini MT, Ferretti P, Tonelli F. Glutathione metabolism in Crohn's disease. *Biochem Med Metab Biol.* 1994 Dec;53(2):87-91.

28. Oeriu S, Tighciu M. Oxidized glutathione as a test of senescence. *Gerontologia.* 1964;49:9-17.

29. James SJ, Melnyk S, Jernigan S, Cleves MA, Halsted CH, Wong DH, Cutler P, Bock K, Boris M, Bradstreet JJ, Baker SM, Gaylor DW. Metabolic endophenotype and related genotypes are associated with oxidative stress in children with autism. *Am J Med Genet B Neuropsychiatr Genet.* 2006 Dec 5;141B(8):947-56.

30. Eisenhauer PB, Harwig SS, Szklarek D, Ganz T, Selsted ME, Lehrer RI. Purification and antimicrobial properties of three defensins from rat neutrophils. *Infect Immun.* 1989 Jul;57(7):2021-7.

31. Salzman NH, Hung K, Haribhai D, Chu H, Karlsson-Sjöberg J, Amir E, Teggatz P, Barman M, Hayward M, Eastwood D, Stoel M, Zhou Y, Sodergren E, Weinstock GM, Bevins CL, Williams CB, Bos NA. Enteric defensins are essential regulators of intestinal microbial ecology. *Nat Immunol.* 2010 Jan;11(1):76-83. Epub 2009 Oct 22.

32. Rowan FE, Docherty NG, Coffey JC, O'Connell PR. Sulphate-reducing bacteria and hydrogen sulphide in the aetiology of ulcerative colitis. *Br J Surg.* 2009 Feb;96(2):151-8.

33. Wehkamp J, Stange EF, Fellermann K. Defensin-immunology in inflammatory bowel disease. *Gastroenterol Clin Biol.* 2009 Jun;33(Suppl 3):S137-S144.

34. Bäckhed F, Ley RE, Sonnenburg JL, Peterson DA, Gordon JI. Host-bacterial mutualism in the human intestine. *Science.* 2005 Mar 25;307(5717):1915-20.

35. Shaw SY, Blanchard JF, Bernstein CN. Association between the use of antibiotics in the first year of life and pediatric inflammatory bowel disease. *Am J Gastroenterol.* 2010 Dec;105(12):2687-92. Epub 2010 Oct 12.

36. Parker W. Reconstituting the depleted biome to prevent immune disorders. *The Evolution & Medicine Review.* October 13, 2010.

37. McKay DM. The beneficial helminth parasite? *Parasitology.* 2006 Jan;132(Pt 1):1-12.

38. Elliott DE, Summers RW, Weinstock JV. Helminths as governors of immune-mediated inflammation. *Int J Parasitol.* 2007 Apr;37(5):457-64. Epub 2006 Dec 28.

39. Summers RW, Elliott DE, Urban JF Jr, Thompson RA, Weinstock JV. *Trichuris suis* therapy for active ulcerative colitis: a randomized controlled trial. *Gastroenterology.* 2005 Apr;128(4):825-32.

40. Bager P, Arnved J, Rønborg S, Wohlfahrt J, Poulsen LK, Westergaard T, Petersen HW, Kristensen B, Thamsborg S, Roepstorff A, Kapel C, Melbye M. *Trichuris suis* ova therapy for allergic rhinitis: a randomized, double-blind, placebo-controlled clinical trial. *J Allergy Clin Immunol*. 2010 Jan;125(1):123-30.e1-3. Epub 2009 Oct 3.

41. La Flamme AC, Canagasabey K, Harvie M, Bäckström BT. Schistosomiasis protects against multiple sclerosis. *Mem Inst Oswaldo Cruz*. 2004;99(5 Suppl 1):33-6. Epub 2004 Oct 13.

42. Sewell DL, Reinke EK, Hogan LH, Sandor M, Fabry Z. Immunoregulation of CNS autoimmunity by helminth and mycobacterial infections. *Immunol Lett*. 2002 Jun 3;82(1-2):101-10.

43. Singer HS, Morris C, Gause C, Pollard M, Zimmerman AW, Pletnikov M. Prenatal exposure to antibodies from mothers of children with autism produces neurobehavioral alterations: A pregnant dam mouse model. *J Neuroimmunol*. 2009 Jun 25;211(1-2):39-48. Epub 2009 Apr 10.

44. Garbett K, Ebert PJ, Mitchell A, Lintas C, Manzi B, Mirnics K, Persico AM. Immune transcriptome alterations in the temporal cortex of subjects with autism. *Neurobiol Dis*. 2008 Jun;30(3):303-11. Epub 2008 Mar 10.

45. Garvey J. Diet in autism and associated disorders. *J Fam Health Care*. 2002;12(2):34-8.

46. Levy SE, Hyman SL. Novel treatments for autistic spectrum disorders. *Ment Retard Dev Disabil Res Rev*. 2005;11(2):131-42.

47. Miele E, Pascarella F, Giannetti E, Quaglietta L, Baldassano RN, Staiano A. Effect of a probiotic preparation (VSL#3) on induction and maintenance of remission in children with ulcerative colitis. *Am J Gastroenterol*. 2009 Feb;104(2):437-43. Epub 2009 Jan 20.

48. Huynh HQ, deBruyn J, Guan L, Diaz H, Li M, Girgis S, Turner J, Fedorak R, Madsen K. Probiotic preparation VSL#3 induces remission in children with mild to moderate acute ulcerative colitis: a pilot study. *Inflamm Bowel Dis*. 2009 May;15(5):760-8.

49. Tursi A, Brandimarte G, Papa A, Giglio A, Elisei W, Giorgetti GM, Forti G, Morini S, Hassan C, Pistoia MA, Modeo ME, Rodino' S, D'Amico T, Sebkova L, Sacca' N, Di Giulio E, Luzza F, Imeneo M, Larussa T, Di Rosa S, Annese V, Danese S, Gasbarrini A. Treatment of relapsing mild-to-moderate ulcerative colitis with the probiotic VSL#3 as adjunctive to a standard pharmaceutical treatment: a double-blind, randomized, placebo-controlled study. *Am J Gastroenterol*. 2010 Oct;105(10):2218-27. Epub 2010 Jun 1.

50. Guandalini S. Update on the role of probiotics in the therapy of pediatric inflammatory bowel disease. *Expert Rev Clin Immunol*. 2010 Jan;6(1):47-54.

51. Ashwood P, Anthony A, Pellicer AA, Torrente F, Walker-Smith JA, Wakefield AJ. Intestinal lymphocyte populations in children with regressive autism: evidence for extensive mucosal immunopathology. *J Clin Immunol*. 2003 Nov;23(6):504-17.

52. Bradstreet JJ, Smith S, Baral M, Rossignol DA. Biomarker-guided interventions of clinically relevant conditions associated with autism spectrum disorders and attention deficit hyperactivity disorder. *Altern Med Rev*. 2010 Apr;15(1):15-32.

53. Eggesbø M, Moen B, Peddada S, Baird D, Rugtveit J, Midtvedt T, Bushel PR, Sekelja M, Rudi K. Development of gut microbiota in infants not exposed to medical interventions. *APMIS*. 2011 Jan;119(1):17-35. Epub 2010 Oct 25.

54. Adlerberth I, Wold AE. Establishment of the gut microbiota in Western infants. *Acta Paediatr.* 2009 Feb;98(2):229-38.

55. Hooper LV, Midtvedt T, Gordon JI. How host-microbial interactions shape the nutrient environment of the mammalian intestine. *Annu Rev Nutr.* 2002;22:283-307. Epub 2002 Apr 4.

56. Khoruts A, Sadowsky MJ. Therapeutic transplantation of the distal gut microbiota. *Mucosal Immunol.* 2011 Jan;4(1):4-7. Epub 2010 Dec 8.

57. Russell G, Kaplan J, Ferraro M, Michelow IC. Fecal bacteriotherapy for relapsing *Clostridium difficile* infection in a child: a proposed treatment protocol. *Pediatrics.* 2010 Jul;126(1):e239-42. Epub 2010 Jun 14.

58. Floch MH. Fecal bacteriotherapy, fecal transplant, and the microbiome. *J Clin Gastroenterol.* 2010 Sep;44(8):529-30.

59. Williams BL, Hornig M, Buie T, Bauman ML, Cho Paik M, Wick I, Bennett A, Jabado O, Hirschberg DL, Lipkin WI. Impaired carbohydrate digestion and transport and mucosal dysbiosis in the intestines of children with autism and gastrointestinal disturbances. *PLoS One.* 2011;6(9):e24585. Epub 2011 Sep 16.

60. Munasinghe SA, Oliff C, Finn J, Wray JA. Digestive enzyme supplementation for autism spectrum disorders: a double-blind randomized controlled trial. *J Autism Dev Disord.* 2010 Sep;40(9):1131-8.

61. Theoharides TC, Doyle R, Francis K, Conti P, Kalogeromitros D. Novel therapeutic targets for autism. *Trends Pharmacol Sci.* 2008 Aug;29(8):375-82. Epub 2008 Jul 6.

CHAPTER SEVEN

GUT MICROBIOTA-BRAIN CONNECTION

By Thomas J. Borody, MD, PhD[1], and Jordana Campbell, BSc[2]

1. Thomas Julius Borody, MD, PhD, Director, Centre for Digestive Diseases, Five Dock NSW 2046 Australia. Thomas J. Borody has a pecuniary interest in the Centre for Digestive Diseases, where fecal microbiota transplantation is a treatment option for patients and has filed patents in this area.

2. Jordana Campbell, BSc, Research Officer, Centre for Digestive Diseases, Five Dock NSW 2046 Australia. Jordana Campbell has no financial interest or affiliation with any institution, organization, or company relating to the manuscript.

Correspondence to:
Jordana Campbell, Research Officer, Centre for Digestive Diseases, Level 1/229 Great North Rd, Five Dock, NSW 2046 Australia.
Phone: (61) 2 9713 4011 Fax: (61) 2 9713 1026
Email: jordana.campbell@cdd.com.au

No support or funding, including pharmaceutical and industry support, was received for work undertaken relating to the manuscript.

Introduction

Autistic disorder is a pervasive developmental disorder manifested in the first three years of life as dysfunction in social interaction, development, and communication. Children either exhibit a failure to advance from birth or, after a period of normal development, suddenly suffer a loss of newly acquired skills (language, eye-to-eye contact, and sociability) referred to as "regressive autism." The latter category appears to be the larger group. Whilst the cause of autism remains unknown, the majority of autism research to date has focused on genetic abnormalities underpinning the disorder, and much of the treatment has relied upon behavioral therapy. However, despite decades of research, scientists are no closer to finding a specific cause of autism or an effective treatment. Recent research calls into question the current genetic theory, with a new report by the Centers for Disease Control and Prevention reporting a 78% increase in autism diagnosis between 2002 and 2008, a figure unexplained by genetic factors which are incapable of altering over a few short years.[1] Similarly, autism concordance of less than 100% in monozygotic twins has been interpreted as evidence that outside factors such as an environmental challenge must work in tandem with a genetic susceptibility.[2] A number of alternate autism etiologies have been proposed, including childhood immunizations, particularly the MMR vaccine, infection, or environmental factors. Interestingly, up to 70% of children with autism suffer from gastrointestinal dysfunction, including diarrhea, constipation, and abdominal pain, with a strong correlation noted between the severity of gastrointestinal symptoms and autism symptom severity.[3] These gastrointestinal symptoms frequently either precede or coincide with the onset of autistic symptoms. In addition, the successful treatment of gastrointestinal symptoms also appears to positively influence autistic behavior, strengthening the link between gut bacterial involvement and the onset of autism.[4]

Gastrointestinal Dysfunction in Autism

Children with autism have been recently shown to have much higher rates of gastrointestinal dysfunction compared with healthy children.[5] Endoscopic and histological findings in autistic spectrum disorders have also revealed unexpected abnormalities, including intestinal inflammation, segmental swelling, hyperemia, superficial erosions, nodularity, and altered intestinal permeability. Goodwin *et al.* first made the observation of gastrointestinal dysfunction in 1971, when he reported on six of fifteen autistic patients who had bulky, odorous, loose or diarrheal stools.[6] Since then, a number of studies have confirmed these findings. Wakefield *et al.* in 1998 reported on 12 children with diagnosed autism (all with regressive-onset autism) who all exhibited a variety of GI ailments, including abdominal pain, diarrhea, and bloating, which had developed coincident with the onset of autistic behavior.[7] Ten of the 12 children displayed ileal lymphoid nodular hyperplasia (LNH) on endoscopy. Eight children also displayed abnormalities in the mucosa, including loss of vascular pattern, erythema, red halo signs, and superficial ulcers, and although the inflammatory changes were patchy, they were distributed throughout the colon. The findings were supported by histological examinations of mucosal biopsies. Cerebral magnetic resonance imaging (MRI) and electroencephalography (EEG) revealed no neurological abnormalities in the children. In a later study, the authors reported on an expanded group of 60 children affected with various developmental disorders.[8] The study cohort consisted of 50 children diagnosed with autism (including the 12 children from the original study) as well as five with Asperger's syndrome and two with disintegrative disorder. All but one of the 60 children had GI symptoms, including abdominal pain, constipation, diarrhea, and bloating. It was observed that ileal LNH presented in 93% of 60 children versus only 14.3% of control children. A further thirty percent had colonic lymphoid nodular hyperplasia. Granularity, loss of vascular pattern, erythema, red halo signs, and superficial ulcers were also described and were distributed throughout the colon. Reactive follicular hyperplasia was present in the ileum of 47 of 51 children with successful ileal biopsies, and histologic signs of chronic colitis were identified in 53 of 60 children (88%). In another study, Horvath *et al.* (2002) reported gastrointestinal symptoms comprising diarrhea, constipation, foul smelling stools, abdominal discomfort, bloating and/or belching in 84.1% of autistic children versus only 31.2% of healthy siblings (*P*<0.0001).[9] Endoscopy and histological assessment was performed to examine the upper GI tract in 36 of the autistic children, which found abnormal findings including reflux esophagitis in 25 of the children (69.4%), chronic gastritis in 15 (41.6%), and chronic duodenitis in 24 (66.6%). Valicenti-McDermott *et al.*, comparing the lifetime prevalence of gut symptoms in autism spectrum disorder (ASD) children versus children with developmental disabilities and those with normal development, found a history of gut symptoms in 70% of autistic children versus only 42% (*p* =.03) in children with developmental disabilities and 29% (*p* <.001) of children with normal development.[10] Parracho *et al.* (2005) also reported that a high proportion of ASD patients suffered from GI disorders (91.4 %).[11] Diarrhea was the most common GI symptom in 58 autistic children (75.6%), followed by excess wind (55.2 %), abdominal pain (46.6 %), constipation (44.8%), and abnormal feces (43.0 %). A number of autistic individuals were recorded to suffer from multiple GI problems, including episodes of alternating diarrhea and constipation. In contrast, only 25% of siblings and none of the healthy unrelated children reported gut symptoms.

Stool clostridia species detected in autism

Several studies have reported more pathogenic intestinal flora in autistic children compared with healthy controls, including distinctive clostridial populations using PCR-based studies. Finegold *et al.* (2002) reported a greater number of clostridial species in the stool of autistic children versus those of healthy children.[12] Nine *Clostridium* species were isolated exclusively from autistic fecal samples, and three species were additionally found uniquely in healthy samples. In a follow-up study, Finegold and colleagues found statistically significant cell count differences of *C. bolteae* and *Clostridium* groups clusters I and XI between autistic and control children using real-time PCR.[13] Mean counts of *C. bolteae* and clusters I and XI in autistic children were 46-fold (P = 0.01), 9.0-fold (P = 0.014), and 3.5-fold (P = 0.004) greater than those in control children, respectively. Parracho *et al.*, employing fluorescence *in situ* hybridization to examine autistic stools versus healthy controls, found a higher incidence of the *Clostridium histolyticum* group (*Clostridium* clusters I and II) in the fecal flora of autistic patients.[11]

Such alterations in the indigenous gut microbiota may reflect colonization with potentially neurotoxin-producing bacteria (including several members of the genus *Clostridium*). Clostridia produce the highest number of toxins of any type of bacteria, and several members of this genus are known to infect humans. Not only do they frequently cause gastrointestinal symptoms, but their metabolic products are also capable of exerting systemic effects. The spore-forming *Clostridium botulinum* is one such example, producing potent neurotoxins that cause constipation and neurological dysfunction, as seen in childhood botulism. Once ingested, the bacterium colonizes the large intestine, producing copious amounts of botulinum toxin in the gastrointestinal lumen, which interferes with impulse transmission, causing constipation, bilateral neuromuscular weakness, paralysis, and impairments of cranial nerve functions (diplopia, dysarthria, and dysphagia). Similarly, *Clostridium tetani* (*C. tetani*), the causative agent of tetanus disease, produces potent neurotoxins including cytotoxin, tetanus neurotoxin (TeNT), and tetanolysin, which interfere with neurotransmitter release. In classical tetanus infection, the neurotoxins move into the cell body and are then transported by transynaptic exchange into the terminals of inhibitory neurons in the spinal cord and brain stem where interruption of neurotransmitter release occurs. This results in increased muscle tone and violent contractions of all major muscle groups. Tetanolysin toxin in tetanus infection promotes the growth of *C. tetani* by increasing intestinal permeability through damage to healthy tissue. Increased intestinal permeability results in food molecules larger than those normally absorbed from the intestinal tract, such as uncleaved proteins (e.g., casein and gluten), entering the bloodstream, which can become antigenic. Interestingly, children with autism frequently develop intolerances to foods containing gluten or casein and are sometimes described as having a "fixed smile," hypertonia, or rigidity, and have difficulty in chewing and swallowing food, a classic symptom of TeNT. Elevated catecholamine (in plasma and urine), tachycardia, profuse sweating, and irregular breathing are all symptoms of autonomic nervous system dysfunction and are documented to occur in both autism and tetanus. These similarities have led Bolte *et al.* (1998) to suggest that autism may occur as a result of subacute, chronic intestinal tetanus infection with subsequent neurotoxin release.[15] Experimental animal studies lend themselves to these claims, with Wells *et al.* (1983) demonstrating that active tetanus toxin and tetani spores persist in the rats' cecum and colon following inoculation of germfree rats with either *C. tetani* spores or vegetative cells.[16] It is through this mechanism that Bolte *et al.* proposes that *C. tetani* neurotoxins exhibit their neurological effects in autism.[15]

Another *Clostridium* species of interest is *Clostridium perfringens* (*C. perfringens*), which produces a large number of toxins, including epsilon toxin that traditionally causes enterotoxemia in sheep, goats, cattle, and horses. Many sheep harbor *C. perfringens* type D in their gastrointestinal tract; however, clinical disease commonly occurs following disruption to the gastrointestinal microbial balance. In young, rapidly growing lambs consuming a high starch diet, the large quantities of starch passing through the small intestine act as a substrate for the proliferation of these saccharolytic bacteria.[17] Here in the intestines, they produce large amounts of epsilon toxin, which results in increased intestinal mucosal permeability, aiding to facilitate its own absorption. Sufficient toxin then enters the bloodstream where it produces neurological dysfunction. Excitement, incoordination, convulsions, or opisthotonos can then be seen. Affected lambs frequently circle or push their heads against fixed objects. Diarrhea sometimes occurs. In adult sheep, the clinical symptoms include diarrhea and neurological signs, including blindness, aimless wandering, ataxia, bruxism, head pressing, nystagmus, posterior paresis, lateral recumbency, opisthotonus, and paddling convulsions. In goats, the course of disease can be peracute, acute, or chronic. The clinical signs include watery diarrhea, sometimes containing blood. Neurologic signs are common. There is little to no information on the effect of epsilon toxin on humans; however, extrapolation from studies with experimentally infected animals suggests that neurologic disease may be possible.

Other potential candidates include *Desulfovibrio* strains. In the case of *Desulfovibrio*, both real-time PCR and culture indicated that at least three species of *Desulfovibrio* (*D. desulfuricans, D. fairfieldensis, and D. piger*) were associated with regressive autism in a significant way.[18] In 14 stool specimens from 30 autistic children, *Desulfovibrio* was found by culture or real-time PCR (46.7%), compared with stools of 7 from siblings of autistic children (28.6%) and zero of 12 stools from healthy controls. There was also a "dose response" with the higher the percent positive by either culture or real-time PCR the more severe the autism.[18]

Clostridial antibiotics in autism

Further supporting a role for clostridia in autism is the proven efficacy of vancomycin in dramatically improving autism symptomatology. Sandler *et al.* (2000), treating a 4½ year old boy with autism and chronic diarrhea with vancomycin, reported a rapid and pronounced symptom improvement that lasted for the length of the treatment.[4] The child had displayed normal motor, cognitive, and social development until the age of 18 months, when he received recurrent antibiotic treatments for otitis media. The patient subsequently developed diarrhea and a gradual decline in motor, cognitive, and social development. Neither conventional (behavioral therapy, speech and play therapy) nor unconventional treatments (e.g., special diets, vitamin megaloading, etc.) showed any positive effect on his autistic symptoms. A 12-week therapeutic trial of vancomycin (125 mg four times per day) was initiated, which resulted in a rapid and significant clinical improvement. The child became affectionate, relatively calm, and promptly achieved toilet training and increased vocabulary. Follow-up behavioral assessments revealed an increase in on-task performance, compliance of parental requests, awareness of environmental surrounds, and persistence when engaging in positive activities. Significant reductions in repetitive and self-stimulatory behaviors were also noted. Following discontinuation of vancomycin therapy, behavioral deterioration was observed, and though still improved over baseline, he eventually lost most of the gains. A follow-up study of ten autistic children treated with short-term oral vancomycin resulted in a short-term benefit in 8/10 patients.[4] However, despite the rapid and significant clinical improvement not seen with other current therapies, the authors abandoned this therapy as efficacy again ceased with cessation of treatment. Not only is vancomycin highly effective against Gram-positive bacteria, particularly clostridia, but oral vancomycin is poorly absorbed systemically, so any effects experienced with its use are likely due to its local action on the gastrointestinal microbiota.

Preliminary success in autism has also been observed at CDD following targeted treatment of the gut microbiota with vancomycin, which is briefly summarized below. Seven patients with severe, regressive autism were successfully treated using 6 – 24 weeks of oral vancomycin. Each patient had followed a typical developmental pattern including language, etc. followed by a rapid loss of these previous gains, resulting in their autism diagnosis. Antibiotic exposure was frequently reported prior to each child's diagnosis, and one patient suffered an abrupt loss of speech and subsequent autism diagnosis after antibiotics but in association with the MMR vaccine. All patients suffered from gastrointestinal symptoms, including diarrhea, constipation, foul-smelling stools and/or flatulence as well as marked behavioral and developmental delays. A CT scan of two children prior to treatment revealed enlarged rectums in association with their constipation. Of the seven patients, four experienced a marked improvement in their autism symptoms as well as their gastrointestinal symptoms whilst on vancomycin therapy, rapidly achieving toilet training, increased word counts, undisturbed sleep, increased sociability, and general behavioral improvements. These observations confirm those of Sandler et al.[4] Given our interest in FMT, we can foresee in the near future a role for an extracted then freeze-dried donor flora as a tool in recolonization of damaged and infected flora of ASD children. This pathway, rather than that of current probiotics, is emphasized because available probiotics are cultured and fail to implant and because it appears we need a large cohort of human flora components to defeat often undiagnosable pathogens. These observations confirm those of Sandler et al.[4]

Microbiota disruption by antibiotics

It has been hypothesised that the early and frequent use of antimicrobial agents in autistic children may disrupt the developing intestinal microbiota and facilitate colonization with opportunistic pathogens. We propose that a toxin-producing Clostridium is the most likely candidate. A large proportion of parents of autistic children report multiple antibiotic courses preceding their child's autism diagnosis. Fallon et al. (2005) in a study of 206 autistic children under the age of three years, found a statistically significant correlation between chronic otitis media and autism diagnosis.[19] A mean number of 9.96 bouts of otitis media were found in the autistic group surveyed and a mean number of 12.04 antibiotic courses; in 206 children, this represents a sum total of 2052 bouts of otitis media and a sum total of 2480 courses of antibiotics. Of the antibiotics, 893 courses were Augmentin, with 362 of these Augmentin courses administered under the age of one year. Parracho *et al.* (2005) supported these findings, reporting extensive and repeated broad-spectrum antibiotic use (>six courses per child), typically for ear infections or respiratory tract disorders in ASD children (34.5%) and their siblings (33.3%), compared with the healthy unrelated group (0%).[11]

Disruption of the intestinal microbiota due to antibiotics has been shown to alter host susceptibility to infection. Nowhere is this most apparent than in *Clostridium difficile* infection (CDI). In CDI, antibiotic-mediated damage to the gut microbiota facilitates colonization with *Clostridium difficile* (*C. difficile*) in an as yet unidentified manner. Following colonization, the bacterium commonly produces two exotoxins: toxin A, an enterotoxin, and toxin B, a cytotoxin that damages intestinal mucosal cells. Both toxins alter intestinal permeability to induce profuse watery diarrhea. Deficiencies in intestinal microbiota constituents including *Bacteroides* and *Firmicutes* species have been demonstrated in patients with initial or recurrent *C. difficile* infection,[20,21] most likely as a result of prior antibiotic damage, and are involved in the infection cycle. *Fecal Microbiota Transplantation* (FMT), first employed in CDI in 1958 by Eiseman *et al.*,[22] is at the stage where it is arguably the most reliable and effective form of *C. difficile* eradication therapy.[23] FMT serves to reintroduce a complete, stable community of gut micro-organisms aimed at repairing or replacing the disrupted native microbiota to correct the underlying imbalance/s and facilitating re-establishment of normal bowel function. Unlike the concept of probiotics, which at best aim to somehow alter the metabolic or immunological activity of the native gut microbiota transiently, FMT results in durable, long-term implantation of donor flora.[24]

Numerous conditions outside of CDI thought to have an unidentified microbiota infection have reported marked benefit from FMT, including ulcerative colitis,[25] Crohn's disease,[26] irritable bowel syndrome,[26] chronic constipation,[27] metabolic syndrome,[28] idiopathic thrombocytopenic purpura,[29] chronic fatigue syndrome,[30] obesity, insulin sensitivity,[28] and multiple sclerosis.[31] There is compelling evidence that the importance of the intestinal microbiota extends beyond the intestine. For many years, gastrointestinal research has highlighted the importance of the gut–brain axis, especially in relation to functional bowel disorders; however, much of this work has previously been predominantly focused on a top-down approach. New work involving the gut microbiota indicates that this communication network is bi-directional and that events occurring in the gut also have an impact on neurological function. Research has shown that this communication occurs via the vagus nerve.[32] Interestingly, a number of neurological conditions report gastrointestinal dysfunction as a primary disease symptom. Up to 80% of patients with Parkinson's disease (PD) report constipation as a primary symptom, one which can, in fact, precede the onset of motor symptoms by up to two decades.[33] In addition, men who experience <1 bowel movement daily have a four-fold increase of developing PD in later life.[34] In 2009, we first presented at the American College of Gastroenterology conference a case report of a 73- year-old male with chronic constipation who was treated with vancomycin, colchicine, and metronidazole targeted against clostridia for his constipation.[35] His baseline motor symptoms included marked pill-rolling hand tremor, micrographia, positive glabellar tap reflex, and cogwheel rigidity. At 21 days on antibiotic treatment, he reported a marked improvement in his constipation symptoms, defecating daily with ease. Surprisingly, he also reported a dramatic improvement in his PD symptoms, with a visible decrease in tremor commencing ten days into therapy. At 6 and 10 months on continuous therapy, he reported resolution of neurological symptoms, including absence of persistent tremors, glabellar tap reflex and no detectable cogwheel rigidity. The remarkable finding of constipation resolution coupled with neurological normalization to antibiotics, two of which are non-absorbed, strongly suggest the gut microbiota is involved in the pathogenesis of this disease. We have also previously reported on the case of a 28-year-old female with myoclonic dystonia and long-standing diarrhea, successfully treated using vancomycin, rifaximin, and metronidazole for her diarrheal illness,[36] as well as the virtually complete and prolonged (>15 years) normalization of previously severe multiple sclerosis symptoms in three patients who underwent FMT for constipation.[31]

Fecal Microbiota Bugs – Future Developments

Given our interest in FMT, we can foresee in the near future a role for an extracted then freeze-dried donor flora as a tool in recolonization of damaged and infected flora of ASD children. This pathway, rather than that of current probiotics is emphasized because available probiotics are cultured and fail to implant and because it appears we need a large cohort of human flora components to eradicate often undiagnosable pathogens.

Conclusion

There is now considerable evidence that the gut microflora plays a role in autism. This role may be central to the etiology and continuation of autism. The gastrointestinal tract has been referred to as the largest (virtual) organ of the body on the basis of its vast cellular composition.[37] It can readily harbor organisms that secrete toxic molecules capable of inflicting neuronal damage. Clostridia bacteria are known neurotoxin producers. Patients with autism have also been shown to have higher numbers of *Desulfovibrio* and *Clostridium* species in their gut. Clinically regressive autistic children can respond remarkably to non-absorbable anti-*Clostridium/Desulfovibrio* antibiotics. Modulation of the gut microbiota via future oral FMT to reduce the number of toxin pathogens through bacteriocin production, capable of eradicating pathogens, as well as stimulating more beneficial gut bacteria and correcting underlying deficiencies (as is the case in *C. difficile* infection – CDI), may more powerfully alleviate the toxin-driven neurological symptoms. The success of vancomycin, a non-absorbed anti-*Clostridium/Desulfovibrio* antibiotic whose action must be via suppression of the diseased microbiota, both clostridia and desulfovibrios, further suggests that these are centrally involved in the pathogenesis of autism and opens the door to the possibility of a cure.

References

1. Baio J. Prevalence of autism spectrum disorders – Autism and developmental disabilities monitoring network, 14 sites, United States, 2008. *Surveillance Summaries* 2012; 61(SS03): 1-19.
2. Bailey A, Le Couteur A, Gottesman I *et al*. Autism as a strongly genetic disorder: evidence from a British twin study. *Psychological Medicine* 1995; 25(1): 63-77.

3. Adams JB, Johanson LJ, Powell LD *et al.* Gastrointestinal flora and gastrointestinal status in children with autism – comparisons to typical children and correlation with autism severity. *BMC Gastroenterology* 2011; 11: 22.

4. Sandler RH, Finegold SM, Bolte ER *et al.* Short term benefit from oral vancomycin treatment of regressive-onset autism. *J Child Neurol* 2000; 15(7): 429-435.

5. Erickson CA, Stigler KA, Corkins MR *et al.* Gastrointestinal factors in autistic disorder: a critical review. *J Autism Dev Disord* 2005; 35(6): 713-727.

6. Goodwin MS, Cowen MA, Goodwin TC. Malabsorption and cerebral dysfunction: a multivariate and comparative study of autistic children. *J Autism Child Schizophr* 1971; 1:48-62.

7. Wakefield AJ, Murch SH, Anthony A *et al.* Ileal-lymphoid-nodular hyperplasia, non-specific colitis, and pervasive developmental disorder in children. *Lancet* 1998; 351(9103): 637-41.

8. Wakefield AJ, Anthony A, Murch SH *et al.* Enterocolitis in children with developmental disorders. *Am J Gastroenterol* 2000; 95: 2285-2295.

9. Horvath K, Perman JA. Autism and gastrointestinal symptoms. *Curr Gastroenterol Rep* 2002; 4(3): 251-258.

10. Valicenti-McDermott M, McVicar K, Rapin I *et al.* Frequency of gastrointestinal symptoms in children with autistic spectrum disorders and association with family history autoimmune disease. *J Dev Behav Pediatr* 2006; 27(Suppl 2): S128-36.

11. Parracho H, Bingham MO, Gibson GR *et al.* Differences between the gut microflora of children with autistic spectrum disorders and that of healthy children. *J Med Micro* 2005; 54: 987-991.

12. Finegold SM, Molitoris D, Song Y *et al.* Gastrointestinal microflora studies in late-onset autism. *Clin Infect Dis* 2002; 35(Suppl 1): S6-S16.

13. Song Y, Liu C, Finegold SM. Real-time PCR quantitation of clostridia in feces of autistic children. *Appl Environ Microbiol* 2004; 70(11): 6459-6465.

14. Finegold SM, Dowd SE, Gontcharova V *et al.* Pyrosequencing study of fecal microflora of autistic and control children. *Anaerobe* 2010; 16(4): 444-53.

15. Bolte ER. Autism and *Clostridium tetani*. *Med Hypotheses* 1998; 51(2): 133-44.

16. Wells CL, Balish E. *Clostridium tetani* growth and toxin production in the intestines of germfree rats. *Infect Immun* 1983; 41(2): 826-828.

17. Finnie JW. Neurological disorders produced by *Clostridium perfringens* type D epsilon toxin. *Anaerobe* 2004; 10: 145-150.

18. Finegold SM. State of the art; microbiology in health and disease: intestinal bacterial flora in autism. *Anaerobe* 2011; 17: 367-368.

19. Fallon J. Could one of the most widely prescribed antibiotics amoxicillin/clavulanate "augmentin" be a risk factor for autism? *Med Hypothesis* 2005; 64(2): 312-5.

20. Tvede M, Rask-Madsen J. Bacteriotherapy for chronic relapsing *Clostridium difficile* diarrhoea in six patients. *Lancet* 1989; 1: 1156-1160.

21. Khoruts A, Dicksved J, Jansson J *et al.* Changes in the composition of the human fecal microbiome after bacteriotherapy for recurrent *Clostridium difficile*-associated diarrhoea. *J Clin Gastroenterol* 2010; 44: 354-360.

22. Eiseman B, Silen W, Bascom G *et al.* Fecal enema as an adjunct in the treatment of pseudomembranous enterocolitis. *Surgery* 1958; 44: 854-859.

23. Brandt LJ, Borody TJ, Campbell J. Endoscopic fecal microbiota transplantation: "First-line" treatment for severe *Clostridium difficile* infection. *J Clin Gastroenterol* 2011; 45(8): 655-657.

24. Grehan MJ, Borody TJ, Leis SM *et al.* Durable alteration of the colonic microbiota by the administration of donor fecal flora. *J Clin Gastroenterol* 2010; 44: 551-561.

25. Borody TJ, Khoruts A. Fecal microbiota transplantation and emerging applications. *Nat Rev Gastroenterol & Hepatol* 2012; 9: 88-96.

26. Borody TJ, George L, Andrews P *et al.* Bowel-flora alteration: a potential cure for inflammatory bowel disease and irritable bowel syndrome? *Med J Aust* 1989; 150: 604.

27. Andrews PJ, Barnes P, Borody TJ. Chronic constipation reversed by restoration of bowel flora. A case and a hypothesis. *Eur J Gastroenterol & Hepatol* 1992; 4: 245-247.

28. Vrieze A, Holleman F, Serlie MJ *et al.* Metabolic effects of transplanting gut microbiota from lean donors to subjects with metabolic syndrome [abstract A90]. Presented at the European Association for the Study of Diabetes meeting (2010).

29. Borody TJ, Campbell J, Torres M *et al.* Reversal of idiopathic thrombocytopenic purpura (ITP) with fecal microbiota transplantation (FMT). [abstract]. *Am J Gastroenterol* 2011; 106: S352.

30. Borody, T. J. Bacteriotherapy for chronic fatigue syndrome: a long-term follow up study. Presented at the 1995 CFS National Consensus Conference.

31. Borody TJ, Leis S, Campbell J *et al.* Fecal microbiota transplantation (FMT) in multiple sclerosis (MS) [abstract]. *Am J Gastroenterol* 2011; 106: S352.

32. Maier SF, Goehler LE, Fleshner M *et al.* The role of the vagus nerve in cytokine-to-brain communication. *Ann NY Acad Sci* 1998; 1(840): 289-300.

33. Savica R, Carlin JM, Grossardt BR *et al.* Medical records documentation of constipation preceding Parkinson's Disease. *Neurol* 2009; 73(21): 1752-1758.

34. Abbott RD, Petrovich H, White LR *et al.* Frequency of bowel movements and the future risk of Parkinson's Disease. *Neurol* 2001; 57: 456-462.

35. Borody TJ, Torres M, Campbell J *et al.* Treatment of severe constipation improves Parkinson's Disease (PD) symptoms. *Am J Gastroenterol* 2009; S999.

36. Borody TJ, Rosen DM, Torres M *et al.* Myoclonus dystonia-affected by GI microbiota. *Am J Gastroenterol* 2011; 106: S352.

37. Qin J, Li R, Raes J et al. A human gut microbial gene catalogue established by metagenomic sequencing. *Nature* 2010; 464: 59-65.

CHAPTER EIGHT

FMT: A PARENT'S ACCOUNT OF A FECAL MICROBIOTA TRANSPLANTATION DONE FOR A 15-YEAR-OLD FEMALE PRESENTING WITH AUTISM, CHRONIC CONSTIPATION, AND VERY LOW ENERGY LEVELS

By Michael F. Wagnitz

Michael Wagnitz is employed as a chemist in the toxicology section of a public health laboratory. This chapter is his personal account. Michael has spent the last 12 years doing whatever is possible to address the underlying medical problems of children diagnosed with autism spectrum disorders.

In May 2012, I went to the AutismOne conference in Chicago, where I attended a presentation by featured speaker Dr. Thomas Borody, a gastroenterologist from the Centre for Digestive Diseases, Sydney, Australia. His talk was about Fecal Microbiota Transplantation (FMT), something I had never heard of before. FMT involves the transfer of gut flora using a stool sample from a healthy donor to a person with a compromised gastrointestinal system. Imagine my surprise a month later when a local reporter was writing about this procedure being done in one of my hometown hospitals. After reading the article, I immediately made an appointment for my 15-

year-old daughter who had suffered from severe, chronic constipation her entire life. She also has an autism diagnosis and has suffered from low energy metabolism and chronic infections.

The story in the newspaper was about a man who was fighting reoccurring flare-ups of *Clostridium difficile* (*C. difficile*) infections, which he had acquired during a prior hospitalization. These flare-ups were having a serious impact on his quality of life. In addition to feeling very miserable, he always had to stay within a short distance of a bathroom due to severe diarrhea. While his condition did respond initially to antibiotic therapy, the results were temporary and the *C. difficile* continued to return. As a last resort, the FMT procedure was done, and the *C. difficile* was permanently eradicated. The story had a very happy ending that included a full recovery.

So, why did I think this procedure could help my daughter? (I was asked that question repeatably by hospital staff.) To begin with, gastrointestinal issues are well documented in the majority of autistic children. My daughter was born by Caesarian section. Research on human gut flora indicates that kids born by C-section have different, permanent gut flora when compared with kids born naturally.[1] Furthermore, due to a blood clot that my wife developed after giving birth, my daughter was unable to properly breast-feed. The health benefits of breast-fed children versus non breast-fed children are well documented. Also, in her first three years of life, my daughter was prescribed antibiotics over 30 times for sinusitis, infections, and fever. Every time it was a different type of antibiotic, which just made matters worse. I also came across published research that showed that the gut flora of autistic children was much different from that of healthy children.[2] This included nine different types of clostridial species between the two groups.[3] It is well-documented that FMT is very effective in eradicating *C. difficile* infections. Could it also work on the other abnormal clostridial species?

Therefore, my feelings were that there was no way my daughter's flora could be even close to normal. What would happen if we did the FMT procedure and replaced her flora with that from a healthy person?

I set up an appointment for her with the local doctor mentioned in the aforementioned newspaper article. I asked him if he would treat her for chronic constipation, which she had suffered from her entire life. Research I provided him showed that FMT had been helpful in cases involving chronic constipation.[4] After three months of my persistent inquiries of him (and his staff), we had the FMT procedure done on September 28, 2012.

The results were remarkable. Normal, daily bowel movements were achieved for the first time in 15 years. Within 36 hours of the procedure, my daughter was a different kid. She had suffered through a very rough summer that had required her to take antibiotics in July for an illness. By August she had zero energy and was feeling miserable. All she wanted to do was lie down. She started wetting her clothing intentionally in hopes that she would be able to come home to change into clean clothes. She started school in September and was doing this 4-5 times a day. She was extremely sick, tired, and unhappy.

This all changed. She has not had a single issue in school for over three months (at the time of this writing), and the teachers cannot believe how well things have turned around. Her new energy level has been remarkable, and she is extremely happy and eager to go to school every day. Her mother agrees that it has been like night and day before and after this procedure. I decided to observe her for at least 90 days before mentioning anything to anyone about this treatment.

The transplant was accomplished through two enema applications on the same day. The actual procedure took less than 60 seconds to complete for each application. Prior to the procedure, the rectum was cleared by using a common laxative in suppository form. I selected the donor by asking the healthiest person I knew if they were interested in helping out. They agreed. The donor had to make several short visits to the hospital prior to the day of the procedure and was screened thoroughly for infectious disease (blood) and parasites (stool). My daughter was able to retain the donor material for an extended period of time, which may have improved the results. She has had a daily bowel movement ever since. Prior to the procedure, five days between bowel movements was not uncommon. The main benefit we've seen, by far, was renewed energy and health and, thus, a much happier young lady.

References

1. Grölund, Minna-Maija; Lehtonen, Olli-Pekka; Eerola, Erkki; Kero, Pentti: Fecal Microflora in Healthy Infants Born by Different Methods of Delivery: Permanent Changes in Intestinal Flora After Cesarean Delivery. *Journal of Pediatric Gastroenterology & Nutrition.* January 1999, 28,(1):19-25.
2. Parracho HM, Bingham MO, Gibson GR, McCartney AL: Differences between the gut microflora of children with autistic spectrum disorders and that of healthy children. *Journal of Medical Microbiology.* 2005, 54(10):987-991.
3. Finegold SM, Dowd SE, Gontcharova V, Liu C, Henley KE, Wolcott RD, Youn E, Summanen PH, Granpeesheh D, Dixon D, Liu M, Molitoris DR, Green JA: Pyrosequencing study of fecal microflora of autistic and control children. *Anaerobe.* 2010, 16(4):444-53.
4. Andrews P., Borody TJ, Shortis NP, Thompson S. Bacteriotherapy [FMT] for chronic constipation—long term follow-up. *Gastroenterology.* 108 (Suppl. 2), A563 (1995).

CHAPTER NINE

THE ROLE OF INTESTINAL AND OTHER MICROBES IN AUTISM AND OTHER DISEASES AFFECTING THE CENTRAL NERVOUS SYSTEM

By Sydney M. Finegold, MD

Introduction: Bacteria and regressive autism

This chapter will examine the role of intestinal microbes in autism and will consider other diseases affecting the central nervous system (CNS) that also have possible gut involvement. There are many varieties of autism, mostly not well characterized. One of the most distinctive is regressive (late onset) autism. The unique feature of regressive autism is normal development up to the age of 18 months or so, followed by loss of spoken and receptive language skills, loss of ability to socialize well with family and friends, development of repetitive behaviors (often involving spinning), decreased cognition, deterioration of behavior, development of abdominal symptoms, appearance of diarrhea or constipation, and other characteristics typical of autism. Although the epidemiology of these phenomena is not well studied, a number of parents describe a scenario in which the child develops an earache or other infection and is treated with antimicrobial agents, following which there is onset of autism.

Autism spectrum disorder (ASD) is a multisystem disease, and a number of autistic children manifest gastrointestinal abnormalities clinically and pathologically.[1-4] Among the abnormalities noted are abdominal pain or discomfort, bloating, and constipation with or without diarrhea. Often, the core problem in autistic children is constipation; even when the primary symptom is diarrhea, the diarrhea may be a post-obstructive phenomenon.[5] Zoppi and colleagues studied 28 children with chronic functional constipation (no evidence of anatomical disorder) by means of quantitative and qualitative analysis of the fecal flora, comparing the results with those obtained from 14 healthy children.[5] The only statistically significant difference between the two populations had to do with species of *Clostridium* and *Bifidobacterium*. In both cases, these genera had higher counts in the children with constipation, with a more pronounced difference for clostridial species.

It is interesting to note the amazing involvement of the gut microbiota in many functions of the human host. The gut microbiota contributes to developmental programming of epithelial cell barrier function, innate and adaptive immune function, gut homeostasis and angiogenesis, and liver function. Recently, it has been noted that the normal gut microbiota modulates brain development and behavior.[6] Germ-free mice show increased motor activity and reduced anxiety, compared with mice with a normal gut microbiota. There are numerous examples of bacteria being implicated in diseases in which both the gut and the CNS are involved, including D-lactic acidosis, Guillain-Barré syndrome, and others. Three recent papers that review various aspects of the gut microbiota and its relation to the CNS and autoimmune disease are excellent and well worth reading.[7-9] Another important paper focuses on intestinal bacteria and their role in the release of biologically active peptides and the regulation of gastrointestinal endocrine cells.[10]

In the case of autism, published data lend credence to the notion that an alteration in colonic flora contributes to autistic symptoms.[11-13] Potential mechanisms by which an abnormal flora might lead to autism involve production of one or more toxins or toxic metabolic products, an immune-mediated process, or molecular mimicry with host tissue (see Finegold et al.[12] for additional details). Diet and use of antimicrobials are two other major factors that may both contribute to autism or ameliorate it, depending on the specific diet and antimicrobial. Figure 1 summarizes my hypothesis as to how these various factors interact to result in regressive autism. There is (usually) an immune defect that can be either genetic or acquired as a result of environmental exposures to toxic compounds. Diet and exposure to particular antimicrobial

Figure 1. Hypothetical pathogenesis of autism

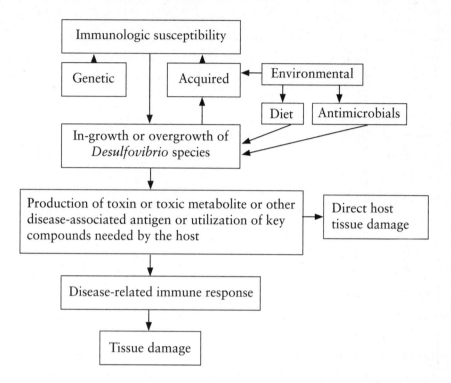

agents set the stage for *Desulfovibrio* species (and perhaps clostridial species) to colonize or increase in numbers. By virtue of *Desulfovibrio*'s lipopolysaccharide (endotoxin), *Desulfovibrio*'s interference with sulfur metabolism, its production of toxic methylmercury from mercury in the environment,[14,15] and other compounds that it produces, colonization by *Desulfovibrio* species can either lead to autism directly or with the help of a weakened immune system. These factors will be discussed at greater length in the remainder of this chapter.

Introduction to gut bacteria

Table 1 lists groups of intestinal bacteria, organized by the various phyla (major divisions) in which they are placed for classification purposes. Although at least 30 phyla have been described, the six listed at the head of each column in Table 1 are the ones involved in the diseases discussed in this chapter, and they are also responsible for the vast

Table 1. Classification of important gut bacteria

	Phyla					
Bacteroidetes	**Firmicutes**	**Actinobacteria**	**Proteobacteria**	**Verrucomicrobia**	**Fusobacteria**
*Bacteroides**	*Clostridium*	*Bifidobacterium**	**Beta group**	*Akkermansia*	*Fusobacterium*
Prevotella	*C. leptum**	*Actinomyces*	*Burkholderia*		
Porphyromonas	*C. coccoides**	*Coriobacteriaceae*	*Oxalobacter*		
Alistipes	*Coprococcus*	*Coriobacterium*	*Alcaligenes*		
Capnocytophaga	*Butyrovibrio*	*Eggerthella*	*Sutterella*		
Anaerostipes	*Staphylococcus*	*Slackia*	**Delta group**		
	Enterococcus	*Atopobium*	*Desulfovibrio*		
	Streptococcus	*Propionibacterium*	*Bilophila*		
	Peptostreptococcus		**Epsilon group**		
	Ruminococcus		*Campylobacter*		
	Blautia		*Helicobacter*		
	Faecalibacterium		**Gamma group**		
	Dialister		*Escherichia*		
	Lactobacillus		*Enterobacter*		
	Eubacterium		*Salmonella*		
	Roseburia		*Yersinia*		
			Serratia		
			Shigella		
			Proteus		
			Pseudomonas		
			Klebsiella		
			Acinetobacter		

*Four dominant groups of fecal microbiota in adults

majority of infections in humans. Virtually all the taxa listed below the phylum level are genera. Each genus may have one or more species. The usual way of designating organisms is with the genus name capitalized and the species name in lower case (for example, *Escherichia coli*).

The *Bacteroidetes*, *Proteobacteria*, *Verrucomicrobia*, and *Fusobacteria* are composed of Gram-negative bacteria, whereas *Firmicutes* and *Actinobacteria* are composed of Gram-positive organisms. The Gram stain, an arbitrary way to classify bacteria that was very helpful before molecular classification schemes, is still useful, particularly in clinical laboratories. It is a two-stain procedure in which Gram-positive organisms take the initial stain (crystal violet) and look purple under the microscope, while Gram-negative organisms lose the initial stain and take the second stain, which is red (either safranin or carbolfuchsin).

Some of the organisms listed are more important in causing true infections in immune-compromised individuals, particularly the aerobic bacteria but also certain virulent anaerobes such as *Clostridium*, *Bacteroides*, and *Actinomyces*. Gram-positive aerobes include *Staphylococcus*, *Enterococcus*, and *Streptococcus* (in the *Firmicutes* phylum). Gram-negative aerobes include *Escherichia*, *Enterobacter*, *Salmonella*, *Yersinia*, *Shigella*, *Serratia*, *Proteus*, *Pseudomonas*, *Klebsiella*, and *Acinetobacter*, all of which are in the gamma group of *Proteobacteria*. In this latter group, *Pseudomonas* is a true aerobe whereas the others are facultative (growing either aerobically or anaerobically). Some organisms, such as *Sutterella*, are microaerophilic, meaning they do not tolerate atmospheric oxygen levels (20%) but may grow well at 2-6% oxygen.

The microscopic morphology of bacteria is rod-shaped (bacillus) or coccoid (coccus, or streptococcus if a chain of cocci). Some of the bacilli (primarily clostridia) form spores, which permit them to survive deleterious influences such as high oxygen content or antibiotics. *Desulfovibrio* is a Gram-negative, non-sporing, curved bacillus that is anaerobic and a major sulfate-reducer. As with clostridia, *Desulfovibrio* is very resistant to harsh environments and can go into a vegetative state without producing spores.

The *Firmicutes/Bacteroidetes* ratio of the human gut microbiome is of interest, and studies have found that the ratio changes at different points in life.[16] In a study comparing infants (defined as 3 weeks to 10 months in age), adults (25 to 45 years old), and the elderly (ages 70 to 90 years), the *Firmicutes/Bacteroidetes* ratio was 0.4 for infants, 10.9 for adults, and 0.6 for the elderly (based on 21, 21, and 20 individuals, respectively).[16] None of the infants had ever received any antibiotics. The adult and elderly subjects had an unrestricted Western-type diet.

Clostridia

Infant botulism illustrates some of the potential mechanisms whereby clostridial species and disease interact. Infant botulism differs from classic (food-borne) botulism in that *Clostridium botulinum* is able to colonize an infant's intestinal tract due to the infant's as yet underdeveloped intestinal flora. Following multiplication of the organism in the gut, elaboration of the neurotoxin occurs *in vivo*.[17] Although diagnosis of infant botulism is rare after 1 year of age,[18] antimicrobial use has been identified as a risk factor for the development of botulism related to intestinal colonization with *C. botulinum* in older children and adults.[19]

In 1998, Bolte published an intriguing hypothesis that *Clostridium tetani* (or other bacteria in the gut) might play a role in late-onset autism.[20] On the basis of this hypothesis, we undertook an open-label 8-week trial of oral vancomycin. In this study,[11] patients with late-onset autism ranged from 43 to 84 months in age. By the Childhood Autism Rating Scale (CARS), six children met the criteria for severe autism, two for moderate autism, and three for mild autism. Notably, there was evidence of a clinical response in 8 of 10 evaluable children, including improvements in behavior, communication, and social skills. Behavior and communication analog rating scales were not done in blinded fashion. However, paired videotapes (30 minutes in a playroom environment) made before and during therapy were evaluated in blinded conditions by a clinical child psychologist who had no personal contact with the children. Patients relapsed to their pre-treatment state within a few weeks of discontinuing the vancomycin because the oral vancomycin suppresses but does not kill the organisms. When the antimicrobial agent (vancomycin) is gone, the bacteria can again multiply and make products that cause disease. This is particularly easy to understand with clostridia, which produce spores that are extremely resistant to deleterious influences. However, as already noted, the non-spore-forming *Desulfovibrio* is also very resistant to such influences.

A second study that we completed on autistic children[12] was entirely microbiologic in nature. The two-part study included 1) fecal flora studies (using pre-treatment specimens from the vancomycin study plus normal controls) and 2) studies of the upper gastrointestinal contents. In both parts of the study, both autistic children (n=13) and control children (n=8) (age- and sex-matched) contributed specimens. Identification of isolates was done by conventional phenotypic tests and by 16S rRNA gene sequencing. In the case of the fecal flora studies, we made the decision to focus primarily on clostridia because of the enormous amount of work involved in doing total flora studies by conventional microbiologic methods. Additional lines of evidence that justify a focus on clostridia include the following:

1. Members of this genus make potent neurotoxins, enterotoxins, and numerous metabolic products.
2. Infant botulism involving *C. botulinum* occurs only at a very young age or in response to antimicrobial administration, and there is involvement of the gastrointestinal tract and the CNS. The organism can survive in the gut because while antibiotics suppress or kill other key elements of the bowel flora, *C. botulinum* is resistant to killing due to its production of spores.
3. Anecdotally, the principal antimicrobial predisposing to late-onset autism used to be the combination of trimethoprim and sulfamethoxazole, to which clostridia are highly resistant. This drug combination is no longer much used; at present, it appears to be the penicillins and cephalosporins that may precipitate autism. This is because clostridia (as well as *Desulfovibrio*) tend to be resistant to these agents, which suppress some of the beneficial flora.
4. As noted, autistic patients respond to oral vancomycin and, anecdotally, to oral metronidazole, which suggests the possibility that a Gram-positive anaerobic organism is involved; however, *Desulfovibrio* is relatively susceptible to vancomycin as well.
5. Unusually high tetanus antitoxin titers have been noted in several children with regressive autism.

We found 23 species of *Clostridium* in the stools of the 13 autistic children and 15 in the stools of the 8 control children studied. The geometric mean count of clostridia was 1 log higher in the stools of autistic children than in the controls. Altogether, there were 25 different species of clostridia encountered, 8 of which had greater than 2% sequence divergence from the closest match in the RDP/GenBank, suggesting that they may have represented novel species not previously encountered.

The upper GI part of the study[12] involved specimens from a subset of 7 children with autism and 4 control children. The cultures were set up to identify any bacterium or yeast that was present. The gastric pH was elevated in 2 of 4 children with autism for whom gastric pH was measured, which is an indicator of hypochlorhydria or low stomach acid. These children had not been on H_2 blockers or proton pump inhibitors. The two children with hypochlorhydria had the most profuse microbial flora present. Even more striking was the total absence of non-spore-forming anaerobic and microaerophilic bacteria from specimens from the control children, whereas such organisms were present in the 4 children with autism whose specimens yielded growth, and 2 children's specimens had 7 to 9 different species. The hypochlorhydria seems to be a part of the autism picture in some children; more work is needed to determine the incidence of this finding and understand its mechanism. How important the non-spore-forming bacteria are also remains to be studied; some non-spore-formers such as *Desulfovibrio* are just as resistant to exposure to air and other potentially harmful substances as are clostridia. However, the methods we used in the study in question[12] would not have detected *Desulfovibrio*, which was not yet on our list of suspects as a potential contributor to autism. Interestingly, among the 3 subjects with autism who had few or no organisms recovered from their specimens, one had never had diarrhea or constipation; a second had had multiple courses of antimicrobials for recurrent sinusitis but none in the month prior to the sampling.

We subsequently tested the fecal specimens using real-time polymerase chain reaction (RT-PCR). We found that cell count differences of *Clostridium bolteae* and *Clostridium* clusters I and XI (but not cluster XIV ab) were statistically significant between autistic and age- and sex-matched control children, with higher bacterial counts in autistic children.[13] Real-time PCR has the advantages of being relatively inexpensive, rapid (2-3 hours), quantitative, and reliable. For example, Rinttilä and colleagues published on an extensive set of 16S rDNA-targeted primers for pathogenic and indigenous bacteria in fecal samples using RT-PCR.[21]

A study by Parracho and colleagues[22] adds important data that back up our earlier work. They compared the fecal flora of autistic children with that of two different control groups—healthy siblings of the autistic children and unrelated healthy children. The study was done using fluorescence *in situ* hybridization (FISH) techniques. The researchers noted a higher incidence of certain clostridia (*Clostridium* clusters I and II) in autistic children than in healthy controls but an intermediate level of these clostridia in the siblings of autistic children. Commenting on the Parracho study, Wang and colleagues note that the greater abundance of *Clostridium histolyticum* reported may not be accurate because 76% of the children had diarrhea and 66% were implementing gluten-free and/or casein-free diets.[23]

Elsewhere, I have pointed out that "*Clostridium clostridioforme*" is actually a mixture of three clinically important species—*C. bolteae*, *C. hathewayi*, and *C. clostridioforme*.[24] Other organisms (*C. citronae* and *C. aldenensis*) also belong to the "*C. clostridioforme* group" which, for a time, was seen as being important in regressive autism (and may yet prove to be).

Also relevant to a consideration of clostridia and autism is a study by MacFabe and colleagues involving injection of propionate into cerebral ventricles of rats.[25] Propionic acid is an end-product of enteric bacterial fermentation, including that of some clostridial species. Haskå and colleagues[26] point out that certain fractions of wheat also increase propionic acid formation in rats. The MacFabe study found that injection of propionic acid induced behaviors resembling autism, such as repetitive dystonic behaviors, retropulsion, seizures, and social avoidance. To the extent that propionic acid is important in "naturally" occurring autism, the production of this compound as an end-product of metabolism of certain organisms such as clostridia means that such organisms also become suspects in the mystery of autism. *Desulfovibrio* does not produce propionic acid in its usual metabolic activities but has other major virulence factors.

I published a hypothesis that clostridial spores are key elements in both therapy and the epidemiology of autism.[27] This hypothesis was based on the model of *Clostridium difficile* (*C. difficile*) infection and outbreaks. The spores of this organism explain the difficulty of eliminating environmental contamination with the organism, the relapse following apparently successful therapy with oral vancomycin, and the selection of resistant *C. difficile* by the use of antimicrobials to which it was resistant. However, spore-forming clostridia may be less important in regressive autism than previously thought in light of our studies demonstrating the likely major importance of *Desulfovibrio*.

My research group took a big step forward when we joined with Scot Dowd (co-owner of a research and testing laboratory in Lubbock, Texas) to employ pyrosequencing techniques, a rapid throughput method that permits examining many more samples in a given time than cultural methods. As with other molecular methods such as RT-PCR, pyrosequencing allows an organism to be identified by matching the DNA with readily available databases. The organisms detected cannot, however, be recovered for other studies such as virulence for animals and antimicrobial susceptibility testing. However, pyrosequencing identifies many organisms that are uncultivable, gives a fairly rough quantitation, and (with proper analysis) provides a much broader picture than is feasible with cultural techniques.

Using pyrosequencing, we were able to determine that the fecal flora of autistic subjects was abnormal when compared with normal controls (Figure 2).[28] Comparing the principal phyla detected by pyrosequencing, we noted that the normal controls had 64% *Firmicutes* and 30% *Bacteroidetes* whereas the corresponding figures were reversed for the autistic subjects (37% *Firmicutes* and 52% *Bacteroidetes*). This is a striking example of an abnormal fecal flora. Siblings were intermediate to the other two groups, suggesting that they may have acquired some flora abnormalities from their association with their autistic sibling. This, if documented, would have profound epidemiological significance and would make the comparison with *C. difficile* colitis more reasonable, given that in the latter entity, there is clearly spread of the offending bacterium from the bowel to surfaces and fomites in the hospital environment and indirect (and probably occasionally direct) contamination of personnel and other patients.

Figure 2. Pyrosequencing results on stools of children with autism, siblings, and normal controls

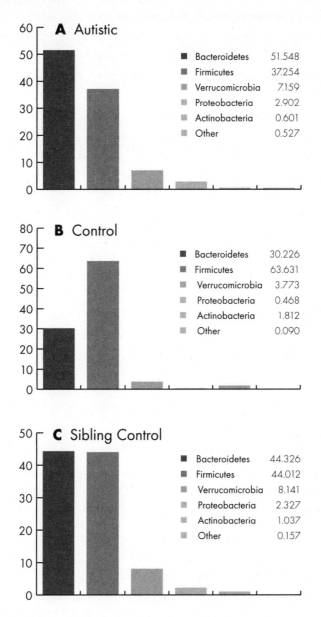

Desulfovibrio

Results of our pyrosequencing study prompted us to suspect that *Desulfovibrio* and *Bacteroides vulgatus*, both significantly more prevalent in autistic subjects than in controls, might play a key role in regressive autism. We proceeded to do selective culture (Table 2) and RT-PCR (Table 3) for both organisms on all of the stools studied previously by pyrosequencing. Although *B. vulgatus* did not show any significant difference between the stool samples from the three groups, the genus *Desulfovibrio* and its five species found in the human gut showed statistically significant differences.[29]

Table 2. Selective medium for *Desulfovibrio* species

	Final Concentration
Water	1 liter
Brucella agar	43 g
Ferric ammonium citrate	0.05%
Pyruvate	1%
$MgSO_4$	0.25%
Hemin (5 mg/ml)	5 µg/ml
Vitamin K_1 (1 mg/ml)	1 µg/ml
Trimethoprim (40 mg/ml)	40 µg/ml
Sulfamethoxazole (76 mg/ml)	76 µg/ml
Vancomycin (10 mg/ml)	10 µg/ml

Table 3. Sequences of oligonucleotide primers and probes

Target organism	Forward primer (5'-3')	Reverse primer (5'-3')	Probe (5'-3')
Bilophila wadsworthia	GGCTGGAAACGGTCGCTAA	GGACTCATCCTTAAGCGATAGC	CGAATACGCTCCCGATTTTATCATTGGG
D. desulfuricans	GGATCGTAAACCTCTGTCAG	CTTTACGCCCAGT(G/A)ATTCC	AACTACGTTGTGCTAATCAGCAGCGT
D. fairfieldensis	GGACTCATCCTCATACGACA	TCGAGTAGAGTGGCGCA	GCAAGCAGAGGCCGTCTTTCCCCT
D. intestinalis	GGATCGTAAACCTCTGTCAG	CTTTACGCCCAGT(G/A)ATTCC	AGAAACCGCACCGTGCTAATCAGCG
D. piger	GGATCGTAAACCTCTGTCAG	CTTTACGCCCAGT(G/A)ATTCC	AAGAAACTAGGGTGTTCTAATCATCATCC
D. vulgaris	GGATCGTAAACCTCTGTCAG	CTTTACGCCCAGT(G/A)ATTCC	CGGTGCTAATCAGCCGTGGTCTG
Desulfovibrio spp.	CCGTAGATATCTGGAGGAACATCAG	ACATCTAGCATCCATCGTTTACAGC	

Interestingly, we noted in the pyrosequencing results that several organisms (including three species of *Bifidobacterium* and three organisms from other genera) were found significantly more often in control stools than in stools obtained from autistic subjects, suggesting that they may play a protective role. We are currently studying all these stools by selective culture and RT-PCR to explore this hypothesis.

I discuss mechanisms by which *Desulfovibrio* might play a role in autism in another *Medical Hypotheses* paper.[30] Notably, although *Desulfovibrio* does not form spores, it behaves very much like a spore-former, with the ability to shut down its metabolism in potentially dangerous circumstances. *Desulfovibrio* can then survive for months in this vegetative state. (For further information, see the work of S. Jill James and Rosemary Waring.[31,32]) One other point that should be made is that lipopolysaccharide (LPS) such as is found in *Desulfovibrio* can penetrate the blood-brain barrier.

Other evidence linking bacteria and autism

Other reports implicate a variety of bowel flora in autism. One report, presented at an International Meeting for Autism Research (IMFAR) by Rosseneu and colleagues[33] from the United Kingdom (UK), described "abnormal" aerobic Gram-negative bacilli (*Enterobacter* and *Citrobacter*) as well as *as Staphylococcus aureus* and *Candida albicans* in "overgrowth" (true quantitation was not done) from rectal and throat swabs from autistic children. The report from this group indicated that 10 children had a good response in an open-label trial with oral polymyxin and oral tobramycin in terms of behavior, social sense, speech, and elimination of the abnormal Gram-negative bacilli. Our own unpublished data found only normal counts of *Escherichia coli* and low counts of *Enterobacter cloacae* and *Klebsiella oxytoca* in autistic children. It seems likely that the very high levels of antimicrobials achieved in the gut with oral administration of polymyxin and tobramycin might lead to elimination of clostridia and other organisms more likely involved in autism than the "abnormal" Gram-negative aerobic bacilli described by the UK group.

A number of other noteworthy studies have explored the relationship between gastrointestinal flora and autism.

- Jeremy Nicholson's group in London[34] studied the urinary metabolic phenotypes of autistic children, their non-autistic siblings, and healthy controls. They found alterations in nicotinic acid metabolism, sulfur and amino acid metabolism, and certain urinary and bacterial co-metabolites in the autistic children.

- Parracho and colleagues, in a later paper,[35] studied probiotics and found that strain *Lactobacillus plantarum* WCSF1 improved behavior and bowel health in autistic subjects.

- Adams and colleagues found a strong correlation of gastrointestinal symptoms with autism severity.[36] The study involved 58 children with ASD and 39 healthy controls. With cultural techniques, they found lower levels of *Bifidobacterium* species and higher levels of *Lactobacillus* species in the autistic group but similar levels of other bacteria and yeast in both groups. However, one-third of the autistic children were taking probiotics; this might well explain the higher *Lactobacillus* presence.

- Wang and colleagues used RT-PCR to study the fecal flora of 23 autistic children (most of whom had the regressive form of autism), 22 siblings of the autistic children, and 9 unrelated healthy controls.[23] Roughly half of the autistic subjects and their siblings had functional GI disease. Using 48-hour stool collections, the researchers found lower relative abundance of *Akkermansia muciniphila* and *Bifidobacterium* species. These authors point out that speciation of *Bifidobacterium* is important because strain *Bifidobacterium longum* NCC3001 has been shown to improve anxiety in mice via the vagal nerve, and other species may be less active or inactive.

- Finally, an elegant study by Williams and colleagues involved 15 autistic children, 13 of whom had regressive behavior, and 7 control children.[37] All samples for study were obtained endoscopically and consisted of 8 mucosal biopsies from each patient (4 from the ileum and 4 from the cecum). Metagenomic analysis of the intestinal bacteria revealed decreases in the *Bacteroidetes*, increases in the ratio of *Firmicutes* to *Bacteroidetes*, and increases in *Betaproteobacteria* in the autistic children. The authors note the discrepancy between their data and the data from our own group's pyrosequencing study, which instead found a decreased ratio of *Firmicutes* to *Bacteroidetes* in the autistic group. These researchers point out that others have reported discrepancies between fecal and mucosal microflora and note that because only about 50% of bacterial cells in feces are viable (the rest being dead or injured), loss of *Bacteroidetes* from mucosal sites could lead to increased numbers in the feces.

Overall, Williams' study[37] demonstrates a relationship between human intestinal gene expression and the bacteria in that region and appears to provide information on the pathophysiology of gastrointestinal symptomatology in children *w*ith regressive autism. Clearly, the GI symptoms commonly seen in children with regressive autism are linked to the autism and are not coincidental. It should be noted that the study also found that disaccharidases and hexose transporters were deficient in the ileum of the autistic children. These enzymatic and transporter deficiencies provide additional substrates for bacterial growth, which can lead to specific changes in composition of the flora. A subsequent paper (In Press, *mBio*) by some of the same authors describes the principal *Proteobacteria* organism in their studies as *Sutterella*.

Autism, infection, and the immune system
The incidence of autism in the offspring of mothers who develop rubella is increased over 200 times.[38,39] Infections with other types of microbes (protozoa and bacteria) are also associated with autism. Studies by Atladottir[40] show significant association of autism with first-trimester maternal viral infection and with second-trimester maternal bacterial infections.

Antibrain antibodies may be found in the blood of autistic children as part of an autoimmune reaction, perhaps due to molecular mimicry, and in the blood of mothers of autistic children. ASD children are more likely than control children to have a family member, particularly a mother, with autoimmune disease or allergy. Variants of MHC (major histocompatibility complex) genes, which are important for immune recognition of infectious diseases, have been found in autism families. Immune cells from the blood of autistic children display a stronger cytokine response to immune stimulation than is true for such cells from neurotypical children.[41] This is especially true of ASD patients who have GI symptoms.

Pardo[42] demonstrated evidence of inflammation in the autistic brain, noting a striking elevation of cytokine titers (particularly IL-6) in the cerebrospinal fluid (CSF). Others have demonstrated the immune-activated state in autism and in a number of areas of the brain.[41] Rather than implying an acute inflammatory episode, this immune-activated state appears to be due to an ongoing subclinical condition that we hypothesize may be due to dysbiosis in the bowel. Levitt of the University of Southern California[43] found that a common variant of the MET gene [met proto-oncogene (hepatocyte growth factor receptor)] increases the risk for autism and has effects on three systems: brain, gut, and the immune system.

Interestingly, intercurrent infection such as a cold or influenza may lead to temporary improvement in the autistic picture due to fever or increased cytokine levels. (In fact, some parents report taking their autistic children to crowded malls hoping they will contract a cold!) Children living on farms, where they undoubtedly encounter germs from the soil and from animals, are less likely to get autoimmune diseases than children raised in urban environments. This has prompted some entrepreneurs to sell hookworms on the Internet to increase people's immunity. A microbiologist friend sent her young autistic son to live with her family on a farm in South America for a year, and when he returned he was remarkably improved.

Implications for prevention and treatment

A vaccine against the LPS or other components of *Desulfovibrio* might be the optimal way to prevent colonization and/or interfere with the virulence of this organism. It could also be useful therapeutically by *ex vivo* production of antibodies for treatment.

A recent paper of ours,[44] accepted for publication as part of a symposium, provides information on susceptibility of *Desulfovibrio* species to various antimicrobials. This data is of interest in terms of considering potential therapies for regressive autism and also in terms of understanding the pathogenesis of the disease and possibilities for prevention. The data must be interpreted with respect to levels of the various drugs achieved in the bowel. The data suggest that penicillins, cephalosporins, trimethoprim/sulfamethoxazole, and fluoroquinolones (which should not be used in young children anyway because of their potential toxicity) may well predispose to regressive autism. This is due to the resistance of *Desulfovibrio* to these antimicrobials and their impact on the bowel flora; their impact permits larger numbers of *Desulfovibrio* to grow after the competition is reduced.

The data also point to other drugs that might be used to treat ear infections, for example, while incurring less risk of major bowel flora changes of the type discussed. Included in this category would be drugs such as the macrolides and tetracyclines. Aztreonam, a monobactam antibiotic that was supplanted by newer drugs after being used for decades, is now being used again in selected situations where Gram-negative bacilli are resistant to many or most other drugs. Although this drug is not supposed to be active against anaerobes, it is moderately active against *Desulfovibrio*. It is susceptible to destruction by beta-lactamases (which it produces itself) but otherwise has a number of good features, such as not being absorbed to any extent when given orally and being well tolerated. Combining aztreonam with sulbactam, a beta-lactamase inhibitor, provides synergistic activity while eliminating the threat posed by the common beta-lactamases.

Diet is clearly important and might provide the best long-term approach to management of autism. It is well established that diet is a major regulator of the human bowel flora. Although appropriate studies have not been done, clearly many autistic children benefit from diets such as the gluten-free/casein-free (GF/CF) diet and the Specific Carbohydrate Diet™. Studies are needed that document and quantitate benefits from these diets and correlate improvement (or lack of improvement) with dietary components, elements removed from a conventional diet, and changes in the bowel flora.

Other modes of therapy that should be evaluated (beyond conventional dietary changes, behavioral therapy, and occupational therapy) are pre- and probiotics. Probiotics are microorganisms that are thought to be beneficial through their suppression of potential pathogens. The principle is a good one, but much more study is needed. Clearly, there must be more tailoring to the specific pathogen that we seek to suppress or eliminate. For example, lactobacilli of one species are not good across the board for all sorts of pathogens, although they are commonly used that way. Because each person's comprehensive situation is unique, as with other regimens under consideration, the best course is to discuss the individual's physiological status and needs for objective laboratory testing and corresponding intervention with their overseeing healthcare professional. Once we determine that a particular organism is responsible for most or all cases of a particular disease entity, such as autism, it may be possible to provide a probiotic that is specifically and solely active against that organism.

Prebiotics are nutritive compounds that can be incorporated in one's diet to stimulate growth of a beneficial bacterium such as *Bifidobacterium*. However, various species of *Bifidobacterium* behave differently, and we have a lot of work to do to determine which particular species may be useful for which disease entities and to be certain that they are not harmful.

Fecal transplant (that is, fecal microbiota transplantation) is another possible mode of therapy that has attracted interest and proved very effective in treating *C. difficile* relapses. Dr. Emma Allen-Vercoe's group at the University of Guelph in Ontario, Canada is studying an artificially produced feces made up of individual species of bacteria normally resident in the bowel flora; these are cultivated outside of the body and put together to produce a group of organisms characteristic of the colonic flora but without any risk of incidental contamination with viruses such as HIV and hepatitis (E. Allen-Vercoe, personal communication).

Other forms of bacterial-CNS interaction
It should be noted that this chapter does *not* cover true infections (in the classical sense) that involve toxin production with CNS implications. Examples of this type of infection would include bacillary dysentery, which has CNS manifestations due to the production of Shiga toxin, and Whipple's disease, in which the *Tropheryma whipplei* DNA may be detected directly in the CSF. Nor does this chapter discuss the common form of food-borne botulism, which typically involves ingestion of

preformed botulinal toxin in a food product; disease results when the toxin migrates up the vagus nerve to reach the CNS. In the same way, if *Clostridium tetani* is introduced into the body by wounds or trauma (via soil or other material), it too will produce toxin that can reach the CNS by migration up the vagus nerve. Gas gangrene clostridia may be introduced by surgery, disease involving the bowel (where the organisms may be found as indigenous flora), or by trauma to skin and soft tissues, including muscle. These situations involving clostridia are often classified as intoxications rather than infections.

Other diseases with microbial and CNS involvement

In addition to autism, the relationship between microbial entities and diseases with CNS involvement is evident for a number of other conditions. Table 4 summarizes some of the key observations pertaining to some of these conditions, and schizophrenia and Alzheimer's disease are discussed following the table. In many of these diseases, including amyotrophic lateral sclerosis (ALS), Gulf War syndrome, and multiple chemical sensitivity, *Desulfovibrio* should be sought as a possible causative agent, along with clostridia and other bacteria. In all of the entities discussed in this section, it may be difficult to determine whether bacteria or other factors in the gut are causing the CNS disease or *vice versa*, or whether both of these may coexist or cycle back and forth.

Table 4. Selected conditions with CNS and possible enteric involvement

---

Amyotrophic lateral sclerosis (ALS) or Lou Gehrig's disease
- A progressive, fatal neurodegenerative disorder[45]
- Cause unknown
- Increased incidence in Gulf War veterans (double that of general population[46-48]) suggests an environmental factor
- Association between ALS and employment in farming or participation in outdoor athletics also consistent with environmental exposure
- Recent paper hypothesized that ALS may be caused by a motor neuron toxin produced by a clostridial species residing in the gut[49]
- ALS involves both upper and lower motor neurons and occasionally bulbar dysfunction

---

- *Desulfovibrio* commonly found around oil wells in the Persian Gulf and elsewhere
- No consequential treatment available

Chronic fatigue syndrome
- Describes sudden onset of profound and prolonged fatigue
- May be preceded by low-grade fever and night sweats, suggesting possibility of a predisposing infection
- Studies have failed to yield consistent results in terms of possible etiology
- Diagnosis based on subjective description of illness by patients
- No reliable laboratory tests for confirmation
- Studies in human subjects and mice suggest an abnormal bowel flora, including low levels of bifidobacteria and small intestinal bacterial overgrowth[50]
- A double-blind, placebo-controlled randomized study reported that administration of *Lactobacillus casei* strain Shirota led to a significant increase in both lactobacilli and bifidobacteria along with a significant decrease in anxiety[51]
- Evidence that parvovirus B19 may be involved in etiology[52]
- Administration of a probiotic consisting of two species of lactobacilli and one of bifidobacteria obtained improvement in neurocognitive function without significant change in the fecal flora; six of the 15 subjects felt that they improved[53]
- Increased numbers of Gram-positive facultative anaerobic bacteria, chiefly enterococci and streptococci, in cases, and a greater percentage of cases versus controls produced d-lactic acid[54]

Depression
- Changes in the gut microbiome have been associated with major depression[8]
- Patients with depression show elevated blood levels of TNF-α and IL-6 cytokines and metabolic disorders related to the gut[55]
- Patients with depression show reduced levels of lactobacilli and bifidobacteria
- Depression associated with low levels of omega-3 fatty acids related to a diet with relatively little fish, nuts, beans, and whole grains

- Low incidence of depression with high intake of seafood[56]
- Administration of the probiotic *Bifidobacterium infantis* to rats with elevated proinflammatory cytokines and elevation of plasma tryptophan levels[57]

D-lactic acidosis

- Rare disease
- Predisposing conditions are extensive small bowel resection following mesenteric infarction and jejunoileal bypass
- In addition to acidosis, patients manifest significant psychiatric and neurologic abnormalities (including hostile behavior, lethargy to stupor or coma, confusion, slurred speech, incoordination, ataxia, asterixis, dizziness, fatigue, weakness, bloating, nausea, diarrhea, foul body odor)
- In a study by our group of two adult patients with D-lactic acidosis,[58] stool cultures showed high counts and marked predominance of Gram-positive, non-spore-forming bacteria, principally bifidobacteria, lactobacilli, and *Eubacterium*
- In contrast with normal controls, neither patient had *Bacteroides* present in counts above 108/gm of stool
- D-lactate produced from appropriate media in significant amounts by many of the bacteria isolated from the two patients but not from any bacteria recovered from normal control subjects
- Good clinical response and normalization of stool flora on oral vancomycin therapy
- Pathogenesis involves exposing intestinal bacteria to carbohydrates, production of both D- and L-lactate from this substrate, lowering of pH by increased luminal lactate, selection of acid-tolerant bacteria (also acid producers) by the low pH, and absorption of the non-metabolizable (by humans) D-lactate
- CNS aberrations do not correlate with the acidosis per se

Fibromyalgia

- Much like chronic fatigue syndrome, with the addition of a diagnostic requirement of needing 11 or more of 18 designated pressure points to demonstrate tenderness to pressure

- A neurogenic origin suggested for the most prominent symptom, chronic widespread pain, with central amplification of pain perception[59]

Guillain-Barré syndrome
- An inflammatory peripheral neuropathy of one type or another that frequently occurs after an enteric infection with *Campylobacter jejuni* or a respiratory infection with *cytomegalovirus* or Epstein-Barr virus
- Spinal fluid unique in that protein levels are elevated but white blood cell counts are not

Gulf War illness or syndrome
- Unexplained illnesses (see ALS above) affect veterans of the Gulf War (Operations Desert Shield and Desert Storm)
- Large numbers of the almost 700,000 servicemen stationed in the first Gulf War have reported a range of chronic symptoms and health problems at rates that exceed those seen in non-deployed veterans
- Symptoms include persistent headaches, joint pain, extreme fatigue, muscle pain, cognitive problems, GI difficulties, and skin abnormalities[60-62]
- VA compensates Gulf War veterans with unexplained illnesses based on objective evidence of disability for at least 6 months due to debilitating symptoms including one or more of those above
- As of February 2005, claims filed by 12,583 Gulf War veterans; of these, 3,265 granted a service connection
- Previous studies proposed bacteria as a factor in Gulf War-related illnesses; Gulf War veterans noted to improve after prolonged course of antibiotics[63]
- Gulf veterans suffering from ALS chronically infected with *Mycoplasma fermentans* according to one report[64]
- Large-scale antibiotic treatment trial that assessed efficacy of doxycycline in improving health of Gulf veterans[65,66] indicated that a 12-month course of doxycycline therapy did not provide significant benefit
- Veterans who received doxycycline therapy showed significantly greater improvement than those taking placebo after three months of therapy, but improvement tapered off by six months

- Findings consistent with doxycycline having effect on bowel flora, as evidenced by initial improvement in symptoms; developing resistance to doxycycline may account for later results

Irritable bowel syndrome (IBS)

- Characterized by chronic or recurrent abdominal pain or distress and irregular defecations, often with abdominal bloating
- Enteric nervous system appears to be involved, accounting for much of the abdominal distress
- Significant percent of patients have depression or anxiety disorder, but the evidence is that IBS is a definite gastrointestinal disorder
- Up to a third of patients with gastroenteritis due to *Salmonella* or *Campylobacter*, or travelers' diarrhea, may be complicated by IBS
- High rates of small intestinal bacterial overgrowth in some studies[67]
- A high-fiber diet may be helpful in patients with constipation
- Probiotics such as *Bifidobacterium* may be helpful, as may rifaximin, a poorly absorbed antibacterial agent
- Cases may be difficult to manage; referral to a competent gastroenterologist may be very helpful

Multiple chemical sensitivity

- Whether or not an infectious agent is involved etiologically is not known – once there is loss of gut wall integrity for whatever reason, chemical and other sensitivities and allergies and other entities discussed here may result
- Chronic fatigue syndrome, fibromyalgia, multiple chemical sensitivity, and posttraumatic stress disorder proposed as overlapping entities, with elevated nitric oxide and peroxynitrite involved in a common etiology[68]
- Xenobiotic detoxification pathways and adverse environmental response should be considered, with emphasis on sulfur-dependent detoxification pathways[69]
- Impaired sulfation and sulfotransferase "starvation" play a role in multiple chemical sensitivity as well as autoimmune and similar diseases, including Alzheimer's disease, Parkinsonism, motor neuron disease, rheumatoid arthritis, delayed food sensitivity, and autism

Multiple sclerosis

- Commensal gut flora, in the absence of pathogens, triggers a relapsing and remitting autoimmune disease[70]
- In animal studies, this does not take place in germfree animals[70,71]
- Recruitment of autoantibody-producing B cells depends on a target autoantigen, myelin oligodendrocyte glycoprotein, and commensal microbiota[70] – in animals, segmented filamentous bacteria that are unculturable can take the place of other commensal flora
- Phosphorylated dihydroceramides, known to be produced by *Bacteroides, Parabacteroides*, and *Prevotella* from the human intestinal tract[72] can enhance murine experimental autoimmune encephalitis, an animal model for MS
- Molecular mimicry may be involved in MS since it is known to play a role in the animal model of brain inflammation, experimental autoimmune encephalomyelitis (EAE)[73-75]
- Vitamin D3 reversibly blocks progression of EAE[76]

Schizophrenia

The relationship of schizophrenia to infectious agents (including rubella, herpes virus, *Toxoplasma*, and bacteria) has been pointed out by various authors. Being born in winter has been documented to lead to an increase in schizophrenia.[77] Mednick and colleagues studied the 1957 influenza outbreak in Finland and found that children born to mothers pregnant during this time had an increased risk of schizophrenia.[78] A study of the role of obstetrical factors in schizophrenia noted exposure to several infectious agents but also commented on fetal exposure to increases in proinflammatory cytokines.[79] Haloperidol, commonly used for treating schizophrenia, is a potent inhibitor of *Toxoplasma gondii*.[80] Interestingly, conditions that had fever as a common thread were noted in the 1880s to induce remarkable remissions in schizophrenic patients.[41]

In his recent book, *Infectious Behavior*,[41] neurobiologist Paul Patterson points out that activation of immune-related genes in schizophrenia is indicative of a subclinical, permanent condition rather than acute infection. Might this not be consistent with a chronic problem such as abnormality of the bowel flora? Five-year follow-up studies with patients initially included in the International Pilot Study of Schizophrenia[81] pointed out that clinical and social outcomes were better in third-world countries than in developed countries; not suggested by the authors were the possibilities that differences in diet, hygiene, and, therefore, intestinal flora might be involved.

In 1966[82] and 1984,[83] Dohan presented striking information on the possible relationship between schizophrenia and eating cereals (especially wheat), perhaps related to celiac disease. During wartime, countries with the greatest rationing of cereals had the lowest incidence of schizophrenia. Japan, which consumed primarily rice (a non-gluten grain) rather than wheat, and Africans, with primarily maize, millet, or sorghum (also gluten-free) as dietary staples, had much less schizophrenia. The benefit of eliminating gluten-containing grains, however, may be limited to a certain subset of schizophrenic patients.[84]

A single case report in a drug-naive schizophrenic reported striking improvement with omega-3 fatty acid supplementation.[85] Animal and preliminary clinical studies indicate that milk (specifically casein, the protein in milk) is linked to both schizophrenia and autism.[86] A high intake of refined sugar led to a worse outcome in schizophrenia.[56]

Alzheimer's disease

This chapter has focused largely on autism, which is diagnosed in early childhood. At the other end of the lifetime continuum, we find Alzheimer's disease (AD). AD is the most common neurodegenerative disease, constituting approximately two-thirds of cases of dementia.[87,88] Clinically, the disease is characterized by progressive impairment in memory, judgment, decision-making, orientation to surroundings, and language as well as a shortened life expectancy.[89] Pathologically, there is neuronal loss, extracellular senile plaques containing the peptide β-amyloid, and neurofibrillary tangles. β-amyloid $A\beta_{42}$ is 42 amino acids long and is of pathogenetic importance because it forms insoluble toxic fibrils and accumulates in the senile plaques. It has been pointed out, however, that the number of amyloid deposits in the brain does not correlate well with the degree of impairment of cognition, and some people without symptoms of AD have many cortical Aβ deposits.[90]

Cholinesterase inhibitors and vitamin E have exhibited benefit in mild to moderately severe cases of AD,[91] and memantine has reduced clinical deterioration in moderate to severe cases.[88] In general, the benefit has been small and has yielded a slowing of deterioration rather than reversal of established disease.[91] Other approaches are under study. Curcumin inhibits β-amyloid fibril (fAβ) formation *in vitro*, as does rifampin,[92] which has antioxidant activity.[93]

Recently, a randomized, controlled trial of doxycycline and rifampin therapy in mild to moderate AD patients was reported.[94] There was significantly less decline in cognition in antimicrobial-treated patients than in placebo controls. This study was undertaken because of the activity of these drugs against *Chlamydia pneumoniae*, which has been suggested as playing an etiologic role in AD. However, there was no difference in detection of this organism between the treatment and control groups. The authors note that both of the antibacterial agents that they used have an effect on cerebral amyloid deposition *in vitro*. Another explanation, not mentioned in this paper, would be an effect of these antibacterial compounds on intestinal flora. Antimicrobial therapy localized to the GI tract offers the promise of determining whether bowel microbial flora are involved in the pathogenesis of AD and may indicate what segment of the flora may be involved. Rifaximin is a rifamycin antimicrobial drug with *in vitro* activity against various elements of the bowel flora. Less than 1% of the drug is absorbed after oral administration. Selection of resistant mutants, a problem with the related drug rifampin, appears to be less common with rifaximin.[95] The drug is FDA-approved and has been used successfully in treating various infections involving the human gut, such as traveler's diarrhea and IBS.[96,97] Moreover, rifaximin is nontoxic and well tolerated.

Let's revisit the question of how an abnormal intestinal flora might predispose to CNS disease, including AD. Possibilities include production of a neurotoxin or other toxic compound by a particular organism, inflammatory response with production of cytokines and free radicals,[98] brain-reactive antibodies, and autoimmunity (not necessarily involving molecular mimicry). Of interest is the production of a variety of amyloid fibers, called curli, by bacteria.[99] Soluble amyloid precursors may be found in human biological fluids. Bacterial amyloid fibers are like eukaryotic amyloid in resisting protease digestion, remaining insoluble when boiled in 1% sodium dodecyl sulfate, and binding to amyloid-specific dyes. It is also interesting to note that the intestinal flora played an important role in amyloid deposition in a transgenic mouse model of familial amyloidotic polyneuropathy.[100]

Why should elderly people develop an intestinal bacterial overgrowth problem? There is no good information available on the incidence of such a problem in elderly individuals, but there are a number of predisposing situations. Dysmotility is probably the principal background factor, perhaps related to diabetes in some patients and perhaps related to nerve cell loss in the myenteric plexus of the small intestine and colon in humans.[101,102] A decrease in IgA antibody in the gut in some patients may contribute to bacterial overgrowth. Achlorhydria or hypochlorhydria is the final factor. Chronic atrophic gastritis is seen in one-third of elderly individuals. Many people in the older age group take proton pump inhibitors, H_2-receptor antagonists, and/or antacids. Why do some people develop AD and others not, assuming that AD is related to bacterial overgrowth? It may be a matter of duration or extent of the overgrowth or due to the presence of one or more particular organisms.

Qu and colleagues note abnormal sulfur metabolism in Alzheimer's disease.[103] That also occurs in autism and may be related to *Desulfovibrio*, which is sulfate-reducing. *Desulfovibrio* and another sulfate-reducing bacterium found in the gut, *Bilophila wadsworthia*, may play a role in AD just as I believe *Desulfovibrio* does in regressive autism. As already noted, *Desulfovibrio* LPS can effect a breakdown in the blood-brain barrier. Qu's group also takes note of cross-talk between hydrogen sulfide and nitric oxide. According to Kamoun, there are only two diseases described with alterations of hydrogen sulfide metabolism: Alzheimer's disease (and I would add regressive autism), with decreased synthesis of hydrogen sulfide in the brain, and Down syndrome (with increased synthesis).[104]

Three important articles with recommendations from the National Institute on Aging and the Alzheimer's Association Workgroup redefine stages and set biomarkers for future research.[105-107]

Conclusions

I believe the material presented in this chapter makes a good case for the interaction of intestinal bacteria, antimicrobial agents, diet, and central nervous system abnormalties summarized very neatly in the title of this book, *Bugs, Bowels, and Behavior.* Regressive autism provides the best evidence for the interactions mentioned. Still, much work remains to be done to convince parents, physicians, and the scientific community that these interrelationships are real and that autism can be treated effectively, at least in younger individuals. Moreover, appropriate studies have yet to be done on older children and adults with ASD and on other forms of autism.

Parents of children with autism should keep accurate log books on what goes on in their children and on the factors that may play a role in their child's disease, without being influenced by those who propose any particular mechanism. Because parents see the entire picture on a daily basis, they are in the best position to provide information on the possible role of antimicrobial agents and to identify the specific agents that may be implicated in precipitating the disease in predisposed children. I have hypothesized that penicillins and cephalosporins are the principal drugs that play this role, based on susceptibility patterns of putative bacterial agents involved and on the flora that might be protective. Thus far, however, we have only anecdotal parental reports. We must also keep an open mind regarding the other disease entities discussed in this chapter and make support available for their further study, given these other entities' equally heavy disease burden.

References

1. D'Eufemia P, Celli M, Finocchiaro R, Pacifico L, Viozzi L, Zaccagnini M, et al. Abnormal intestinal permeability in children with autism. *Acta Paediatr.* 1996;85:1076-9.
2. Horvath K, Papadimitriou JC, Rabsztyn A, Drachenberg C, Tildon JT. Gastrointestinal abnormalities in children with autistic disorder. *J Pediatr.* 1999;135(5):559-63.
3. Melmed RD, Schneider CK, Fabes RA, Phillips J, Reichelt K. Metabolic markers and gastrointestinal symptoms in children with autism and related disorders. *J Pediat Gastroenterol Nutr.* 2000;31(Suppl 2):S31-S32.
4. Torrente F, Ashwood P, Day R, Machado N, Furlano RI, Anthony A, et al. Small intestinal enteropathy with epithelial IgG and complement deposition in children with regressive autism. *Mol Psychiatr.* 2002;7:375-82.
5. Zoppi G, Cinquetti M, Luciano A, Benini A, Muner A, Bertazzoni Minelli E. The intestinal ecosystem in chronic functional constipation. *Acta Paediatr.* 1998;87:836-41.
6. Heijtz RD, Wang S, Anuar F, Qian Y, Bjorkholm B, Samuelsson A, et al. Normal gut microbiota modulates brain development and behavior. *Proc Natl Acad Sci U S A.* 2011;108(7):3047-52.

7.	Sekirov I, Russell SL, Antunes LC, Finlay BB. Gut microbiota in health and disease. *Physiol Rev.* 2010;90(3):859-904.

8.	Ochoa-Reparaz J, Mielcarz DW, Begum-Haque S, Kasper LH. Gut, bugs, and brain: role of commensal bacteria in the control of central nervous system disease. *Ann Neurol.* 2011;69(2):240-7.

9.	Rook GA. Hygiene hypothesis and autoimmune diseases. *Clin Rev Allergy Immunol.* 2011 Nov 17. [Epub ahead of print]

10.	Uribe A, Alam M, Johansson O, Midtvedt T, Theodorsson E. Microflora modulates endocrine cells in the gastrointestinal mucosa of the rat. *Gastroenterology.* 1994;107(5):1259-69.

11.	Sandler RH, Finegold SM, Bolte ER, Buchanan CP, Maxwell AP, Vaisanen ML, et al. Short-term benefit from oral vancomycin treatment of regressive-onset autism. *J Child Neurol.* 2000;15(7):429-35.

12.	Finegold SM, Molitoris D, Song Y, Liu C, Väisänen M-L, Bolte E, et al. Gastrointestinal microflora studies in late-onset autism. *Clin Infect Dis.* 2002;35(Suppl 1):S6-S16.

13.	Song Y, Liu C, Finegold SM. Real-time PCR quantitation of clostridia in feces of autistic children. *Appl Environ Microbiol.* 2004;70(11):6459-65.

14.	Choi SC, Chase T Jr, Bartha R. Enzymatic catalysis of mercury methylation by *Desulfovibrio desulfuricans* LS. *Appl Environ Microbiol.* 1994;60(4):1342-6.

15.	Choi SC, Bartha R. Cobalamin-mediated mercury methylation by *Desulfovibrio desulfuricans* LS. *Appl Environ Microbiol.* 1993;59(1):290-5.

16.	Mariat D, Firmesse O, Levenez F, Guimaraes V, Sokol H, Dore J, et al. The Firmicutes/Bacteroidetes ratio of the human microbiota changes with age. *BMC Microbiol.* 2009;9:123.

17.	Wilcke BW Jr, Midura TF, Arnon SS. Quantitative evidence of intestinal colonization by *Clostridium botulinum* in four cases of infant botulism. *J Infect Dis.* 1980;141:419-23.

18.	Cherington M. Clinical spectrum of botulism. *Muscle Nerve.* 1998;21(6):701-10.

19.	Shapiro RL, Hatheway C, Swerdlow DL. Botulism in the United States: a clinical and epidemiological review. *Ann Intern Med.* 1998;129(3):221-8.

20.	Bolte ER. Autism and *Clostridium tetani. Med Hypotheses.* 1998;51:133-44.

21.	Rinttila T, Kassinen A, Malinen E, Krogius L, Palva A. Development of an extensive set of 16S rDNA-targeted primers for quantification of pathogenic and indigenous bacteria in faecal samples by real-time PCR. *J Appl Microbiol.* 2004;97(6):1166-77.

22.	Parracho HM, Bingham MO, Gibson GR, McCartney AL. Differences between the gut microflora of children with autistic spectrum disorders and that of healthy children. *J Med Microbiol.* 2005;54(Pt 10):987-91.

23.	Wang L, Christophersen CT, Sorich MJ, Gerber JP, Angley MT, Conlon MA. Low relative abundances of the mucolytic bacterium *Akkermansia muciniphila* and *Bifidobacterium* spp. in feces of children with autism. *Appl Environ Microbiol.* 2011;77(18):6718-21.

24.	Finegold SM, Song Y, Liu C, Hecht DW, Summanen P, Kononen E, et al. *Clostridium clostridioforme*: a mixture of three clinically important species. *Eur J Clin Microbiol Infect Dis.* 2005;24(5):319-24.

25.	MacFabe DF, Rodriguez-Capote K, Hoffman JE, Franklin AE, Mohammad-Asef Y, Taylor AR, et al. A novel rodent model of autism: intraventricular infusions of propionic acid increase locomotor activity and induce neuroinflammation and oxidative stress in discrete regions of adult rat brain. *Am J Biochem Biotech.* 2008;4(2):146-66.

26. Haska L, Andersson R, Nyman M. A water-soluble fraction from a by-product of wheat increases the formation of propionic acid in rats compared with diets based on other by-product fractions and oligofructose. *Food Nutr Res.* 2011;55.

27. Finegold SM. Therapy and epidemiology of autism--clostridial spores as key elements. *Med Hypotheses.* 2008;70(3):508-11.

28. Finegold SM, Dowd SE, Gontcharova V, Liu C, Henley KE, Wolcott RD, et al. Pyrosequencing study of fecal microflora of autistic and control children. *Anaerobe.* 2010;16(4):444-53.

29. Finegold SM. State of the art; microbiology in health and disease. Intestinal bacterial flora in autism. *Anaerobe.* 2011;17(6):367-8.

30. Finegold SM. *Desulfovibrio* species are potentially important in regressive autism. *Med Hypotheses.* 2011;77(2):270-4.

31. James SJ, Cutler P, Melnyk S, Jernigan S, Janak L, Gaylor DW, et al. Metabolic biomarkers of increased oxidative stress and impaired methylation capacity in children with autism. *Am J Clin Nutr.* 2004;80(6):1611-7.

32. Waring RH, Klovrza LV. Sulphur metabolism in autism. *J Nutr Environ Med.* 2000;10:25-32.

33. Rosseneu SLM, van Saene HKF, Heusckel R, Murch SH. Abnormal throat and gut flora in children with regressive autism. Presented at International Meeting for Autism Research (IMFAR), 2002.

34. Yap IK, Angley M, Veselkov KA, Holmes E, Lindon JC, Nicholson JK. Urinary metabolic phenotyping differentiates children with autism from their unaffected siblings and age-matched controls. *J Proteome Res.* 2010;9(6):2996-3004.

35. Parracho HMRT, Gibson GR, Knott F, Bosscher D, Kleerebezem M, McCartney AL. A double-blind, placebo-controlled, crossover-designed probiotic feeding study in children diagnosed with autistic spectrum disorders. *International Journal of Probiotics and Prebiotics.* 2010;5(2):69-74.

36. Adams JB, Johansen LJ, Powell LD, Quig D, Rubin RA. Gastrointestinal flora and gastrointestinal status in children with autism--comparisons to typical children and correlation with autism severity. *BMC Gastroenterol.* 2011;11:22.

37. Williams BL, Hornig M, Buie T, Bauman ML, Cho PM, Wick I, et al. Impaired carbohydrate digestion and transport and mucosal dysbiosis in the intestines of children with autism and gastrointestinal disturbances. *PLoS ONE.* 2011;6(9):e24585.

38. Chess S. Follow-up report on autism in congenital rubella. *J Autism Child Schizophr.* 1977;7(1):69-81.

39. Chess S. Autism in children with congenital rubella. *J Autism Child Schizophr.* 1971;1(1):33-47.

40. Atladottir HO, Thorsen P, Ostergaard L, Schendel DE, Lemcke S, Abdallah M, et al. Maternal infection requiring hospitalization during pregnancy and autism spectrum disorders. *J Autism Dev Disord.* 2010;40(12):1423-30.

41. Patterson PH. *Infectious Behavior: Brain-Immune Connections in Autism, Schizophrenia, and Depression,* 1st ed. Cambridge, MA: The MIT Press, 2011.

42. Pardo CA, Vargas DL, Zimmerman AW. Immunity, neuroglia and neuroinflammation in autism. *Int Rev Psychiatry.* 2005;17(6):485-95.

43. Campbell DB, Warren D, Sutcliffe JS, Lee EB, Levitt P. Association of MET with social and communication phenotypes in individuals with autism spectrum disorder. *Am J Med Genet B Neuropsychiatr Genet.* 2010;153B(2):438-46.

44. Finegold SM, Downes J, Summanen PH. Microbiology of regressive autism. *Anaerobe* 2011 Dec 22. [Epub ahead of print]

45. Rowland LP, Shneider NA. Amyotrophic lateral sclerosis. *N Engl J Med.* 2001;344(22):1688-1700.

46. Haley RW. Excess incidence of ALS in young Gulf War veterans. *Neurology.* 2003;61(6):750-6.

47. Horner RD, Kamins KG, Feussner JR, Grambow SC, Hoff-Lindquist J, Harati Y, et al. Occurrence of amyotrophic lateral sclerosis among Gulf War veterans. *Neurology.* 2003;61(6):742-9.

48. Coffman CJ, Horner RD, Grambow SC, Lindquist J. Estimating the occurrence of amyotrophic lateral sclerosis among Gulf War (1990-1991) veterans using capture-recapture methods. *Neuroepidemiology.* 2005;24(3):141-50.

49. Longstreth WT Jr, Meschke JS, Davidson SK, Smoot LM, Smoot JC, Koepsell TD. Hypothesis: a motor neuron toxin produced by a clostridial species residing in gut causes ALS. *Med Hypotheses.* 2005;64(6):1153-6.

50. Logan AC, Rao AV, Irani D. Chronic fatique syndrome: lactic acid bacteria may be of therapeutic value. *Med Hypotheses.* 2003;60(6):915-23.

51. Rao AV, Bested AC, Beaulne TM, Katzman MA, Iorio C, Berardi JM, et al. A randomized, double-blind, placebo-controlled pilot study of a probiotic in emotional symptoms of chronic fatigue syndrome. *Gut Pathog.* 2009;1(1):6.

52. Fremont M, Metzger K, Rady H, Hulstaert J, De MK. Detection of herpesviruses and parvovirus B19 in gastric and intestinal mucosa of chronic fatigue syndrome patients. *In Vivo.* 2009;23(2):209-13.

53. Sullivan A, Nord CE, Evengard B. Effect of supplement with lactic-acid producing bacteria on fatigue and physical activity in patients with chronic fatigue syndrome. *Nutr J.* 2009;8:4.

54. Sheedy JR, Wettenhall RE, Scanlon D, Gooley PR, Lewis DP, McGregor N, et al. Increased d-lactic acid intestinal bacteria in patients with chronic fatigue syndrome. *In Vivo.* 2009;23(4):621-8.

55. Dowlati Y, Herrmann N, Swardfager W, Liu H, Sham L, Reim EK, et al. A meta-analysis of cytokines in major depression. *Biol Psychiatry.* 2010;67(5):446-57.

56. Peet M. International variations in the outcome of schizophrenia and the prevalence of depression in relation to national dietary practices: an ecological analysis. *Br J Psychiatry.* 2004;184:404-8.

57. Desbonnet L, Garrett L, Clarke G, Bienenstock J, Dinan TG. The probiotic *Bifidobacteria infantis*: an assessment of potential antidepressant properties in the rat. *J Psychiatr Res.* 2008;43(2):164-74.

58. Stolberg L, Rolfe R, Gitlin N, Merritt J, Mann L, Jr., Linder J, et al. d-Lactic acidosis due to abnormal gut flora: diagnosis and treatment of two cases. *N Engl J Med.* 1982;306(22):1344-8.

59. Clauw DJ, Arnold LM, McCarberg BH. The science of fibromyalgia. *Mayo Clin Proc.* 2011;86(9):907-11.

60. Kang HK, Mahan CM, Lee KY, Magee CA, Murphy FM. Illnesses among United States veterans of the Gulf War: a population-based survey of 30,000 veterans. *J Occup Environ Med.* 2000;42(5):491-501.

61. Kang HK, Ma BL, Mahan CM, Eisen SA, Engel CC. Health of US veterans of 1991 Gulf War: a follow-up survey in 10 years. *J Occup Environ Med.* 2009;51(4):401-10.

62. Fukuda K, Nisenbaum R, Stewart G, Thompson WW, Robin L, Washko RM. et al. Chronic multisymptom illness affecting Air Force veterans of the Gulf War. *JAMA.* 1998;280(11):981-8.

63. Nicolson GL, Rosenberg-Nicolson NL. Doxycycline treatment and Desert Storm. *JAMA*. 1995;273(8):618-9.

64. Nicolson GL, Nasralla MY, Haier J, Pomfret J. High frequency of systemic mycoplasmal infections in Gulf War veterans and civilians with Amyotrophic Lateral Sclerosis (ALS). *J Clin Neurosci*. 2002;9(5):525-9.

65. Collins JF, Donta ST, Engel CC, Baseman JB, Dever LL, Taylor T, et al. The antibiotic treatment trial of Gulf War veterans' illnesses: issues, design, screening, and baseline characteristics. *Control Clin Trials*. 2002;23(3):333-53.

66. Donta ST, Engel CC, Jr., Collins JF, Baseman JB, Dever LL, Taylor T, et al. Benefits and harms of doxycycline treatment for Gulf War veterans' illnesses: a randomized, double-blind, placebo-controlled trial. *Ann Intern Med*. 2004;141(2):85-94.

67. Pimentel M, Chow EJ, Lin HC. Eradication of small intestinal bacterial overgrowth reduces symptoms of irritable bowel syndrome. *Am J Gastroenterol*. 2000;95(12):3503-6.

68. Pall ML, Satterlee JD. Elevated nitric oxide/peroxynitrite mechanism for the common etiology of multiple chemical sensitivity, chronic fatigue syndrome, and posttraumatic stress disorder. *Ann N Y Acad Sci*. 2001;933:323-9.

69. McFadden SA. Phenotypic variation in xenobiotic metabolism and adverse environmental response: focus on sulfur-dependent detoxification pathways. *Toxicology*. 1996;111(1-3):43-65.

70. Berer K, Mues M, Koutrolos M, Rasbi ZA, Boziki M, Johner C, et al. Commensal microbiota and myelin autoantigen cooperate to trigger autoimmune demyelination. *Nature*. 2011;479(7374):538-41.

71. Lee YK, Menezes JS, Umesaki Y, Mazmanian SK. Proinflammatory T-cell responses to gut microbiota promote experimental autoimmune encephalomyelitis. *Proc Natl Acad Sci U S A*. 2011;108(Suppl 1):4615-22.

72. Nichols FC, Yao X, Bajrami B, Downes J, Finegold SM, Knee E, et al. Phosphorylated dihydroceramides from common human bacteria are recovered in human tissues. *PLoS ONE*. 2011;6(2):e16771.

73. Westall FC. Molecular mimicry revisited: gut bacteria and multiple sclerosis. *J Clin Microbiol*. 2006;44(6):2099-104.

74. Ebringer A, Rashid T, Wilson C. Bovine spongiform encephalopathy, multiple sclerosis, and creutzfeldt-jakob disease are probably autoimmune diseases evoked by *Acinetobacter bacteria*. *Ann N Y Acad Sci*. 2005;1050:417-28.

75. Steinman L, Utz PJ, Robinson WH. Suppression of autoimmunity via microbial mimics of altered peptide ligands. *Curr Top Microbiol Immunol*. 2005;296:55-63.

76. Cantorna MT, Hayes CE, Deluca HF. 1,25-Dihydroxyvitamin D3 reversibly blocks the progression of relapsing encephalomyelitis, a model of multiple sclerosis. *Proc Natl Acad Sci U S A*. 1996;93(15):7861-4.

77. O'Callaghan E, Gibson T, Colohan HA, Walshe D, Buckley P, Larkin C, et al. Season of birth in schizophrenia. Evidence for confinement of an excess of winter births to patients without a family history of mental disorder. *Br J Psychiatry*. 1991;158:764-9.

78. Mednick SA, Huttunen MO, Machon RA. Prenatal influenza infections and adult schizophrenia. *Schizophr Bull*. 1994;20(2):263-7.

79. Mittal VA, Ellman LM, Cannon TD. Gene-environment interaction and covariation in schizophrenia: the role of obstetric complications. *Schizophr Bull*. 2008;34(6):1083-94.

80. Jones-Brando L, Torrey EF, Yolken R. Drugs used in the treatment of schizophrenia and bipolar disorder inhibit the replication of *Toxoplasma gondii*. *Schizophr Res*. 2003;62(3):237-44.

81. Leff J, Sartorius N, Jablensky A, Korten A, Ernberg G. The International Pilot Study of Schizophrenia: five-year follow-up findings. *Psychol Med*. 1992;22(1):131-45.

82. Dohan FC. Cereals and schizophrenia data and hypothesis. *Acta Psychiatr Scand*. 1966;42(2):125-52.

83. Dohan FC, Harper EH, Clark MH, Rodrigue RB, Zigas V. Is schizophrenia rare if grain is rare? *Biol Psychiatry*. 1984;19(3):385-99.

84. Kalaydjian AE, Eaton W, Cascella N, Fasano A. The gluten connection: the association between schizophrenia and celiac disease. *Acta Psychiatr Scand*. 2006;113(2):82-90.

85. Puri BK, Richardson AJ, Horrobin DF, Easton T, Saeed N, Oatridge A, et al. Eicosapentaenoic acid treatment in schizophrenia associated with symptom remission, normalisation of blood fatty acids, reduced neuronal membrane phospholipid turnover and structural brain changes. *Int J Clin Pract*. 2000;54(1):57-63.

86. Fridl M. University of Florida researchers cite possible link between autism, schizophrenia and diet. *Science Daily*. March 16, 1999. Available online at: http://www.sciencedaily.com/releases/1999/03/990316103010.htm

87. Nussbaum RL, Ellis CE. Alzheimer's disease and Parkinson's disease. *N Engl J Med*. 2003;348:1356-64.

88. Reisberg B, Doody R, Stoffler A, Schmitt F, Ferris S, Mobius HJ. Memantine in moderate-to-severe Alzheimer's disease. *N Engl J Med*. 2003;348:1333-41.

89. Selkoe D. Alzheimer disease: mechanistic understanding predicts new therapies. *Ann Intern Med*. 2004;140:627-38.

90. Hardy J, Selkoe DJ. The amyloid hypothesis of Alzheimer's disease: progress and problems on the road to therapeutics. *Science*. 2002;297:353-6.

91. Clark CM, Karlawish JHT. Alzheimer disease: current concepts and emerging diagnostic and therapeutic strategies. *Ann Intern Med*. 2003;138:400-10.

92. Ono K, Hasegawa K, Naiki H, Yamada M. Curcumin has potent anti-amyloidogenic effects for Alzheimer's beta-amyloid fibrils in vitro. *J Neurosci Res*. 2004;75(6):742-50.

93. Grundman M, Delaney P. Antioxidant strategies for Alzheimer's disease. *Proc Nutr Soc*. 2002;61:191-202.

94. Loeb MB, Molloy D, Smieja M, Standish T, Goldsmith CH, Mahony J, et al. A randomized, controlled trial of doxycycline and rifampin for patients with Alzheimer's disease. *J Am Geriatr Soc*. 2004;52(3):381-7.

95. Huang DB, DuPont HL. Rifaximin--a novel antimicrobial for enteric infections. *J Infect*. 2005;50(2):97-106.

96. Gerard L, Garey KW, DuPont HL. Rifaximin: a nonabsorbable rifamycin antibiotic for use in nonsystemic gastrointestinal infections. *Expert Rev Anti Infect Ther*. 2005;3(2):201-11.

97. Scarpignato C, Pelosini I. Rifaximin, a poorly absorbed antibiotic: pharmacology and clinical potential. *Chemotherapy*. 2005;51(Suppl 1):36-66.

98. Prasad KN, Hovland AR, La Rosa FG, Hovland PG. Prostaglandins as putative neurotoxins in Alzheimer's disease. *Proc Soc Exp Biol Med*. 1998;219(2):120-5.

99. Chapman MR, Robinson LS, Hultgren SJ. *Escherichia coli's* how-to guide for forming amyloid. *ASM News*. 2003;69(3):121-6.

100. Noguchi H, Ohta M, Wakasugi S, Noguchi K, Nakamura N, Nakamura O, et al. Effect of the intestinal flora on amyloid deposition in a transgenic mouse model of familial amyloidotic polyneuropathy. *Exp Anim.* 2002;51(4):309-16.

101. de Souza RR, Moratelli HB, Borges N, Liberti EA. Age-induced nerve cell loss in the myenteric plexus of the small intestine in man. *Gerontology.* 1993;39(4):183-8.

102. Gomes OA, de Souza RR, Liberti EA. A preliminary investigation of the effects of aging on the nerve cell number in the myenteric ganglia of the human colon. *Gerontology.* 1997;43(4):210-7.

103. Qu K, Lee SW, Bian JS, Low CM, Wong PT. Hydrogen sulfide: neurochemistry and neurobiology. *Neurochem Int.* 2008;52(1-2):155-65.

104. Kamoun P. Endogenous production of hydrogen sulfide in mammals. *Amino Acids.* 2004;26(3):243-54.

105. McKhann GM, Knopman DS, Chertkow H, Hyman BT, Jack CR Jr, Kawas CH, et al. The diagnosis of dementia due to Alzheimer's disease: recommendations from the National Institute on Aging-Alzheimer's Association workgroups on diagnostic guidelines for Alzheimer's disease. *Alzheimers Dement.* 2011;7(3):263-9.

106. Jack CR Jr, Albert MS, Knopman DS, McKhann GM, Sperling RA, Carrillo MC, et al. Introduction to the recommendations from the National Institute on Aging-Alzheimer's Association workgroups on diagnostic guidelines for Alzheimer's disease. *Alzheimers Dement.* 2011;7(3):257-62.

107. Albert MS, DeKosky ST, Dickson D, Dubois B, Feldman HH, Fox NC, et al. The diagnosis of mild cognitive impairment due to Alzheimer's disease: recommendations from the National Institute on Aging-Alzheimer's Association workgroups on diagnostic guidelines for Alzheimer's disease. *Alzheimers Dement.* 2011;7(3):270-9.

CHAPTER TEN

GASTROINTESTINAL BALANCE AND NEUROTRANSMITTER FORMATION

By Amy Yasko, PhD, AMD, FAAIM, and Nancy Mullan, MD

The complexity of the gastrointestinal tract

Over the past few decades, research has significantly changed the way that scientists understand gastrointestinal (GI) function and dysfunction. We have come to recognize that the GI tract is, in fact, far more subtle and complex than initially thought. Studies have illuminated how the complex interaction of the immune system, the neuroendocrine system, and the microbial environment within the gut affects not only GI function but also the function of other organs and systems in the body, most notably the brain and nervous system. We now understand that body systems and organs function within a web of physiology and biochemistry, and we no longer consider each system as discrete and isolated from the others.

During this same time period, autism spectrum disorders (ASDs)—consisting of autism, pervasive developmental disorder (PDD), attention-deficit disorder (ADD), and attention-deficit/hyperactivity disorder (ADHD)—have been acknowledged as multifactorial conditions. A number of causal factors must come together to create the constellation of symptoms that result in a diagnosis of one or several of these conditions. Prominent among these factors is GI dysfunction.[1-3] The investigation of how the gastrointestinal environment and its function influence the central nervous system and other neurologic functions is, therefore, particularly pertinent.

Bäckhed and colleagues[4] describe the human gut microbiome (the microbial community that resides in the intestine) as follows:

The adult human intestine is home to an almost inconceivable number of microorganisms. The size of the population—up to 100 trillion—far exceeds that of all other microbial communities associated with the body's surfaces and is ~10 times greater than the total number of our somatic and germ cells. Thus, it seems appropriate to view ourselves as a composite of many species and our genetic landscape as an amalgam of genes embedded in our Homo sapiens genome and in the genomes of our affiliated microbial partners (the microbiome).

Our gut microbiota can be pictured as a microbial organ placed within a host organ. It is composed of different cell lineages with a capacity to communicate with one another and the host; it mediates physiologically important chemical transformations; and it can manage and repair itself through self-replication. The gut microbiome, which may contain >100 times the number of genes in our genome, endows us with functional features that we have not had to evolve ourselves. (p. 1915)

Colonization of the newborn's GI tract starts immediately after birth. The earliest bacteria colonized can modulate the expression of genes in the host epithelial cells, thus creating a favorable environment for themselves. This can prevent the growth of other bacteria introduced at a later time. Therefore, this initial colonization is very relevant to the final composition of the adult individual's flora.[5] The predominant intestinal mucosa-associated bacterial community is host-specific and significantly different from the fecal bacterial community.[6]

Gastrointestinal mucus serves as a matrix for the flora contained in the GI tract.[7] The integrity of the mucosal barrier is maintained by a single layer of tightly fitted epithelial cells called enterocytes that comprise a surface area greater than 400 square meters, which is 200 times greater than the surface of the skin. Approximately 70 percent of the body's immune system is present in specialized lymphatic compartments within the GI mucosa and in the intercellular spaces along its epithelium. Experimental evidence demonstrates that the gastrointestinal mucosal immune system functions separately from the bloodborne (e.g., white blood cells and immunoglobulins) immune system.[8] It is significant to note that the gastrointestinal tract houses a separate immune system – the enteric immune system.

In the remainder of this chapter, we discuss factors contributing to chronic microbial imbalance in the gastrointestinal tract and review some of the microorganisms (such as clostridia, streptococci, and *Helicobacter pylori*) that can have far-reaching effects when out of balance. We focus, in particular, on the influence of pathogenic organisms on neurotransmitter formation because of the essential role of neurotransmitters as the body's chemical messengers.

What causes chronic microbial imbalance

Gut mucosal integrity can be compromised by a number of factors, including chronic microbial imbalance (dysbiosis), inflammation, and immune system dysregulation. Dysbiosis can produce mucosal damage, and the accompanying inflammatory processes may lead to a disruption in microvilli function and gut permeability. These, in turn, can manifest as gluten, casein, and/or lactose intolerance; food allergies or intolerance; abdominal pain and discomfort; or abnormal bowel function. Non-GI-related symptoms can also appear, such as headaches, skin irritations, chronic joint pain, anxiety, or depression.

Imbalances in the flora of the GI tract may begin as early as birth. Maternal streptococci, for example, can be transmitted from the mother to the neonate during delivery. Although researchers originally believed that transmission occurred solely via vaginal delivery,[9] more recent data suggest that streptococcal infection can also occur in infants who have been delivered via cesarean section.[10] The rate of mother-to-infant transmission of streptococci during vaginal delivery is between 20 and 30 percent.

Increased gut acidity also can predispose to microbial imbalance. Some of the factors that contribute to increased gut acidity and gut flora imbalances include vitamin B12 deficiency, decreased pancreatic or liver function, genetics/blood type, and antibiotic use.

Vitamin B12 deficiency: Intrinsic factor, a substrate produced by the gastric lining, is necessary for the uptake of vitamin B12 by the small intestine. Sufficient stomach acid is necessary for intrinsic factor activation. The secretion of stomach acid and the secretion of intrinsic factor parallel one another,[11] and loss of gastric secreting cells decreases both intrinsic factor and stomach acid.[12] Proton pump inhibitors, a group of drugs widely used for peptic ulcer disease and other hyperacidic conditions, antagonize stomach acid levels and lead to decreases in intrinsic factor and decreased uptake of B12.[13] A significant lack of B12 has been found in autism, irrespective of age.[14] Efforts by the body to increase B12 levels lead to increased intrinsic factor and would be expected to increase stomach acid.[13,15] While the growth of many bacteria is inhibited in an acidic (low pH) environment, streptococci are among those bacteria that can survive and flourish at a lower pH.[16] Increased stomach acid secondary to B12 deficiency, therefore, leads to a gut environment that predisposes to the growth of streptococci and other pathogenic bacteria that can survive in an acid milieu, such as *Escherichia coli* (*E. coli*).[16,17]

Decreased pancreatic or liver function: One of the roles of bile is to neutralize stomach acid. Lack of bile due to decreased pancreatic or liver function contributes to an acidic gut environment. Impairments in liver or pancreatic function due to toxin overload or infectious diseases such as rubella (which is known to infect the pancreas), therefore, decrease the body's ability to neutralize excess acid.

Genetics and blood type: Genetics and blood type can predispose to colonization with streptococci. For example, single nucleotide polymorphisms (SNPs) that decrease the level of B12 in the body can contribute to an environment that is conducive to the growth of streptococci. Blood type also appears to play a role, which may be related in part to the increased acidity seen in those with blood type O.[18] Effects of different carbohydrate groupings on the surface of blood cells of varying blood types may also have an impact on the ability of streptococci to aggregate in the system.[19]

Antibiotics: Normal flora help to protect the gut from the growth of pathogenic organisms. Antibiotic use is well known to cause imbalances in normal gut flora. The use of antibiotics without concurrent addition of probiotics, therefore, can predispose to the growth of streptococci as well as other pathogenic organisms such as clostridia. Fecal flora studies of children with ASD have found that the number of clostridial species are greater and the clostridial counts higher in ASD children when compared with controls.[1,3]

Clostridial and other species

Clostridia are spore-forming, Gram-positive anaerobes. The growth of anaerobes is inhibited or significantly slowed in the presence of oxygen. The dearth of oxygen in the lumen of the small and large intestines predisposes this environment to the growth of anaerobic organisms. There are more than 50 species of clostridia, a number of which cause significant illness. To name only a few examples, *Clostridium botulinum* (*C. botulinum*) causes botulism, *C. perfringens* causes gas gangrene and food poisoning, *C. tetani* causes tetanus, and *C. difficile* causes pseudomembranous colitis. Table 1 provides a more comprehensive list of the many conditions associated with clostridial infection.

C. *difficile* is most often found in the gut and is part of the normal GI flora in 2-10 percent of humans.[20] However, the suppression of normal GI flora that accompanies oral antibiotic use allows *C. difficile* to proliferate and produce cytopathic toxins and enterotoxins that are disruptive to cells and the intestine. The range of symptoms that C. *difficile* infection can cause is significant. Symptoms vary from diarrhea alone to marked diarrhea and necrosis of the GI mucosa with accumulation of inflammatory cells and fibrin.[20]

The *C. difficile* organism is resistant to most commonly used antibiotics. This is because many antibiotics work by interrupting an aspect of the target organism's growth cycle, and this kind of antibiotic is less effective with slow-growing organisms such as C. *difficile*. Although laboratories are required to label some growth of the C. *difficile* organism as "normal," if it is growing in an individual who does not have sufficient methionine and folate cycle activity to produce T and B cells for adaptive immune function, then any growth of C. *difficile* can be pathogenic. This also includes individuals who are immunocompromised, have heavy metal toxicity, or who have viruses, bacteria, and fungi in their systems.

Similar patterns hold true for organisms other than clostridia. Many organisms normally found in the gut can become pathogenic in the face of poor methionine and folate cycle function, insufficient

Table 1. Selected conditions associated with clostridial infections

Agent	Condition	Toxin
C. perfringens	Soft-tissue infection: crepitant cellulitis, myositis, clostridial myonecrosis	α-toxin (others)
	Hemolysis	Phospholipase C α-toxin
	Muscle necrosis	θ-toxin
Enteric diseases		
C. perfringens type A	Food poisoning	Enterotoxin
C. perfringens type C	Enteritis necroticans	β-toxin
C. difficile	Antibiotic-associated colitis	Toxin A
C. septicum (others)	Neutropenic enterocolitis	Unknown, possibly β-toxin
C. septicum	Colorectal malignancy	
	Hemolysis by septicolysine	δ-toxin
	Tissue necrosis	α-toxin
	DNA lysis by DNase	β-toxin
	Hyaluronan lysis by hyaluronilase	γ-toxin
Neurologic syndromes		
C. tetani	Tetanus	Tetanospasmin
C. botulinum	Botulism	Botulinal toxins A-G
C. perfringens, C. ramosum (many others)	Abdominal infections: Cholecystitis, peritonitis, ruptured appendix, bowel perforation, neutropenic enterocolitis	β-toxin

Source: Beers MH, Berkow R (Eds.). Anaerobic bacteria: clostridial infections. *In The Merck Manual of Diagnosis and Therapy*, 17th edition (section 13, page 1176). West Point, PA: Merck & Co., Inc., 1999.

immune function, and high total toxic burden. For example, some streptococci are normally present in the gut, but because of the host's physiologic status, the organism's presence may become pathogenic.

Impact of clostridial and other species on neurotransmitter formation
It is hard to overstate the negative impact of bacterial infection on the formation of neurotransmitters. Chronic infections induce T cell activation, cytokine formation, and macrophage activation, increasing oxidative stress, which impairs neurotransmitter formation (Figure 1).

Dihydroxyphenylpropionic acid (DHPPA) is a marker for bacterial infection with clostridial species,[21] *Pseudomonas* species,[22] and *E. coli.*[23] The production of DHPPA that results from infection with these bacteria may reduce formation of the neurotransmitter dopamine through its depletion of the enzyme tyrosinase.[24] There are two pathways for

Figure 1. The impact of infection on neurotransmitter formation

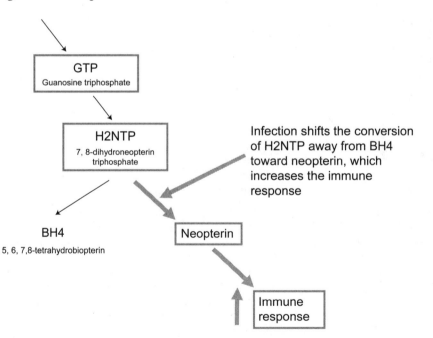

The effect of infection overall is to increase oxidative stress, which in itself impairs the production of BH4 and hence neurotransmitters. Beyond this, the consequence of the T cell activation, cytokine production, and macrophage activation that accompany infection is to shift the conversion of H2NTP from BH4 to neopterin, which increases the immune response.

dopamine synthesis in the body. In the primary pathway, phenylalanine is hydroxylated to tyrosine in a reaction catalyzed by phenylalanine hydroxylase. This reaction is dependent on tetrahydrobiopterin (BH4) (see Figure 2). The resulting tyrosine is hydroxylated to L-DOPA (3,4-dihydroxyphenylalanine) by the enzyme tyrosine hydroxylase in a second BH4-dependent reaction. L-DOPA is then decarboxylated in a reaction catalyzed by aromatic acid decarboxylase to synthesize dopamine. Dopamine is the substrate for the subsequent synthesis of the catecholamines norepinephrine and epinephrine.

This primary pathway for dopamine synthesis can be compromised by a number of factors. For example, microbes can increase the serum phenylalanine-tyrosine ratio, which inhibits the first step in the pathway. Besides inhibiting this pathway, high levels of phenylalanine may also cause a drop in serotonin and/or GABA (gamma-aminobutyric acid), which may result in obsessive-compulsive disorder (OCD) behaviors.[25]

Figure 2. The primary pathway for dopamine synthesis

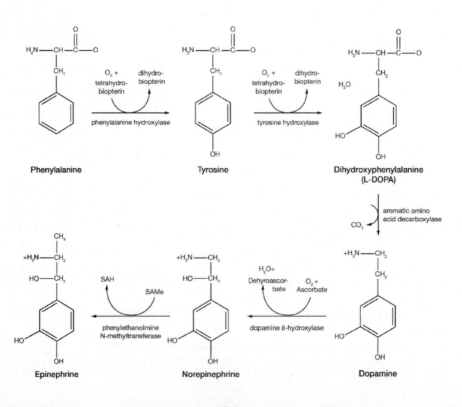

The exigencies of tyrosine hydroxylase activity also have an impact on this dopamine synthesis pathway.[26-28] If levels of norepinephrine and epinephrine increase as the result of stressors (including infections), feedback inhibition on tyrosine hydroxylase will result. Increased glutamate also decreases tyrosine hydroxylase activity. Glutamate (via NMDA receptors) and dopamine (via D2 receptors) decrease tyrosine hydroxlase phosphorylation by decreasing cAMP, a messenger derived from adenosine triphosphate (ATP) that is important in many biological processes. Because tyrosine hydroxylase activity is stimulated by phosphorylation, a situation of decreased tyrosine hydroxylase phosphorylation leads to decreased enzyme activity and lower levels of dopamine.[29]

The levels of BH4 in the body are critical to both dopamine and serotonin synthesis. However, BH4 is a vulnerable molecule and can be deficient for a number of reasons, some of which involve gut bacteria. As a substrate for various reactions, BH4 is especially subject to depletion. Biopterin deficiency will reduce available BH4, as will oxidative stress. In addition, the presence of aluminum or lead inhibits the activity of dihydrobiopterin reductase, which catalyzes BH4 synthesis from dihydrobiopterin (BH2). BH4 levels also are profoundly decreased by infection because the body's immune response produces neopterin, which reduces the production of BH4 (see Figure 1). Finally, individuals with MTHFR A1298C mutations may have a reduced ability to synthesize BH4.[30] The product of the MTHFR enzyme reaction, 5-methyltetrahydrofolate, has been shown to be directly related to BH4 levels[31-33] and to be reversible, with BH4 production being the outcome of the reverse reaction.[34-36]

Although the primary sequence for dopamine production is through the pathway shown in Figure 2, this pathway may not always function. Alternatively, the enzyme tyrosinase can act on tyrosine to produce L-DOPA in a one-step process,[37] following which aromatic acid decarboxylase can act on L-DOPA to produce dopamine. This alternative pathway is able to circumvent the blockages that can result from problems with phenylalanine levels, tyrosine hydroxylase activity, lack of BH4, or oxidative stress. With the depletion of tyrosinase that results from bacterial infection-induced production of DHPPA, however, both the primary and the secondary pathways for the production of dopamine can be compromised. In addition, the production of norepinephrine and epinephrine are likely to be decreased because dopamine subsequently converts to norephinephrine and ephinephrine.

Biofilms and streptococci

A biofilm is a community of one or several diverse species of organisms that firmly fix to a surface and grow within a self-produced polymer matrix. Ultimately, the group of organisms begins to function as a unit. The community aspect of biofilm formations offers a number of advantages, including protection from hostile environmental conditions and the opportunity to sequester nutritional resources. In addition, a microbial community offers the possibility for a variety of different organisms (bacteria, fungi, viruses, and single-celled parasites) to live together, exchange genetic information, communicate through chemical signaling, act cooperatively, and, in so doing, enhance their own survival and the survival of the collective. It has come to be recognized that the formation of biofilms is the preferred form of growth for organisms, whereas growth of planktonic (single-celled or free-floating) organisms is an artifact of *in vitro* culture.[38] Certain organisms have evolved genetically to be viable only in a biofilm.[39] The take-home message here is that organisms don't really live on their own in nature – they live in communities.

Biofilms can form quickly. In a human body that is experiencing nutrient depletion or high oxidative stress, *E. coli* bacteria can activate genes that form biofilms in a variety of environments within 24 hours.[40-42] In ASD patients, in particular, the GI tract is a natural place for biofilms to form; the lack of cell-mediated immunity in these patients predisposes them to biofilm growth. Moreover, the range of GI symptoms caused by biofilms is clearly identifiable in the ASD population.[2]

Among many other organisms, streptococci have been identified in biofilms. This form of organization gives streptococci an adaptational advantage and the capacity to thrive in a wide range of pH conditions and environments in which they otherwise would not survive.[43] Generally, bacteria elicit a B-cell-mediated immune response and viruses a T-cell-mediated immune response. Streptococci, however, prompt the elaboration of a large number of extracellular toxins, all of which have the ability to nonspecifically stimulate T cells. Once an immune response is mounted against streptococcal species, therefore, the response involves both B cells and T cells, resulting in a major inflammatory reaction. In addition, streptococcal infection increases the production of hydrogen peroxide (H2O2), thereby increasing oxidative stress in the body, and depletes the peroxidase enzyme necessary for the production of thyroid hormone, possibly reducing levels of thyroxine (T4) and triiodothyronine (T3).[44] This and other consequences of streptococcal infection are summarized in Figure 3.

Figure 3. Consequences of streptococcal infection

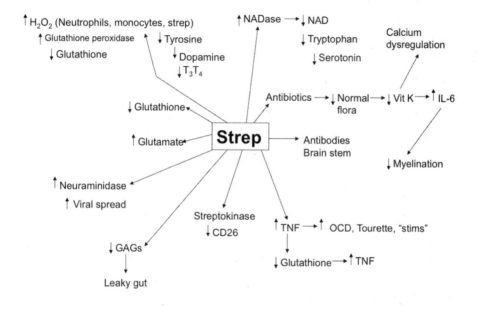

Several species of streptococci are well characterized as causing neuropsychiatric symptoms[45] and contributing to disorders such as autism and anorexia nervosa.[46] Autoantibodies to group A streptococcal sugar moieties are implicated in OCD, Tourette syndrome, chronic tic disorders, ADHD, and Sydenham chorea, a neuropsychiatric complication of rheumatic fever.[47,48] Sydenham chorea is one of the best examples of postinfectious autoimmunity produced by molecular mimicry (when molecules are similar and the body confuses an invader with the body's own tissue) between host and antigen. Following a pharyngeal infection with group A *Streptococcus*, chorea antibodies produced in response to a group A streptococcal carbohydrate target the surface of human neuronal cells, producing abrupt, spontaneous movements of the face and extremities, OCD behaviors, hyperactivity, emotional lability, and other psychiatric symptoms.[47] The binding of cross-reacting antibodies to human basal ganglia results in changes to neuronal signaling transduction and neurotransmitter synthesis and release.[46]

Infection with group A beta-hemolytic *Streptococcus* (GABHS) can result in a pediatric syndrome labeled as pediatric autoimmune neuropsychiatric disorders associated with streptococcal infections (PANDAS). Individuals with PANDAS develop tics, OCD symptoms, and, in some cases, psychosis, without the comorbid chorea component. When sera from GABHS-immunized mice were tested for immunoreactivity to mouse brain, a subset was found to be immunoreactive to several brain regions, including the deep cerebellar nuclei (DCN), the globus pallidus (one of three nuclei that make up the basal ganglia), and the thalamus (involved in sensory perception and regulation of motor functions).[48] GABHS mice showing serum immunoreactivity to DCN also had increased IgG deposits in the DCN and exhibited abnormal behavior. The motoric and behavioral disturbances that result from an immune response to GABHS suggest that anti-GABHS antibodies cross-reacting with brain components are part of the pathophysiology of these disturbances.[48]

Streptococcal infection leads to elevated levels of the inflammatory cytokines TNF-alpha and NF-kB. High levels of TNF-alpha have been implicated in Tourette syndrome, facial tics, OCD behavior, and schizophrenia. The increased TNF-alpha levels that occur with streptococcal infection cause increased levels of glutamate, an excitatory neurotransmitter. When the normal processes that regulate glutamate levels malfunction and toxic levels build up in the synaptic junctions, glutamate toxicity can produce neuron loss. Moreover, the neuroinflammatory response in and of itself also contributes to glutamate excitotoxicity and neuronal loss. The two pathogenic mechanisms, glutamate excitotoxicity and neuroinflammation, seem to be linked.[49]

To remove excess glutamate, the brain requires sufficient levels of oxygen and energy. However, glutamate release leads to the release of insulin, which results in decreased glucose levels. Because the amount of glucose in the brain regulates the removal of excess glutamate from the synapses, a drop in blood glucose disrupts the removal process and allows a buildup of toxic glutamate. (Hypoglycemia or low calorie/ starvation conditions can induce a similar cycle involving glutamate release, insulin release, decreased glucose, and inability to remove excess glutamate from the brain.) Excess glutamate is problematic because it depletes glutathione. Glutathione is one of the body's most powerful antioxidants and helps to protect neurons from damage. Glutathione depletion consequently leads to the death of additional neurons. If glutamate itself were not already reducing glutathione levels, the high TNF-alpha levels resulting from streptococcal infection also would result in decreased glutathione because TNF-alpha levels are inversely correlated with glutathione levels.

The association between chronic bacterial infection and neurologic and psychiatric disorders can additionally be explained by the fact that streptococcal and other bacterial infections cause the breakdown of tryptophan, a direct precursor of serotonin. States of persistent immune activation diminish the availability of free serum tryptophan and compromise serotonin production. As immune activation accelerates tryptophan degradation, tryptophan depletion, in turn, may downregulate the immune response. In addition, a breakdown product of tryptophan degradation, quinolinic acid, begins to accumulate. Quinolinic acid is another excitotoxin and may contribute to the development of the neuropsychiatric disorders seen in the presence of chronic infection and serotonin depletion.[50]

Gut imbalances and heavy metals

Bacterial infection promotes accumulation and retention of heavy metals in the body,[51-56] which contributes to oxidative stress and impairs neurotransmitter formation. Metals may be retained in the body through several mechanisms.[51-56] We have documented the sequestration of aluminum and lead in the organisms of the microbiome and the impacts of retention of these metals at length elsewhere.[57,58] The elimination of abnormal gastrointestinal flora and excretion of the metals they retain, therefore, may be essential for proper function of the biochemical pathways in the body, along with maintenance of proper balance among the organisms that should be present in the gastrointestinal tract.[58]

Streptoccal infections act in a number of ways to retain heavy metals in the body, including sequestering metals within the cell walls of the bacteria. Another mechanism related to metal retention involves sulfhydryl groups, which ordinarily bind and eliminate toxic and heavy metals. *Streptococcus* produces an extracellular enzyme called sulfhydryl protease that is capable of cleaving these sulfhydryl groups, leading to a deficiency of sulfur-containing moieties in the body. Streptococci proliferate in the presence of iron[59] and reduce the capacity of the body to excrete this heavy metal. Iron, in turn, increases the virulence of many bacteria, including streptococci. In addition, iron is necessary for biofilm formation.[60-63] Excess iron can increase microbial imbalances in the body, including but not limited to streptococcal infections.

Aluminum is a well-documented and undisputed neurotoxin that is associated with cognitive, psychological, and motor abnormalities. Both clinical observation and animal experiments have documented neurotoxicity from excess brain exposure to aluminum,[64] which has been found in elevated levels in the brains of patients with Parkinsonism,[65-67] amyotrophic lateral sclerosis (ALS),[66,67] and Alzheimer-type dementia.[68-72] Aluminum induces encephalopathy[67,73,74] and causes neuroanatomical and neurochemical changes in the brain, including neurofilament disturbances[65,69,75-77] followed by nerve cell loss.[73,78] Primate studies have provided evidence of aluminum's ability to induce seizures.[79-82]

While staphylococci are especially prone to retaining aluminum,[54] it is likely that other bacteria also can do so. Moreover, aluminum may increase the propensity for bacteria to form a biofilm, in part because of its pro-oxidant activity.[83] It has been characterized as having direct effects on biofilm activity in other systems.[84]

Helicobacter pylori in autism spectrum disorders

Helicobacter pylori (H. pylori) is a Gram-negative, spiral-shaped bacterium that lives in the stomach and duodenum. This ulcer-causing gastric pathogen is able to colonize in the harsh acidic environment of

Figure 4. *Helicobacter pylori*

Figure 5. *H. pylori* invasion

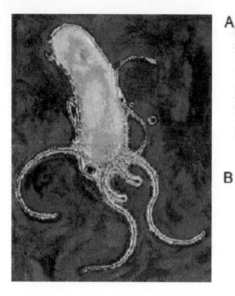

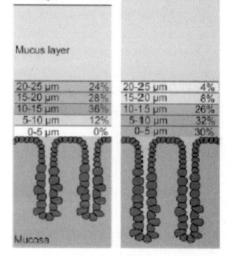

Distribution of *H. pylori* and *H. felis* in the mucus layer of mice and Mongolian gerbils. *(A)* The tissue surface of the *H. pylori*-infected gerbil depicted from the luminal side of the antrum. Several focus planes have been digitally combined, the *H. pylori* in the mucus layer subsequently highlighted in red. *(B)* The gastric mucosa and mucus of the *H. felis*-infected mouse and the *H. pylori*-infected gerbil are shown as schematic cross sections. The first 25 µm of the mucus layer on the tissue side ("juxtamucosal" mucus) are subdivided into 5 µm sections. The numbers represent the percentage of bacteria present within each section. The first 10 µm from the luminal surface is referred to as "luminal mucus," the rest of the mucus layer as "central mucus." *H. felis* was found located between 5 and 25 µm from the tissue surface. *H. pylori*, however, colonizes the whole section 0-25 µm from the tissue surface. Some *H. pylori* were attached to cells.

Source: Schreiber S, Konradt M, Groll C, Scheid P, Hanauer G, Werling HO, et al. The spatial orientation of *Helicobacter pylori* in the gastric mucus. *PNAS*. 2004;101(14):5024–9.

the human stomach. Although the stomach is protected from its own gastric juice by a thick layer of mucus that covers the stomach lining, *H. pylori* takes advantage of this protection by living in the mucus lining itself. It does so using long, whip-like flagella that facilitate locomotion through the mucus layer (see Figure 4). Although the organism is best known for its etiologic role in ulcers and impaired digestion, it also can induce vasovagal symptoms after eating, including weakness, skin pallor, profuse sweating, and sensations of loss of consciousness that resolve after eradication of the infection.[85]

In the mucus lining, *H. pylori* survives the stomach's acidic conditions by producing urease, an enzyme that catalyzes hydrolysis of urea into ammonia and bicarbonate. As strong bases, ammonia and bicarbonate produce a cloud of alkalinity around the bacterium, making it impossible for the body's normal defenses (such as T cells, natural killer cells, and other white blood cells) to get to it in the gastric mucus layer. Polymorphs, white blood cells containing a segmented nucleus that are first responders to infection sites, release superoxide radicals on stomach lining cells in an increasing inflammatory response. Other factors that contribute to *H. pylori* colonization of the gastric mucosa include adhesins, molecules that make the bacteria adhere to the mucosa, and genes encoding proteins with chemotaxis into the mucus.[86,87] Incidentally—but importantly— *H. pylori* infection increases TNF-alpha levels. The organism binds to the mucin and uses it to burrow into the cells lining the mucosal layer to create an infection.[88] It very deeply infects those cells and is distributed evenly throughout (see Figure 5).

H. pylori uses the gastric mucus pH gradient for chemotactic orientation.[89] When there is a low pH at the gastric mucosal surface, the bacterium orients itself toward the mucosa. When the gradient is eliminated, the bacterium loses its orientation (Figure 6). Binding of *H. pylori* has been found to be 4 times higher at an acidic pH of 5.4 than at a more alkaline pH of 7.4.[90] Using betaine hydrochloride to facilitate digestion may, therefore, be counterproductive because it actually creates a gastric environment in which *H. pylori* has improved binding capacities.

Because *H. pylori* burrows into the mucus layer of the stomach and is very persistent there, it is difficult to get a positive test for it even

Figure 6. Loss of *H. pylori* orientation

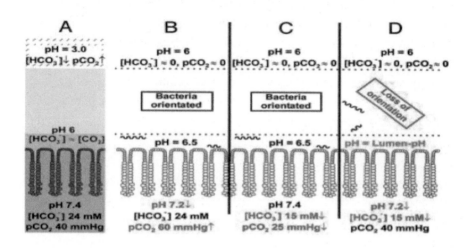

pH and bicarbonate/CO_2 gradients. Shown are the alterations made in the interdependent pH, bicarbonate, and CO_2 concentrations in the mucus layer. *(A)* The normal conditions with a low luminal pH of 3 in either the infected or the uninfected mucosa. This luminal pH induces a pH of 6 in the juxtamucosal mucus. Under these conditions, secreted bicarbonate and diffused CO_2 have the same concentration in the juxtamucosal mucus, whereas at the luminal side of the mucus layer, the bicarbonate concentration is low and the pCO_2 high. The neutralization of the juxtamucosal mucus to pH 6 is caused by active bicarbonate secretion and a neutral pH in the newly secreted mucus. *(B-D)*. To eliminate the pH bicarbonate/CO_2 gradient, the luminal pH was neutralized to 6, and three different constellations of arterial pH, bicarbonate and CO_2 were tested. *(B)*. The first alteration of the gradient was achieved by doubling the inspiratory CO_2 fraction, bicarbonate concentrations maintained at normal values through dialysis. This caused a low arterial pH with a normal bicarbonate concentration. *(C)*. In the second constellation, a reduced arterial bicarbonate concentration was combined with a normal pH. This was achieved by reducing the arterial pCO_2 through hyperventilation and lowering the bicarbonate concentration through dialysis. Neither the first nor the second alteration affected bacterial orientation. *(D)*. However, a combined reduction of arterial pH and bicarbonate concentration through dialysis caused a loss of bacterial orientation, the bacteria spreading over the entire mucus layer.

Source: Schreiber S, Konradt M, Groll C, Scheid P, Hanauer G, Werling HO, et al. The spatial orientation of *Helicobacter pylori* in the gastric mucus. *PNAS*. 2004;101(14):5024–9.

when it is present. In addition, *H. pylori* can remain for long periods of time and is extremely difficult to eradicate. One of us (Yasko) has developed laboratory indicators and biochemical markers for this organism, which show that *H. pylori* is positive in a high percentage of ASD and other chronically ill patients. *H. pylori* is, in fact, a critical piece of the ASD puzzle. Many factors that we have been dealing with in autism for a long time are related to *H. pylori*, including problems with gluten and casein, breakdown of glutathione, excess stomach acid, and the high norepinephrine seen in ADD and ADHD. All of these factors can be accounted for by the presence of *H. pylori* and, additionally, can act to increase *H. pylori* in the GI tract (see Figure 7). *H. pylori* has so many insidious effects on the body (described in the paragraphs that follow) that it has become a key part of what we look at in our therapeutic protocol. *H. pylori* connects a lot of dots by virtue of its numerous biochemical impacts.

Figure 7. Pleiotropic effects of *H. pylori* in the body

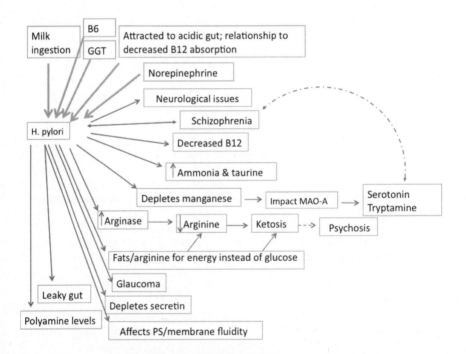

Neurotransmitters: *H. pylori* affects neurotransmitters and brain neurochemistry, creating neurological symptoms that include psychotic disorders related to imbalances in serotonin and tryptamine levels (see *Tryptamine* below). It also affects acetylcholine release and levels of epinephrine and norepinephrine.

Intestinal permeability: The GI epithelium is protected by a mucosal barrier that separates it from the contents of the GI lumen (Figure 8). This mucosal barrier is formed by the interactions of various mucosal secretions.[5] *H. pylori* activates claudins (intercellular adhesion molecules)

Figure 8. The mucosal barrier

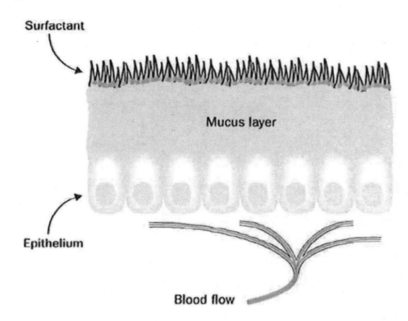

The mucosal barrier separates the internal milieu from the luminal environment. The function of the barrier depends on the integrity of the mucosa—from the endothelium through to the epithelial cell lining—and the reactivity of dynamic defensive factors such as mucosal blood flow, epithelial secretions, and immunocompetent cells. The mucus layer is formed by the interaction of various mucosal secretions, including mucin glycoproteins, trefoil peptides, and surfactant phospholipids. However, resident bacteria are the crucial line of resistance by exogenous microbes.

Source: Guarner F, Malagelada JR. Gut flora in health and disease. *Lancet.* 2003 Feb 8;361(9356):512-9.

that insert themselves in between the epithelial cells, thereby increasing epithelial permeability.[91] Interestingly, duplication of the claudin genes, which effectively increases their activity, also produces apraxia.[92]

Food allergies: *H. pylori* infection increases the incidence of food allergy by facilitating the passage of intact proteins across the gastric epithelial barrier. This increases the presentation of food antigens, which may cause immune reactions and clinical symptoms of disease.[93]

Secretin: Secretin, one of the hormones that controls digestion, was a hot topic some years ago. We now know that *H. pylori* depletes secretin, which may explain some of its effects on the gut and speech.[94]

Arginine and ketosis: Arginine makes urea to neutralize stomach acid or, alternatively, makes intermediates (such as nitric oxide) that relax blood vessels (Figure 9). When *H. pylori* infection is present, it induces arginine to produce urea as opposed to nitric oxide because urea provides the alkalinity necessary for its survival. In this way, *H.*

Figure 9. Arginine metabolism: enzymology, nutrition, and clinical significance

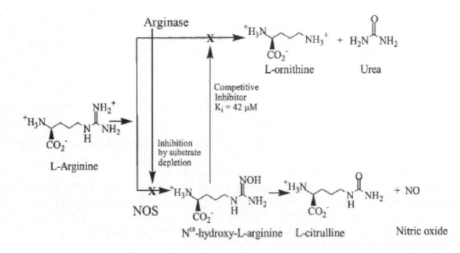

Source: Ash DE. Structure and function of arginases. *J Nutr.* 2004;134(10 Suppl):2760S-2764S.

pylori depletes arginine through its overuse of the enzyme arginase, and the two manganese molecules that are in arginase are wasted.[86] Frequently, there is persistent low manganese in spite of what should be ample manganese supplementation in patients with *H. pylori*. The *H. pylori* bacterium upregulates host arginase II in macrophages in both mouse and human gastric tissues and increases *H. pylori*-mediated apoptosis.[95,96]

The depletion of arginine impacts the mitochondria, reducing mitochondrial energy production from glucose. *H. pylori* uses pyruvate as opposed to glucose. Sugars are not major substrates for this organism.[97] As fat (rather than sugars or glucose) is broken down for energy, energy production shifts to produce three ketone bodies (acetone, betahydroxybutyrate, and acetoacetate). High rates of fatty acid oxidation generate large amounts of acetyl-CoA, leading to the synthesis in the liver of the three ketone bodies. This reduces the metabolic efficiency of the Krebs cycle (which uses glucose), and ketones spill into the circulation, causing serum levels to rise several fold. The ketones then are used as an energy source in extrahepatic tissues, including the brain.[98] Additionally, breakdown of fats may lead to the subsequent depletion of carnitine, further affecting an individual's ability to utilize the Krebs cycle.

Abnormalities in the production of ketone bodies have been studied in individuals with mental disease for over 60 years. Observations record abnormally high ketone body formation in schizophrenia and other mental disorders.[99] When *H. pylori* is present, a ketogenic diet may exacerbate mental symptoms, and even without *H. pylori* infection, a shift to using fat for energy may create psychosis. Excess ketones secondary to *H. pylori*, inefficient ACAT enzyme activity, or starvation, can create psychological and emotional disorders.[100] The state of ketosis induced by *H. pylori* may also be involved with language delay and apraxia.[101] However, some practitioners find the ketogenic diet helpful for seizures. Physiological situations are highly individual, so it is always advisable to check with the patient's overseeing physician.

Tryptamine: Tryptamine is a trace amine that is found in very low concentrations in the mammalian central nervous system, is localized in neurons, and which exhibits a very high turnover and short half-life. Tryptamine has been posited by some to be a neuromodulator,[102] perhaps opposing the actions of serotonin, otherwise known as 5-hydroxytryptamine (5-HT). As shown in Figure 10, the serotonin and tryptamine molecules are very closely chemically related. Given this close relationship, tryptamine may be involved in the regulation of mood, emotion, sleep, and appetite, which are the cardinal functions of serotonin.

Ketosis increases tryptamine levels in animal models. Elevated tryptamine urinary excretion has been observed in schizophrenic patients, suggesting that tryptamine may be involved in the pathophysiology of schizophrenia.[103] Due to the delicate balance in the body between serotonin metabolites, melatonin, 5-hydroxyindoleacetic acid (5-HIAA), and tryptamine, factors such as *H. pylori* infection can disturb the balance of these metabolites. This may cause neurologically-based symptoms affecting mood, appetite, emotions, sleep, OCD behaviors, and psychosis. In fact, the psychotic impact of tryptamine has been compared to LSD and mescaline. Tryptamine-induced symptoms include vegetative states, athetoid move-ments, delusions, hallucinations, autistic-like behavior, language disturbances, spatial and temporal perception disturbances, euphoria, and anxiety.[103-105]

Phospholipids and membrane fluidity: When *H. pylori* infection is present, it changes the way functionally important phospholipids are positioned in the neuronal cell membrane. Direct contact of *H. pylori* with epithelial cells induces externalization of the inner leaflet enriched host phospholipid, phosphatidylserine (PS), to the outer leaflet of the host plasma membrane. When cells begin to undergo apoptosis, a collapse of lipid asymmetry occurs with concomitant exposure of PS at the outer leaflet of the plasma membrane, which serves as an "eat me" signal for phagocytes, thus inciting neuronal cell death.[106]

Other effects: *H. pylori* also decreases levels of B12 in the body, decreases iron levels, increases ammonia and taurine, and can produce glaucoma in young individuals that resolves when the *H. pylori* is treated.

H. pylori infection is not just an immediate acute infection. Rather, it is a long-term chronic problem that may take months or years to eradicate. Chronic *H. pylori* gastritis alters feeding behaviors, delays

Figure 10. Serotonin and tryptamine molecules

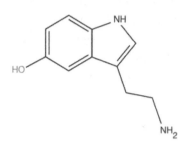

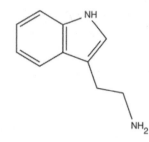

5-Hydroxytryptamine   Tryptamine

(Serotonin)

gastric emptying, alters gastric neuromuscular function, impairs acetylcholine release, produces greater antral muscle relaxation upon electrical field stimulation, and increases the density of SP- and CGRP-containing nerves in a mouse model. These effects can persist for months after the infection has been eradicated.[107] Multiple mechanisms, including persistent immune gut activation and altered brain neurochemistry, may be responsible for the maintenance of abnormal feeding behaviors, providing an explanation for the lack of apparent symptom resolution following the eradication of *H. pylori*.[108] An extended period may be necessary before gastric physiology can return to normal after successful *H. pylori* treatment.[109]

Treatment considerations

Many organisms normally found in the gut can become pathogenic in the face of poor methionine and folate cycle function, insufficient immune function, and a high toxic burden. Therefore, it is essential to treat imbalanced gut flora whenever these conditions are present. Although organisms such as *E. coli* and streptococci often are reported on stool analyses as normal flora, any such organisms appearing on the stool culture of an immunocompromised individual should be considered possible pathogens. These organisms' potential pathogenic impacts in significantly immunocompromised individuals are amply documented, even if mainstream opinion continues to consider them nonpathogenic.

Our treatment approach emphasizes specialty nutritional products developed for the purpose of rebalancing. The use of prescription antibiotics often leads to further depletion of normal flora and additional imbalances, whereas herbal agents and specialty nutritional products can be utilized more safely.

Where iron is concerned, we do not give iron for documented or imagined iron deficiency, such as a low red blood cell count. We regard laboratory findings of iron deficiency or iron excretion from the body as an indication for lactoferrin and/or other specialty nutritional products designed to place iron appropriately in the body.

Vitamin D plays a critical role in mucosal barrier homeostasis by preserving the integrity of tight junction complexes and the healing capacity of the colonic epithelium. Vitamin D deficiency, therefore, may compromise the mucosal barrier.[110] Vitamin D also seems to decrease levels of NF-kB, a cytokine that when elevated is linked to symptomatic behavior as well as inflammation associated with GI infections and PANDAS.[111] We, therefore, consider supplementation with vitamin D3 when indicated by laboratory testing.

As we hope to have demonstrated, addressing GI balance plays a vital role in enhancing neurotransmitter balance and overall function. Appropriate support with probiotic flora can lay the groundwork for an internal GI environment more conducive to normal bacterial growth. Additional steps to optimize the GI environment include focusing on pH levels, reducing hyperacidity, using digestive enzymes, reaching ideal B12 levels, and implementing other GI supports appropriate to the individual. All of these measures can help to promote the growth of beneficial flora rather than favor dysbiosis. For example, achieving sufficient levels of B12 will preclude the increase in acid formation that occurs when the body stimulates production of intrinsic factor in an attempt to raise B12 stores.

It is important to directly address dysbiotic and imbalanced flora in immunocompromised individuals. Treatment of streptococci and *H. pylori*, along with clostridia, *Pseudomonas* species, *E. coli*, and *Klebsiella*, among others, should be strongly emphasized no matter whether they are reported as normal or imbalanced. Getting the gut environment in balance, populating it with appropriate normal flora, and eradicating symptom-producing dysbiotic and imbalanced flora are key steps to achieving gastrointestinal health, gut epithelial wall integrity, neurotransmitter balance, and symptom resolution.

References

1. Parracho HM, Bingham MO, Gibson GR, McCartney AL. Differences between the gut microflora of children with autistic spectrum disorders and that of healthy children. *J Med Microbiol.* 2005;54(10):987-91.
2. Hicks J. Biofilm: a cause of chronic gastrointestinal issues in ASD. *Autism Science Digest.* 2011, Issue 2, pp. 47-53.
3. Finegold SM, Molitoris D, Song Y, Liu C, Vaisanen ML, Bolte E, et al. Gastrointestinal microflora studies in late-onset autism. *Clin Infect Dis.* 2002;35(Suppl 1):S6-S16.
4. Bäckhed F, Ley RE, Sonnenburg JL, Peterson DA, Gordon JI. Host-bacterial mutualism in the human intestine. *Science.* 2005;307(5717):1915-20.
5. Guarner F, Malagelada JR. Gut flora in health and disease. *Lancet.* 2003; 361(9356):512-9.
6. Zoetendal EG, von Wright A, Vilpponen-Salmela T, Ben-Amor K, Akkermans AD, de Vos WM. Mucosa-associated bacteria in the human gastrointestinal tract are uniformly distributed along the colon and differ from the community recovered from feces. *Appl Environ Microbiol.* 2002;68(7):3401-7.
7. Bengmark S. Immunonutrition: role of biosurfactants, fiber, and probiotic bacteria. *Nutrition.* 1998;14(7-8):585-94.
8. Takahashi I, Kiyono H. Gut as the largest immunologic tissue. *J Parenter Enteral Nutr.* 1999;23(5 Suppl):S7-S12.
9. Kowalska B, Niemiec KT, Drejewicz H, Polak K, Kubik P, Elmidaoui A, et al. Prevalence of group B streptococcal colonization in pregnant women and their newborns based on the results of examination of patients in the obstetric and gynecology department of the National Research Institute of Mother and Child—a pilot study. *Ginekol Pol.* 2003;74(10):1223-7.
10. Krasnianin E, Skret-Magierlo J, Witalis J, Barnas E, Kluz T, Koziel A, et al. The incidence of *Streptococcus* group B in 100 parturient women and the transmission of pathogens to the newborn. *Ginekol Pol.* 2009;80(4):285-9.
11. Ardeman S, Chanarin I. Intrinsic factor secretion in gastric atrophy. *Gut.* 1966;7(1):99-101.
12. Giorgini GL Jr, Iannuccilli E, Leduc LP, Thayer WR Jr. Control of intrinsic factor secretion in rats. Relation of vitamin B12 deficiency and gastric hormonal secretion. *Am J Dig Dis.* 1973;18(4):332-6.
13. Kapadia C. Cobalamin (vitamin B12) deficiency: is it a problem for our aging population and is the problem compounded by drugs that inhibit gastric acid secretion? *J Clin Gastroenterol.* 2000;30(1):4-6.
14. Zimmer MH, Hart LC, Manning-Courtney P, Murray DS, Bing NM, Summer S. Food variety as a predictor of nutritional status among children with autism. *J Autism Dev Disord.* 2011 May 10.
15. Smith CD, Herkes SB, Behrns KE, Fairbanks VF, Kelly KA, Sarr MG. Gastric acid secretion and vitamin B12 absorption after vertical Roux-en-Y gastric bypass for morbid obesity. *Ann Surg.* 1993;218(1):91-6.
16. Cotter PD, Hill C. Surviving the acid test: responses of gram-positive bacteria to low pH. *Microbiol Mol Biol Rev.* 2003;67(3):429-53.

17. Berry ED, Cutter CN. Effects of acid adaptation of *Escherichia coli* O157:H7 on efficacy of acetic acid spray washes to decontaminate beef carcass tissue. *Appl Environ Microbiol.* 2000;66(4):1493-8.

18. Roberts JA. Blood groups and susceptibility to disease: a review. *Brit J Prev Soc Med.* 1957;11(3):107-25.

19. Ligtenberg AJ, Veerman EC, de Graaff J, Nieuw Amerongen AV. Saliva-induced aggregation of oral streptococci and the influence of blood group reactive substances. *Arch Oral Biol.* 1990;35 Suppl:141S-143S.

20. Brooks G, Carroll KC, Butel J, Morse S, Mietzner T. Jawetz, *Melnick & Adelberg's Medical Microbiology*, twenty-fifth edition. New York, NY: McGraw-Hill Medical, 2010.

21. Bralley JA, Lord RS. *Laboratory Evaluations in Molecular Medicine: Nutrients, Toxicants, and Cell Regulators.* Norcross, GA: Institute for Advances in Molecular Medicine, 2001.

22. Shukla OP. Microbial transformation of quinoline by a *Pseudomonas* sp. *Appl Environ Microbiol.* 1986;51(6):1332-42.

23. Burlingame R, Chapman PJ. Catabolism of phenylpropionic acid and its 3-hydroxy derivative by *Escherichia coli. J Bacteriol.* 1983;155(1):113-21.

24. Kahn V, Ben-Shalom N, Zakin V. P-hydroxy-phenylpropionic acid (PHPPA) and 3,4-dihydroxy-phenylpropionic acid (3,4-DPPA) as substrates for mushroom tyrosinase. *J Food Biochem.* 1999;23(1):75-94.

25. Wannemacher RW Jr, Klainer AS, Dinterman RE, Beisel WR. The significance and mechanism of an increased serum phenylalanine-tyrosine ratio during infection. *Am J Clin Nutr.* 1976;29(9):997-1006.

26. Alterio J, Ravassard P, Haavik J, Le Caer JP, Biguet NF, Waksman G, et al. Human tyrosine hydroxylase isoforms: inhibition by excess tetrahydropterin and unusual behavior of isoform 3 after cAMP-dependent protein kinase phosphorylation. *J Biol Chem.*1998;273(17):10196-201.

27. Dogan MD, Sumners C, Broxson CS, Clark N, Tümer N. Central angiotensin II increases biosynthesis of tyrosine hydroxylase in the rat adrenal medulla. *Biochem Biophys Res Commun.* 2004;313(3):623-6.

28. Gabor R, Regunathan S, Sourkes TL. Central regulation of adrenal tyrosine hydroxylase: interaction between dopamine and GABA systems. *Neuropharmacology.*1989;28(5):521-7.

29. Lindgren N, Xu ZD, Herrera-Marschitz M, Haycock J, Hökfelt T, Fisone G. Dopamine D2 receptors regulate tyrosine hydroxylase activity and phosphorylation at Ser40 in rat striatum. *Eur J Neurosci.* 2001;13(4):773-80.

30. Yasko A. *Genetic Bypass: Using Nutrition to Bypass Genetic Mutations.* New York, NY: Matrix Development Publishing, 2005.

31. Leeming RJ, Harpey JP, Brown SM, Blair JA. Tetrahydrofolate and hydroxycobalamin in the management of dihydropteridine reductase deficiency. *J Ment Defic Res.* 1982;26(1):21-5.

32. Griffith TM, Chaytor AT, Bakker LM, Edwards DH. 5-methyltetrahydrofolate and tetrahydrobiopterin can modulate electrotonically mediated endothelium-dependent vascular relaxation. *Proc Natl Acad Sci USA.* 2005;102(19):7008-13.

33. Hamon CG, Blair JA, Barford PA. The effect of tetrahydrofolate on tetrahydrobiopterin metabolism. *J Ment Defic Res.* 1986;30(2):179-83.

34. Matthews RG, Kaufman S. Characterization of the dihydropterin reductase activity of pig liver methylenetetrahydrofolate reductase. *J Biol Chem.* 1980;255(13):6014-7.

35. Robien K, Ulrich CM. 5,10 methylenetetrahydrofolate reductase polymorphisms and leukemia risk: a HuGE minireview. *Am J Epidemiol.* 2003;157(7):571-82.

36. Bottiglieri T, Hyland K, Laundy M, Godfrey P, Carney MW, Toone BK, et al. Folate deficiency, biopterin and monoamine metabolism in depression. *Psychol Med.* 1992;22(4):871-6.

37. Rios M, Habecker B, Sasaoka T, Eisenhofer G, Tian H, Landis S, et al. Catecholamine synthesis is medicated by tryosinase in the absence of tyrosine hydroxylase. *J Neurosci.* 1999;19(9):3519-26.

38. Jefferson KK. What drives bacteria to produce a biofilm? *FEMS Microbiol Lett.* 2004;236(2):163-73.

39. Li YH, Lau PC, Lee JH, Ellen RP, Cvitkovitch DG. Natural genetic transformation of *Streptococcus mutans* growing in biofilms. *J Bacteriol.* 2001;183(3):897-908.

40. Cho H, Jönsson H, Campbell K, Melke P, Williams JW, Jedynak B, et al. Self-organization in high-density bacterial colonies: efficient crowd control. *PLoS Biol.* 2007;5(7):e302.

41. Vieira HL, Freire P, Arraiano CM. Effect of *Escherichia coli* morphogene bolA on biofilms. *Appl Environ Microbiol.* 2004;70(9):5682-4.

42. Aldea M, Hernandez-Chico C, de la Campa AG, Kushner SR, Vicente M. Identification, cloning and expression of boIA, an ftsZ-dependent morphogene of *Escherichia coli*. *J Bacteriol.* 1988;170(11):5169-76.

43. Cvitkovitch DG, Li YH, Ellen RP. Quorum sensing and biofilm formation in streptococcal infections. *J Clin Invest.* 2003;112(11):1626-32.

44. Doran KS, Nizet V. Molecular pathogenesis of neonatal group B streptococcal infection: no longer in its infancy. *Mol Microbiol.* 2004;54(1):23-31.

45. Mell LK, Davis RL, Owens D. Association between streptococcal infection and obsessive-compulsive disorder, Tourette's syndrome, and tic disorder. *Pediatrics.* 2005;116(1);56-60.

46. Fujinami RN, Sweeten TL. Letting antibodies get to your head. *Nat Med.* 2003;9(7):823-5.

47. Kirvan CA, Swedo SE, Heuser JS, Cunningham MW. Mimicry and autoantibody-mediated neuronal cell signaling in Sydenham chorea. *Nat Med.* 2003;9(7):914-20.

48. Hoffman KL, Hornig M, Yaddanapudi K, Jabado O, Lipkin WI. A murine model for neuropsychiatric disorders associated with group A beta-hemolytic streptococcal infection. *J Neurosci.* 2004;24(7):1780-91.

49. Tolosa L, Caraballo-Miralles V, Olmos G, Lladó J. TNF-alpha potentiates glutamate-induced spinal cord motoneuron death via NF-kB. *Mol Cell Neurosci.* 2011;46(1):176-86.

50. Wirleitner B, Neurauter G, Schröcksnadel K, Frick B, Fuchs D. Interferon-gamma-induced conversion of tryptophan: immunologic and neuropsychiatric aspects. *Curr Med Chem.* 2003;10(16):1581-91.

51. Gadd GM. Heavy metal accumulation by bacteria and other microorganisms. *Cell Mol Life Sci.* 1990;46(8):834-40.

52. Perdrial N, Liewig N, Delphin JE, Elsass F. TEM evidence for intracellular accumulation of lead by bacteria in subsurface environments. *Chem Geol.* 2008;253(3-4):196-204.

53. Summers AO, Silver S. Microbial transformations of metals. *Ann Rev Microbiol.* 1978;32:637-72.

54. Bradley TJ, Parker MS. Binding of aluminum ions by *Staphylococcus aurens* 893. *Experientia.* 1968;24(11):1175-6.

55. Wood JM, Wang HK. Microbial resistance to heavy metals. *Environ Sci Technol.* 1983;17(12):582A-592A.

56. Strandberg GW, Shumate SE II, Parrott JR Jr. Microbial cells as biosorbents for heavy metals: accumulation of uranium by *Saccharomyces cerevisiae* and *Pseudomonas aeruginosa. Appl Environ Microbiol.* 1981;41(1):237-45.

57. Yasko A, Mullan N. How bacterial imbalances may predispose to seizure disorder. *Autism File Global.* 2010, Issue 38, pp. 86-90.

58. Yasko A. *Autism: Pathways to Recovery.* Bethel, Maine: Neurological Research Institute, 2009.

59. Crichton R. *Iron Metabolism: From Molecular Mechanisms to Clinical Consequences*, 3rd edition. Hoboken, NJ: John Wiley & Sons, 2009.

60. Griffiths E. Iron and bacterial virulence--a brief overview. *Biol Met.* 1991;4(1):7-13.

61. Wooldridge KG, Williams PH. Iron uptake mechanisms of pathogenic bacteria. *FEMS Microbiol Rev.* 1993;12(4):325-48.

62. Payne SM, Finkelstein RA. The critical role of iron in host-bacterial interactions. *J Clin Invest.* 1978;61(6):1428-40.

63. Payne SM. Iron acquisition in microbial pathogenesis. *Trends Microbiol.* 1993;1(2):66-9.

64. Agency for Toxic Substances and Disease Registry. Toxicological profile for aluminum. Atlanta, GA: ATSDR, September 2008.

65. Garruto RM, Fukatsu R, Yanagihara R, Gajdusek DC. Hook G, Fiori CE. Imaging of calcium and aluminum neurofibrillary tangle-bearing neurons in Parkinsonism-dementia of Guam. *Proc Natl Acad Sci USA.* 1984;81(6):1875-9. Correction: *Proc Natl Acad Sci USA.* 1984;81(13):4240.

66. Perl DP, Gajdusek DC, Garruto RM, Yanagihara RT, Gibbs CJ. Intraneuronal aluminum accumulation in amyotrophic lateral sclerosis and Parkinsonism-dementia of Guam. *Science.* 1982;217(4564):1053-5.

67. Nayak P, Chatterjee AK. Effects of aluminum exposure on brain glutamate and GABA systems: an experimental study in rats. *Food Chem Toxicol.* 2001;39(12):1285-9.

68. Deloncle R, Guillard O. Mechanism of Alzheimer's disease: arguments for a neurotransmitter-aluminium complex implication. *Neurochem Res.*1990;15(12):1239-45.

69. Crapper DR, Krishnan SS, Quittkat S. Aluminium, neurofibrillary degeneration and Alzheimer's disease. *Brain.* 1976;99(1):67-80.

70. Flaten TP. Aluminium as a risk factor in Alzheimer's disease, with emphasis on drinking water. *Brain Res Bull.* 2001;55(2):187-96.

71. McDermott JR, Smith AI, Iqbal K, Wisniewski HM. Brain aluminum in aging and Alzheimer's disease. *Neurology.* 1979;29(6):809-14.

72. Swegert CV, Dave KR, Katyare SS. Effect of aluminium-induced Alzheimer like condition on oxidative energy metabolism in rat liver, brain and heart mitochondria. *Mech Ageing Dev.* 1999;112(1):27-42.

73. Ghetti B, Musicco M, Norton J, Bugiani O. Nerve cell loss in the progressive encephalopathy induced by aluminum powder. A morphologic and semiquantitative study of the Purkinje cells. *Neuropathol Appl Neurobiol.* 1985;11(1):31-53.

74. Gulya K, Rakonczay Z, Kasa P. Cholinotoxic effects of aluminum in rat brain. *J Neurochem.* 1990;54(3):1020-6.

75. Perl DP, Brody AR. Alzheimer's disease: X-ray spectrometric evidence of aluminum accumulation in neurofibrillary tangle-bearing neurons. *Science.*

1980;208(4441):297-9.

76. Simpson J, Yates CM, Whyler DK, Wilson H, Dewar AJ, Gordon A. Biochemical studies on rabbits with aluminum induced neurofilament accumulations. *Neurochem Res.* 1985;10(2):229-38.

77. Yates CM, Simpson J, Russell D, Gordon A. Cholinergic enzymes in neurofibrillary degeneration produced by aluminum. *Brain Res.* 1980;197(1):269-74.

78. Bilkei-Gorzó A. Neurotoxic effect of enteral aluminium. *Food Chem Toxicol.* 1993;31(5):357-61.

79. Faeth WH, Walker AE, Kaplan AD, Warner WA. Threshold studies on production of experimental epilepsy with alumina cream. *Proc Soc Exp Biol Med.* 1955;88(3):329-31.

80. Kopeloff LM, Chusid JG, Kopeloff N. Chronic experimental epilepsy in Macaca mulatta. *Neurology.*1954;4(3):218-27.

81. Lockard JS, Wyler AR. The influence of attending on seizure activity in epileptic monkeys. *Epilepsia.* 1979;20(2):157-68.

82. Mayanagi Y. Alumina cream-induced temporal lobe epilepsy in the monkey as an experimental model. *Folia Psychiatr Neurol Jpn.* 1979;33(3):457-62.

83. Exley C. The pro-oxidant activity of aluminum. *Free Radic Biol Med.* 2004;36(3):380-7.

84. Sonak S, Bhosle NB. Observations on biofilm bacteria isolated from aluminium panels immersed in estuarine waters. *Biofouling.* 1995;8:243-54.

85. Lugon JR, Moreira MD, de Almeida JMR, Silva AS, Esberard ECB, Bousquet-Santos K, et al. Cardiovascular autonomic response to food ingestion in patients with gastritis: a comparison between *Helicobacter pylori*-positive and -negative patients. *Helicobacter.* 2006;11:173-80.

86. De Reuse H, Skouloubris S. Nitrogen metabolism. In HLT Mobley, GL Mendz, SL Hazell (Eds.), *Helicobacter pylori: Physiology and Genetics* (Chapter 11). Washington, DC: ASM Press, 2001.

87. Celli JP, Turner BS, Afdhal NH, Keates S, Chiran I, Kelly C, et al. *Helicobacter pylori* moves through mucus by reducing mucin viscoelasticity. *PNAS.* 2009;106(34):14321-6.

88. Yea SS, Yang YI, Jang WH, Lee YJ, Bae HS, Paik KH. Association between TNF-alpha promoter polymorphism and *Helicobacter pylori* cagA subtype infection. *J Clin Pathol.* 2001;54(9):703-6.

89. Schreiber S, Konradt M, Groll C, Scheid P, Hanauer G, Werling HO, et al. The spatial orientation of *Helicobacter pylori* in the gastric mucus. *PNAS.* 2004;101(14):5024–9.

90. Corthésy-Theulaz I, Porta N, Pringault E, Racine L, Bogdanova A, Kraehenbuhl JP, et al. Adhesion of *Helicobacter pylori* to polarized T84 human intestinal cell monolayers is pH dependent. *Infect Immun.* 1996;64(9):3827-32.

91. Fedwick JP, Lapointe TK, Meddings JB, Sherman PM, Buret AG. *Helicobacter pylori* activates myosin light-chain kinase to disrupt claudin-4 and claudin-5 and increase epithelial permeability. *Infect Immun.* 2005;73(12):7844-52.

92. Sommerville MJ, Mervis CB, Young EJ, Seo EJ, del Campo M, Bamforth S, et al. Severe expressive-language delay related to duplication of the Williams-Beuren locus. *N Engl J Med.* 2005;353(16):1694-701.

93. Matysiak-Budnik T, Heyman MJ. Food allergy and *Helicobacter pylori*. *J Pediatr Gastroenterol Nutr.* 2002;34(1):5-12.

94. Love JW. Peptic ulceration may be a hormonal deficiency disease. *Med Hypotheses.* 2008;70(6):1103-7.

95. Ash DE. Structure and function of arginases. *J Nutr.* 2004;134(10 Suppl):2760S-2764S.

96. Das P, Lahiri A, Lahiri A, Chakravortty D. Modulation of the arginase pathway in the context of microbial pathogenesis: a metabolic enzyme moonlighting as an immune modulator. *PLoS Pathog.* 2010;6(6):e1000899.

97. Chalk PA, Roberts AD, Blows WM. Metabolism of pyruvate and glucose by intact cells of Helicobacter pylori studied by 13C NMR spectroscopy. *Microbiology.* 1994;140(Pt 8):2085-92.

98. Hartman AL, Gasior M, Vining EP, Rogawski MA. The neuropharmacology of the ketogenic diet. *Pediatr Neurol.* 2007;36(5):281-92.

99. Kitays JI, Altschule MD. Blood ketone concentration in patients with mental and emotional disorders. *AMA Arch Neurol Psychiatry.* 1952;68(4):506-9.

100. Tyni T, Palotie A, Viinikka L, Valanne L, Salo MK, von Döbein U, et al. Long-chain 3-hydroxyacyl-coenzyme A dehydrogenase deficiency with the G1528C mutation: clinical presentation of thirteen patients. *J Pediatr.* 1997;130(1):67-76.

101. Watanabe C, Oishi T, Yamamoto T, Sasaki K, Tosaka M, Sata T, et al. Chorea and Broca aphasia induced by diabetic ketoacidosis in a type 1 diabetic patient diagnosed as Moyamoya disease. *Diabetes Res Clin Pract.* 2005;67(2):180-5.

102. Yu AM, Granvil CP, Haining RL, Krausz KW, Corchero J, Küpfer A, et al. The relative contribution of monoamine oxidase and cytochrome P450 isozymes to the metabolic deamination of the trace amine tryptamine. *J Pharmacol Exp Ther.* 2003;304(2):539-46.

103. Szara S. The comparison of the psychotic effect of tryptamine derivatives with the effects of mescaline and LSD-25 in self-experiments. In S Garattini, V Ghetti (Eds.), *Psychotropic Drugs* (pp. 460-7). New York: Elsevier, 1957.

104. Yilmaz Y, Gul CB, Arabul M, Eren MA. *Helicobacter pylori*: a role in schizophrenia? *Med Sci Monit.* 2008;14(7):HY13-16.

105. De Hert M, Hautekeete M, De Wilde D, Peuskens J. High prevalence of *Helicobacter pylori* in institutionalized schizophrenia patients. *Schizophr Res.* 1997;26(2-3):243-4.

106. Murata-Kamiya N, Kikuchi K, Hayashi T, Higashi H, Hatakeyama M. *Helicobacter pylori* exploits host membrane phosphatidylserine for delivery, localization, and pathophysiological action of the CagA oncoprotein. *Cell Host Microbe.* 2010;7(5):399-411.

107. Bercik P, Verdú EF, Foster JA, Lu J, Scharringa A, Kean I, et al. Role of gut-brain axis in persistent abnormal feeding behavior in mice following eradication of *Helicobacter pylori* infection. *Am J Physiol Regul Integr Comp Physiol.* 2009;296(3):R587-R594.

108. Zheng H, Patterson LM, Phifer CB, Berthoud HR. Brain stem melanocortinergic modulation of meal size and identification of hypothalamic POMC projections. *Am J Physiol Regul Integr Comp Physiol.* 2005;289(1):R247–R258.

109. Ladas SD, Katsogridakis J, Malamou H, Giannopoulou H, Kesse-Elia M, Raptis SA. *Helicobacter pylori* may induce bile reflux: link between *H pylori* and bile induced injury to gastric epithelium. *Gut.* 1996;38(1):15-8.

110. Kong J, Zhang Z, Musch MW, Ning G, Sun J, Hart J, et al. Novel role of the vitamin D receptor in maintaining the integrity of the intestinal mucosal barrier. *Am J Physiol Gastrointest Liver Physiol.* 2008;294(1):G208-G216.

111. Cohen-Lahav M, Shany S, Tobvin D, Chaimovitz C, Douvdevani A. Vitamin D decreases NFkB activity by increasing IkBα levels. *Nephrol Dial Transplant.* 2006;21:889-97.

CHAPTER ELEVEN

INTERRELATIONSHIPS AMONG THE GUT, MITOCHONDRIAL FUNCTION, AND NEUROLOGICAL SEQUELAE

By Daniel A. Rossignol, MD, FAAFP

Evidence of a gut-brain connection

Over the last century, a connection between gastrointestinal (GI) abnormalities and problems outside of the GI tract has become evident. For example, an association between GI problems and arthritis was described in 1910.[1] Over time, a relationship between the GI tract and the brain (a gut-brain connection) also has emerged. As long ago as 1889, researchers reported "an exhaustional-confusional form of insanity proceeding from a dilated and over-filled colon."[2] Colonic irrigation was commonly used in the late 1800s and early 1900s, with some investigators reporting that colon cleansing improved certain mental diseases.[3]

Notwithstanding this history, it is only in the last decade or so that the gut-brain connection has become more widely acknowledged. Research in this area has greatly increased. While this chapter's overall focus is on the interaction between the gut and the brain, it highlights mitochondrial function as one of the critical bridges between these two body systems. I first examine some potential mechanisms of a gut-brain connection. Next, I discuss mitochondrial function in detail and assess how problems with mitochondrial function (mitochondrial dysfunction) can contribute to both GI abnormalities and neurological sequelae. In the context of abnormal GI function, I also review the potential adverse effects on mitochondrial function of bacterial imbalances in the GI tract and discuss how this can adversely affect the gut-brain connection. I conclude with a discussion of the potential role of hyperbaric oxygen therapy (HBOT) in improving mitochondrial dysfunction as well as GI and brain function.

Potential mechanisms of a gut-brain connection

Over time, a number of ideas have been developed to explain potential mechanisms of action for the gut-brain connection. One idea derives from evidence demonstrating that the central nervous system (CNS) and the GI tract share similar cells, including glial cells. In the GI tract, astrocyte-like glia are partly responsible for the proper functioning of the intestinal barrier and help to prevent larger food particles and other molecules from entering the circulatory system. Abnormalities in the GI glial cells may contribute to autoimmune diseases, enterocolitis, diabetes, irritable bowel syndrome (IBS), and inflammatory bowel disease (IBD).[4]

The second body of evidence supporting a gut-brain connection comes from recent studies focusing on the bacteria in the GI tract. Whereas approximately 30,000 genes are found in the average human, more than 3 million genes from GI tract bacteria are present. The GI tract contains tenfold more bacteria (10^{14}) than the average number of cells (10^{13}) in a human body, and these bacteria serve important purposes. For example, the symbiotic relationship that exists between humans and their intestinal microbial flora is crucial for nutrient assimilation and important for the development of the innate immune system. Exposure to "good" bacteria in the GI tract programs the immune system to more effectively fight infections.[5] While it was already established that bacteria communicate with each other through a process known as quorum sensing,[6] it is now apparent that the bacteria in the human GI tract also communicate with human cells through hormonal signals.[7] This communication is important because bacteria and humans share metabolic pathways that are essential for health.[8]

The third idea supporting a gut-brain connection comes from evidence that GI tract abnormalities may adversely affect brain function. Dysbiosis is the term used to refer to either an increase in the number of abnormal bacteria or a disruption in the type of bacteria in the GI tract. Although the idea that dysbiosis may contribute to abnormalities *inside* the GI tract (such as diarrhea and constipation) is fairly straightforward, it is increasingly apparent that dysbiosis also has effects *outside* the GI tract, including effects on brain function. Recent evidence has demonstrated that atypical levels and types of bacteria in the GI tract contribute to metabolic abnormalities reported in neurological and psychiatric conditions such as autism spectrum disorders (ASDs).[9] The pathogenic metabolites produced by these bacteria in the GI tract may contribute to the brain dysfunction and metabolic problems that have been observed. As other examples, hydrogen sulfide produced in part by GI bacteria has been shown to play a role in blood pressure regulation,[10] and the unique makeup of the microbial community in the GI tract also may help determine a person's weight by influencing fat storage regulation.[11] Even a decade ago, the idea that the bacteria in the GI tract might influence blood pressure regulation or weight would have seemed untenable.

Fourth, dietary factors also point to a gut-brain connection. Perhaps nowhere is this more apparent than in the case of celiac disease, a condition defined by intestinal damage resulting from gluten reactivity. Unfortunately, it has taken centuries for humans to realize that gluten exposure also can impair brain function in some people[12] and lead to conditions such as ataxia and schizophrenia. Interestingly, the prevalence of celiac disease is 3.5 times higher in children with ASD than in the general population.[13] However, recent studies reveal that the general prevalence of celiac disease remains under-recognized.[12]

Exposure to foods other than gluten-containing foods may also impair brain function. For example, a one-month study reported disruptive behaviors in an 8-year-old boy with autism after exposure to a number of common foods.[14] Staff collected frequency data on behaviors such as object throwing, scratching, biting, and screaming. The study included periods of a normal American diet, a fasting period, and a period during which individual foods were reintroduced one by one. During the latter phase, it was observed that mushrooms, dairy products, wheat, corn, tomatoes, and sugar all provoked behavioral problems.[14] Some children will manifest similar types of sensitivities. These reactions point to a connection between food that is ingested and effects in the brain, which then result in certain behavioral changes.

Exposure to cow's milk may also impair brain function in some people, including individuals with cerebral folate deficiency (CFD).

CFD is a newly described neurodevelopmental disorder typified by low cerebrospinal fluid (CSF) levels of 5-methyltetrahydrofolate (5MTHF) (the metabolically active form of folic acid) in spite of normal systemic folic acid (folate) levels.[15] 5MTHF is normally transported into the CNS through endocytosis by the cerebral folate receptor-alpha (FRα) in a process that is dependent on cellular energy.[15] The most common cause of CFD is circulating autoantibodies that bind to the cerebral FRα and inhibit the transport of 5MTHF into the CSF. Lowered levels of 5MTHF in the CSF can lead to neurological abnormalities, including spastic paraplegia, cerebellar ataxia, dyskinesia, seizures, acquired microcephaly, and developmental regression that can occur as early as 4 months of age.[15,16] Central visual disturbances (optic atrophy and blindness) and hearing loss also have been described at later ages.[15] To date, seven studies have reported CFD in children with ASD,[15,17-22] and several studies have described CFD in Rett syndrome.[23-25] CFD has also been reported in individuals with mitochondrial disease,[26,27] perhaps because mitochondria are integral for providing the energy needed for the transport of 5MTHF into the brain. Treatment with oral folinic acid can lead to partial or complete recovery in some children.[15,17] In one such case, a 12-year-old girl with progressive spasticity, abnormal gait, and speech problems who had been diagnosed as paraplegic recovered from this condition after she was discovered to have CFD and was treated with oral folinic acid.[28]

Cow's milk contains soluble folate receptor antigen, which is 91% homologous to the FRα. Autoantibodies to the FRα cross-react with the soluble folate receptor antigen in cow's milk, which causes an increase in the circulating autoantibody concentration. Exposure to cow's milk has been shown to increase the concentration of the folate receptor autoantibody and lead to worsening of CFD symptoms, while elimination of cow's milk has been reported to lower the autoantibody concentration and improve CFD symptoms.[20] Moreover, re-exposure to cow's milk after a period of being cow's milk-free substantially worsens the condition and increases the autoantibody concentration.[20] These findings may help explain why some parents of children with ASD report improvements in their child on a cow's milk-free diet.[29] Exposure to cow's milk also has been associated with constipation in children with ASD.[30]

Figure 1.

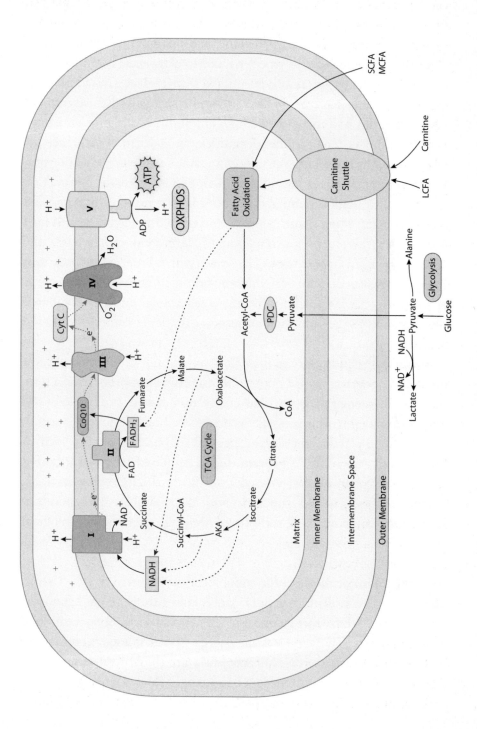

Besides the potential effect of dietary exposures on brain function, toxic byproducts produced by certain bacteria can also negatively affect brain function, especially in the face of liver dysfunction. For example, in individuals with hepatic encephalopathy, the intake of large amounts of protein can contribute to abnormal brain function. This occurs because protein is eventually broken down into ammonia, which is directly toxic to brain cells and can easily diffuse into the CNS from the bloodstream.[31] High ammonia levels are associated with neuropsychological abnormalities in patients with hepatic encephalopathy.[32] Because the mitochondria in the liver are responsible for the detoxification of ammonia, it is apparent that liver dysfunction contributes to high ammonia. Ammonia is also produced by bacteria in the GI tract. High protein intake and dysbiosis in the face of liver dysfunction, therefore, can contribute to elevated ammonia levels and subsequent brain impairment. The important role of dysbiosis in this impairment is further illustrated by the finding that use of an antibiotic (rifaximin) reduces the risk of hepatic encephalopathy when compared with a placebo by eliminating ammonia-producing bacteria in the GI tract.[33]

From this section, we can infer that mitochondrial function plays at least two important roles in maintaining a proper gut-brain connection. First, mitochondria help to detoxify certain toxins produced by GI bacteria that may otherwise adversely affect brain function. Second, mitochondria provide the energy needed to pump nutrients such as 5MTHF into the brain, a process that is impaired by autoantibodies that increase upon exposure to cow's milk. In the following sections, I review mitochondrial function and discuss how mitochondrial dysfunction can contribute to both GI abnormalities and neurological sequelae.

Overview of mitochondrial function

Mitochondria are distinct cellular organelles that generate adenosine triphosphate (ATP) from adenosine diphosphate (ADP) by oxidizing glucose and fatty acids. ATP is the energy carrier in most mammalian cells. In the simplest terms, mitochondria are the powerhouses of the cell, generating energy from the breakdown of food. Figure 1 depicts a mitochondrion and shows the pathways involved when mitochondria break down food and use oxygen to create ATP (the energy source for the body, analogous to gasoline for a car). (For a more detailed review of mitochondrial function, see Haas and coauthors.[34])

As seen in Figure 1, the structure of the mitochondrion consists of outer and inner membranes, with a space (the intermembrane space) in between. The matrix is the innermost part of the mitochondria where many biochemical reactions occur, including the tricarboxylic acid (TCA) cycle (also known as the Krebs cycle or citric acid cycle). The inner mitochondrial membrane contains 5 complexes (known as complexes I through V) that make up the electron transport chain (ETC). On the bottom of the figure, you can see glucose, which is eventually broken down into pyruvate through the process of glycolysis. Pyruvate is then transported into the mitochondria and eventually is broken down into acetyl-CoA, which enters the TCA cycle.

Fatty acid metabolism is shown on the bottom right-hand corner of the figure. Short-chain fatty acids (SCFA) and medium-chain fatty acids (MCFA) can diffuse directly into the mitochondria, whereas long-chain fatty acids (LCFA) are transported into the mitochondria by attaching to carnitine, which shuttles these fatty acids across the inner and outer mitochondrial membranes. Once inside the mitochondria, the fatty acids, like pyruvate, are broken down and converted into acetyl-CoA, which feeds into the TCA cycle. However, some of the electrons released from burning fatty acids (fatty acid oxidation) can feed into complex II through FADH2, bypassing complex I in the process (which may partially explain why a ketogenic diet, which involves a high intake of fats, might be helpful for treating mitochondrial dysfunction).[35]

The three dotted lines with arrows coming off of the TCA cycle are electrons (negatively charged particles) that are transferred through NADH into complex I. Complex I then transfers these electrons to coenzyme Q10 (CoQ10) which, in turn, transfers the electrons to complex III. When the electrons pass through complex I, NADH is converted to NAD+. Hydrogen protons (positively charged hydrogen particles, H+) are pumped from the matrix (the innermost part of the mitochondria) through the inner membrane and into the intermembrane space, where they build up and form an electrochemical gradient. The electrons that passed to complex III are now transferred by cytochrome C (Cyt C) to complex IV. This process also pumps more hydrogen protons into the intermembrane space through complexes III and IV. During this process, oxygen is converted into water in complex IV. The hydrogen protons in the intermembrane space then diffuse back into the matrix through complex V (ATP synthase), and this generates ATP through a process known as oxidative phosphorylation.

Mitochondrial dysfunction

The concept of mitochondrial dysfunction is relatively new, and mitochondrial medicine is a rapidly evolving field of medicine. Mitochondrial disease, once thought uncommon, is now considered the most recognized cause of metabolic disease,[36] with the minimum birth prevalence of an ETC defect estimated at 1 in 7634 individuals.[37] If the ETC in the mitochondrion does not work properly (is blocked), metabolites begin to back up. Elevations can then occur in TCA cycle metabolites, fatty acids, and pyruvate. Moreover, pyruvate transportation can be slowed, and pyruvate can convert into elevated levels of lactate (also known as lactic acid) and alanine.

Mitochondrial disease has a broad phenotypic presentation: children with mitochondrial disease can have normal intelligence, mental retardation, or developmental delay.[38] One recent study reported that approximately 5% of children with ASD have mitochondrial disease.[39] It is important to note that illness or stress will generally place mitochondria under more stress and increase dysfunction.[39] Thus, stressors such as dehydration, fever, and infection can lead to a functional decline and neurodegenerative regression in individuals with mitochondrial disease.[18,40]

To evaluate possible mitochondrial dysfunction, it is important to examine a patient's clinical history. Occasionally, there will be a family history of mitochondrial disease. Other clinical history that is often observed in mitochondrial dysfunction includes developmental regression (loss of previously acquired skills), seizures, fatigue or lethargy, ataxia (lack of coordination of muscle movements), motor delays, GI abnormalities (such as reflux, constipation, diarrhea, and inflammation), and cardiomyopathy (significant heart problems). Elevations in the various metabolites described previously are laboratory markers of mitochondrial dysfunction, making laboratory testing a helpful tool for identifying mitochondrial dysfunction. Generally, the higher the elevations and the more metabolites affected, the more likely it is that mitochondrial dysfunction exists.

The tests in question are typically covered by insurance and can be performed by any standard laboratory. The laboratory tests (ideally performed in the morning after fasting for 8-10 hours) may include those listed in Table 1. If the test results are abnormal, they may need to be repeated for confirmation. If the results are normal but mitochondrial dysfunction is still suspected, then repeating the tests when the child is sick or under stress may help unmask and identify mitochondrial dysfunction.

Table 1. Laboratory markers of mitochondrial dysfunction

- Lactate (lactic acid)
- Pyruvate
- Carnitine (free and total)
- Acylcarnitine panel (fatty acids attached to carnitine)
- *Quantitative* plasma amino acids (for measuring alanine and lysine)
- Ubiquinone (also known as CoQ10)
- Ammonia
- Creatine kinase (CK)
- AST (aspartate aminotransferase) and ALT (alanine aminotransferase)
- CO_2 and glucose

Mitochondrial dysfunction, neurological sequelae, and GI abnormalities
Since mitochondria are predominantly responsible for energy production, organs with the highest energy demand are most adversely affected by mitochondrial dysfunction. Low-energy cells (such as skin cells) have fewer mitochondria, while cells with higher energy needs contain more mitochondria. Cells that have high energy demands and, thus, many mitochondria include muscle, liver, brain, cerebrovascular endothelium, and GI cells.[39] Neural synapses (areas of high energy consumption[41]) are especially dependent on mitochondrial function.[42] This helps explain how mitochondrial dysfunction can lead to impaired brain function.

Mitochondria are concentrated in the dendritic and axonal termini, where they play an important role in ATP production, calcium homeostasis, and synaptic plasticity.[43,44] Mitochondrial dysfunction can lead to reduced synaptic neurotransmitter release. Neurons that have high firing rates, such as GABAergic interneurons, may be the most adversely affected.[45] Mitochondria also play an important role in cellular lipid metabolism, signaling, and repair.[46,47]

The ETC is the predominant source and the major target of reactive oxygen species (ROS).[48,49] ROS (also called free radicals) are molecules with an unpaired electron that can cause damage to cells and tissues by removing an electron from a surrounding compound or molecule. This damage is termed oxidative stress. Oxidative stress has been reported in many neurological disorders.[48,50] The ETC is protected from the damage caused by ROS by a mitochondrial-specific superoxide dismutase and by antioxidants such as glutathione (GSH).[49] Under normal circumstances, GSH, the body's main antioxidant, can donate an electron to the free radical and quench the free radical before it can cause damage. Unfortunately, mitochondria lack the enzymes to synthesize GSH and, therefore, are dependent on cytosolic GSH production.[51,52] When the GSH in mitochondria is depleted, cells are more vulnerable to oxidative stress and damage from ROS originating from the mitochondria.[53] Additionally, some factors can increase ROS production, including environmental toxins, infections, and autoimmune disease, which can directly and indirectly lead to impairments in ETC activity,[45,54,55] GSH depletion,[54] and activation of mitochondrial and non-mitochondrial-dependent biochemical cascades that result in programmed cell death (apoptosis).[56]

Certain mammalian cells, such as neuronal and non-neuronal brain cells, are particularly vulnerable to oxidative stress. Moreover, the high rate of oxygen delivery and consumption in the brain provides the oxygen molecules necessary to generate ROS. The brain's ability to withstand oxidative stress is limited for the following reasons:

a. a high content of substrates (such as polyunsaturated fatty acids) that are easily oxidized
b. relatively low levels of antioxidants, such as GSH and antioxidant enzymes

c. the endogenous generation of ROS via several specific reactions
d. the endogenous generation of nitric oxide (NO), a compound that readily transforms into reactive nitrogen species
e. non-replicating cells that, if damaged, may become permanently dysfunctional or committed to apoptosis[54,56]

Not surprisingly, mitochondrial dysfunction has been implicated in many neurological and psychiatric diseases, including neurodegenerative diseases such as Huntington's disease, Friedreich's ataxia,[48] Parkinson's disease, and amyotrophic lateral sclerosis (ALS).[57] Less obviously, mitochondrial dysfunction can also contribute to GI problems. For example, children with mitochondrial diseases are more likely to have GI abnormalities when compared with controls,[39] and unexplained GI problems have been associated with mitochondrial disease.[58] Constipation is a common symptom in children with mitochondrial disease[38] as is the more severe condition of obstipation (an inability to produce stool and gas).[59] Given the high energy demands of both the GI tract and the cerebrovascular endothelium, it is apparent that mitochondrial dysfunction may contribute to barrier dysfunction in both the brain and GI tract.[39]

Dysbiosis, mitochondrial dysfunction, and neurological sequelae
The type of bacteria present in the GI tract may have a significant impact on the development of the brain and, eventually, on adult behavior. For example, the bacteria in the GI tract influence how the body uses vitamin B6, which then can affect the health of nerve cells. GI tract bacteria also have an influence on autoimmune diseases such as multiple sclerosis. A newly developed biochemical test that may help identify autism is based on the end products of GI bacterial metabolism.[9]

Bacteria in the GI tract have been shown to influence anxiety. In one study,[60] mice lacking normal gut microflora were compared with mice with normal gut bacteria. Investigators looked at behavior, brain development, and brain chemistry. Illustrating one way in which the composition of the gut flora affect brain function, the animals lacking normal gut microflora actually had less anxiety as measured by some behavioral-related tests and displayed increased motor activity when compared with mice with normal gut flora. Two genes that may play a role in increasing anxiety—brain-derived neurotrophic factor (BDNF) and nerve growth factor-inducible clone A (NGF1-A)—were downregulated in the animals lacking the normal flora. In addition, the study demonstrated how the gut bacteria shape brain function by influencing brain cells to turn gene expression on or off, which in this instance affected the expression of almost 40 genes found in five different areas of the brain. These findings indicate that some brain-directed behaviors are influenced by the makeup of the GI flora.[60]

Interestingly, some bacteria in the GI tract produce metabolites that may be potentially harmful. One example is propionic acid, an enteric short-chain fatty acid that is a fermentation end product of enteric bacteria. Propionic acid has been shown to inhibit mitochondrial fatty acid metabolism and function,[61-65] contribute to seizure activity,[39] and produce evidence of neuroinflammation, including reactive astrogliosis and activated microglia.[61] Clostridia, which are anaerobic, spore-forming Gram-positive rod bacteria, are known to produce propionic acid,[61] and a derivative of propionic acid recovered in the urine of individuals with ASD has been reported as a marker of clostridia.[66] A recent rat model of ASD demonstrated that the administration of propionic acid induced mitochondrial dysfunction and led to brain, behavioral, and metabolic changes consistent with ASD, including clinical features such as repetitive behaviors, social interaction problems, hyperactivity, oxidative stress, lowered GSH levels, microglial activation, and altered carnitine levels.[61-65] Furthermore, significantly elevated concentrations of clostridia in the GI tract have been reported in some children with ASD when compared with controls[67-70] and in children with constipation when compared with controls.[71] Treatment of clostridia improves brain function in children with ASD[70,72] and has been shown to decrease hyperactivity and hypersensitivity as well as increase social interaction, eye contact, and vocalizations.[70] Interestingly, clostridia levels increase with age and may lead to increased production of toxins that may affect liver function and play a role in cancer.[73,74]

My clinical experience confirms that a number of children with ASD have evidence of clostridia. Symptoms commonly associated with increased clostridia include hyperactivity, irritability, aggressiveness, increased self-stimulatory behavior, and obsessive behavior. Treatment of clostridia is often associated with a reduction in these behaviors, usually within several days to a week. In the context of clostridia in children with ASD, treatment with carnitine may be particularly helpful. This is because carnitine deficiency has been implicated in ASD,[75,76] some studies have reported improvements with the use of carnitine in ASD,[77-83] and carnitine may lower the toxicity[84] of propionic acid produced by clostridia. Carnitine has also been reported to improve mitochondrial function.[85]

HBOT and mitochondrial dysfunction

Although treatments for mitochondrial dysfunction remain relatively limited,[39] one treatment that has garnered interest in recent years is HBOT. HBOT involves inhaling up to 100% oxygen at a pressure greater than one atmosphere in a pressurized chamber.[86] Since hypoxia is known to impair mitochondrial function,[87] and because only approximately 0.3% of inhaled oxygen is ultimately delivered to mitochondria,[88] increasing oxygen delivery to dysfunctional mitochondria through HBOT might aid in improving function.[89,90]

Both animal and human studies have examined the effects of HBOT on mitochondrial function. In a mouse model with an intrinsic impairment of mitochondrial complex IV, HBOT at 2 atmospheres "significantly ameliorate[d] mitochondrial dysfunction" and delayed the onset of motor neuron disease when compared with control mice.[89] In other animal studies, HBOT increased the amount of work done by mitochondria,[91] improved mitochondrial function after brain injury,[90] and prevented mitochondrial deterioration[92] when compared with room air pressure and 100% oxygen levels. HBOT has also been reported to increase sperm motility by augmenting mitochondrial oxidative phosphorylation in fructolysis-inhibited sperm cells from rats. Fructose is the sugar used by sperm for energy production.[93] In rats, HBOT prevented apoptosis and improved neurological recovery after cerebral ischemia by opening mitochondrial ATP-sensitive potassium channels.[94] In another animal model, hypoxia and ischemia led to diminished ATP and phosphocreatine production; the addition of HBOT restored these levels to near normal and increased energy utilization when compared with room air oxygen and pressure levels.[95]

In an animal model, HBOT was recently shown to activate mitochondrial DNA transcription and replication and increase the biogenesis of mitochondria in the brain.[96] It is possible that HBOT could be used to increase the production of mitochondria in humans. Although biogenesis has not yet been proven to occur in humans, I have had two patients with severe mitochondrial disease and abnormal mitochondrial function (as measured by muscle biopsy) who have improved clinically with HBOT at 1.3 to 1.5 atmospheres and who now have normal mitochondrial function (again as measured by muscle biopsy).

In a recent human study of 69 patients with severe traumatic brain injury, HBOT at 1.5 atmospheres and 100% oxygen significantly increased brain oxygen levels, increased cerebral blood flow, and decreased CSF lactate levels. It also improved brain metabolism and mitochondrial function when compared with both room air treatment and 100% oxygen given at normobaric pressure.[97]

HBOT and GI function

Because HBOT possesses potent anti-inflammatory properties,[98,99] it may be useful in ameliorating inflammatory conditions of the GI tract. Several published animal models of IBD have demonstrated that HBOT can significantly lower inflammation in the GI tract and improve IBD.[99-104] Other studies have reported improvements using HBOT for Crohn's disease[105-108] and ulcerative colitis.[109-111] In addition, HBOT can kill clostridial species, because these bacteria are anaerobic.[112] In my clinical experience, children with evidence of clostridia often have significant improvements in GI function (especially in diarrhea) with the use of HBOT.

HBOT and brain function

HBOT may help improve brain function in certain conditions. In animal models, HBOT improves learning and memory.[113] In healthy young adults, the addition of 100% oxygen when compared with room air significantly enhances memory,[114] cognitive performance (including word recall and reaction time),[115] attention, and picture recognition.[116] Several studies have shown improvements in traumatic or chronic brain injury with HBOT.[117-120] In a recent study of 16 individuals who had traumatic brain injury, individuals exhibited significant improvements with the use of HBOT at 1.5 atmospheres and 100% oxygen in their neurological exam, IQ, memory, post-traumatic stress symptoms, depression, and anxiety; they also displayed objective improvements in brain perfusion.[121] Studies also have reported behavioral improvements in children with ASD using HBOT at 1.3 to 1.5 atmospheres.[122-126] HBOT may bring about improvements even in conditions where permanent brain problems are thought to be present, including cerebral palsy[127,128] and fetal alcohol syndrome.[129]

Conclusions

The evidence for a gut-brain connection has become stronger over time. Abnormalities in the GI tract, including dysbiosis, and abnormalities caused by intake of gluten and cow's milk proteins may contribute to abnormal brain function. Mitochondria play an important role in the gut-brain connection, and abnormalities in mitochondrial function are found in many neurological and psychiatric disorders. Mitochondrial dysfunction can lead to GI abnormalities and brain dysfunction. Ultimately, mitochondrial dysfunction can have adverse effects on the gut-brain connection. Treatment of mitochondrial dysfunction with modalities such as carnitine and HBOT may be beneficial in maintaining and/or improving the gut-brain connection. Additional studies examining the gut-brain connection in neurological and psychiatric disorders are warranted.

References

1.   Marshall HW. Arthritis of gastrointestinal origin, its diagnosis and treatment. *JAMA*. 1910;55(22):1871.
2.   Moyer HN. Insanity proceeding from the colon. *JAMA*. 1889;13(7):230.
3.   Marshall HK, Thompson CE. Colon irrigation in the treatment of mental disease. *New Engl J Med*. 1932;207(10):454-7.
4.   Savidge TC, Sofroniew MV, Neunlist M. Starring roles for astroglia in barrier pathologies of gut and brain. *Lab Invest*. 2007;87(8):731-6.
5.   Clarke TB, Davis KM, Lysenko ES, Zhou AY, Yu Y, Weiser JN. Recognition of peptidoglycan from the microbiota by Nod1 enhances systemic innate immunity. *Nat Med*. 2010;16(2):228-31.
6.   Hughes DT, Sperandio V. Inter-kingdom signalling: communication between bacteria and their hosts. *Nat Rev Microbiol*. 2008;6(2):111-20.
7.   Sperandio V, Torres AG, Jarvis B, Nataro JP, Kaper JB. Bacteria-host communication: the language of hormones. *Proc Natl Acad Sci USA*. 2003;100(15):8951-6.

8. Nicholson JK, Holmes E, Lindon JC, Wilson ID. The challenges of modeling mammalian biocomplexity. *Nat Biotechnol.* 2004;22(10):1268-74.

9. Yap IK, Angley M, Veselkov KA, Holmes E, Lindon JC, Nicholson JK. Urinary metabolic phenotyping differentiates children with autism from their unaffected siblings and age-matched controls. *J Proteome Res.* 2010;9(6):2996-3004.

10. Yang G, Wu L, Jiang B, Yang W, Qi J, Cao K *et al.* H2S as a physiologic vasorelaxant: hypertension in mice with deletion of cystathionine gamma-lyase. *Science.* 2008;322(5901):587-90.

11. Bäckhed F, Ding H, Wang T, Hooper LV, Koh GY, Nagy A *et al.* The gut microbiota as an environmental factor that regulates fat storage. *Proc Natl Acad Sci USA.* 2004;101(44):15718-23.

12. Hadjivassiliou M, Grunewald RA, Davies-Jones GA. Gluten sensitivity as a neurological illness. *J Neurol Neurosurg Psychiatry.* 2002;72(5):560-3.

13. Barcia G, Posar A, Santucci M, Parmeggiani A. Autism and coeliac disease. *J Autism Dev Disord.* 2008;38(2):407-8.

14. O'Banion D, Armstrong B, Cummings RA, Stange J. Disruptive behavior: a dietary approach. *J Autism Child Schizophr.* 1978;8(3):325-37.

15. Ramaekers VT, Blau N. Cerebral folate deficiency. *Dev Med Child Neurol.* 2004;46(12):843-51.

16. Ramaekers VT, Hausler M, Opladen T, Heimann G, Blau N. Psychomotor retardation, spastic paraplegia, cerebellar ataxia and dyskinesia associated with low 5-methyltetrahydrofolate in cerebrospinal fluid: a novel neurometabolic condition responding to folinic acid substitution. *Neuropediatrics.* 2002;33(6):301-8.

17. Ramaekers VT, Blau N, Sequeira JM, Nassogne MC, Quadros EV. Folate receptor autoimmunity and cerebral folate deficiency in low-functioning autism with neurological deficits. *Neuropediatrics.* 2007;38(6):276-81.

18. Shoffner J, Hyams L, Langley GN, Cossette S, Mylacraine L, Dale J *et al.* Fever plus mitochondrial disease could be risk factors for autistic regression. *J Child Neurol.* 2010;25(4):429-34.

19. Ramaekers VT, Rothenberg SP, Sequeira JM, Opladen T, Blau N, Quadros EV *et al.* Autoantibodies to folate receptors in the cerebral folate deficiency syndrome. *N Engl J Med.* 2005;352(19):1985-91.

20. Ramaekers VT, Sequeira JM, Blau N, Quadros EV. A milk-free diet downregulates folate receptor autoimmunity in cerebral folate deficiency syndrome. *Dev Med Child Neurol.* 2008;50(5):346-52.

21. Moretti P, Peters SU, Del Gaudio D, Sahoo T, Hyland K, Bottiglieri T *et al.* Brief report: autistic symptoms, developmental regression, mental retardation, epilepsy, and dyskinesias in CNS folate deficiency. *J Autism Dev Disord.* 2008;38(6):1170-7.

22. Moretti P, Sahoo T, Hyland K, Bottiglieri T, Peters S, del Gaudio D *et al.* Cerebral folate deficiency with developmental delay, autism, and response to folinic acid. *Neurology.* 2005;64(6):1088-90.

23. Ramaekers VT, Hansen SI, Holm J, Opladen T, Senderek J, Hausler M *et al.* Reduced folate transport to the CNS in female Rett patients. *Neurology.* 2003;61(4):506-15.

24. Ramaekers VT, Sequeira JM, Artuch R, Blau N, Temudo T, Ormazabal A *et al.* Folate receptor autoantibodies and spinal fluid 5-methyltetrahydrofolate deficiency in Rett syndrome. *Neuropediatrics.* 2007;38(4):179-83.

25. Perez-Duenas B, Ormazabal A, Toma C, Torrico B, Cormand B, Serrano M *et al.* Cerebral folate deficiency syndromes in childhood: clinical, analytical, and etiologic aspects. *Arch Neurol.* 2011;68(5):615-21.

26. Ramaekers VT, Weis J, Sequeira JM, Quadros EV, Blau N. Mitochondrial complex I encephalomyopathy and cerebral 5-methyltetrahydrofolate deficiency. *Neuropediatrics*. 2007;38(4):184-7.

27. Garcia-Cazorla A, Quadros EV, Nascimento A, Garcia-Silva MT, Briones P, Montoya J *et al*. Mitochondrial diseases associated with cerebral folate deficiency. *Neurology*. 2008;70(16):1360-2.

28. Hansen FJ, Blau N. Cerebral folate deficiency: life-changing supplementation with folinic acid. *Mol Genet Metab*. 2005;84(4):371-3.

29. Whiteley P, Haracopos D, Knivsberg AM, Reichelt KL, Parlar S, Jacobsen J *et al*. The ScanBrit randomised, controlled, single-blind study of a gluten- and casein-free dietary intervention for children with autism spectrum disorders. *Nutr Neurosci*. 2010;13(2):87-100.

30. Afzal N, Murch S, Thirrupathy K, Berger L, Fagbemi A, Heuschkel R. Constipation with acquired megarectum in children with autism. *Pediatrics*. 2003;112(4):939-42.

31. Cagnon L, Braissant O. Hyperammonemia-induced toxicity for the developing central nervous system. *Brain Res Rev*. 2007;56(1):183-97.

32. Weissenborn K, Ennen JC, Schomerus H, Ruckert N, Hecker H. Neuropsychological characterization of hepatic encephalopathy. *J Hepatol*. 2001;34(5):768-73.

33. Bass NM, Mullen KD, Sanyal A, Poordad F, Neff G, Leevy CB *et al*. Rifaximin treatment in hepatic encephalopathy. *N Engl J Med*. 2010;362(12):1071-81.

34. Haas RH, Parikh S, Falk MJ, Saneto RP, Wolf NI, Darin N *et al*. Mitochondrial disease: a practical approach for primary care physicians. *Pediatrics*. 2007;120(6):1326-33.

35. Kang HC, Lee YM, Kim HD, Lee JS, Slama A. Safe and effective use of the ketogenic diet in children with epilepsy and mitochondrial respiratory chain complex defects. *Epilepsia*. 2007;48(1):82-8.

36. Zeviani M, Bertagnolio B, Uziel G. Neurological presentations of mitochondrial diseases. *J Inherit Metab Dis*. 1996;19(4):504-20.

37. Skladal D, Halliday J, Thorburn DR. Minimum birth prevalence of mitochondrial respiratory chain disorders in children. *Brain*. 2003;126(Pt 8):1905-12.

38. Nissenkorn A, Zeharia A, Lev D, Watemberg N, Fattal-Valevski A, Barash V *et al*. Neurologic presentations of mitochondrial disorders. *J Child Neurol*. 2000;15(1):44-8.

39. Rossignol DA, Frye RE. Mitochondrial dysfunction in autism spectrum disorders: a systematic review and meta-analysis. *Mol Psychiatry*. 2011 Jan 25.

40. Edmonds JL, Kirse DJ, Kearns D, Deutsch R, Spruijt L, Naviaux RK. The otolaryngological manifestations of mitochondrial disease and the risk of neurodegeneration with infection. *Arch Otolaryngol Head Neck Surg*. 2002;128(4):355-62.

41. Ames A, 3rd. CNS energy metabolism as related to function. *Brain Res Brain Res Rev*. 2000;34(1-2):42-68.

42. Mattson MP, Liu D. Energetics and oxidative stress in synaptic plasticity and neurodegenerative disorders. *Neuromolecular Med*. 2002;2(2):215-31.

43. Chen H, Chan DC. Mitochondrial dynamics--fusion, fission, movement, and mitophagy--in neurodegenerative diseases. *Hum Mol Genet*. 2009;18(R2):R169-76.

44. Li Z, Okamoto K, Hayashi Y, Sheng M. The importance of dendritic mitochondria in the morphogenesis and plasticity of spines and synapses. *Cell*. 2004;119(6):873-87.

45. Anderson MP, Hooker BS, Herbert MR. Bridging from cells to cognition in autism pathophysiology: biological pathways to defective brain function and plasticity. *Am J Biochem Biotech*. 2008;4(2):167-76.

46. Marin-Garcia J, Goldenthal MJ. Heart mitochondria signaling pathways: appraisal of an emerging field. *J Mol Med*. 2004;82(9):565-78.

47. Goldenthal MJ, Marin-Garcia J. Mitochondrial signaling pathways: a receiver/integrator organelle. *Mol Cell Biochem*. 2004;262(1-2):1-16.

48. Trushina E, McMurray CT. Oxidative stress and mitochondrial dysfunction in neurodegenerative diseases. *Neuroscience*. 2007;145(4):1233-48.

49. Fernandez-Checa JC, Garcia-Ruiz C, Colell A, Morales A, Mari M, Miranda M *et al*. Oxidative stress: role of mitochondria and protection by glutathione. *Biofactors*. 1998;8(1-2):7-11.

50. Chauhan A, Chauhan V. Oxidative stress in autism. *Pathophysiology*. 2006;13(3):171-81.

51. Enns GM. The contribution of mitochondria to common disorders. *Mol Genet Metab*. 2003;80(1-2):11-26.

52. James SJ, Rose S, Melnyk S, Jernigan S, Blossom S, Pavliv O *et al*. Cellular and mitochondrial glutathione redox imbalance in lymphoblastoid cells derived from children with autism. *FASEB J*. 2009;23(8):2374-83.

53. Fernandez-Checa JC, Kaplowitz N, Garcia-Ruiz C, Colell A, Miranda M, Mari M *et al*. GSH transport in mitochondria: defense against TNF-induced oxidative stress and alcohol-induced defect. *Am J Physiol*. 1997;273(1 Pt 1):G7-17.

54. Calabrese V, Lodi R, Tonon C, D'Agata V, Sapienza M, Scapagnini G *et al*. Oxidative stress, mitochondrial dysfunction and cellular stress response in Friedreich's ataxia. *J Neurol Sci*. 2005;233(1-2):145-62.

55. Munnich A, Rustin P. Clinical spectrum and diagnosis of mitochondrial disorders. *Am J Med Genet*. 2001;106(1):4-17.

56. Roberts RA, Laskin DL, Smith CV, Robertson FM, Allen EM, Doorn JA *et al*. Nitrative and oxidative stress in toxicology and disease. *Toxicol Sci*. 2009;112(1):4-16.

57. Martin LJ. Mitochondriopathy in Parkinson disease and amyotrophic lateral sclerosis. *J Neuropathol Exp Neurol*. 2006;65(12):1103-10.

58. Verma A, Piccoli DA, Bonilla E, Berry GT, DiMauro S, Moraes CT. A novel mitochondrial G8313A mutation associated with prominent initial gastrointestinal symptoms and progressive encephaloneuropathy. *Pediatr Res*. 1997;42(4):448-54.

59. Skladal D, Sudmeier C, Konstantopoulou V, Stockler-Ipsiroglu S, Plecko-Startinig B, Bernert G *et al*. The clinical spectrum of mitochondrial disease in 75 pediatric patients. *Clin Pediatr (Phila)*. 2003;42(8):703-10.

60. Heijtz RD, Wang S, Anuar F, Qian Y, Bjorkholm B, Samuelsson A *et al*. Normal gut microbiota modulates brain development and behavior. *Proc Natl Acad Sci USA*. 2011;108(7):3047-52.

61. MacFabe DF, Cain DP, Rodriguez-Capote K, Franklin AE, Hoffman JE, Boon F *et al*. Neurobiological effects of intraventricular propionic acid in rats: possible role of short chain fatty acids on the pathogenesis and characteristics of autism spectrum disorders. *Behav Brain Res*. 2007;176(1):149-69.

62. MacFabe DF, Rodríguez-Capote K, Hoffman JE, Franklin AE, Mohammad-Asef Y, Taylor AR *et al*. A novel rodent model of autism: intraventricular infusions of propionic acid increase locomotor activity and induce neuroinflammation and oxidative stress in discrete regions of adult rat brain. *Am J Biochem Biotech*. 2008;4(2):146-66.

CHAPTER TWELVE

MILK: EFFECTS & IMPLICATIONS FOR AUTISM AND OTHER DISORDERS

By Krystal D. Dubé and Richard C. Deth PhD

Northeastern University, Bouvé College of Health Sciences, School of Pharmacy, Boston, Massachusetts, USA

Background: Autism is a developmental disorder of unknown etiology. The prevalence of autism has drastically increased over the past few decades and there are numerous theories regarding the cause.

Objective: An overview of current research into the possible cause(s) of autism with a focus on milk and its potential role will be provided.

Findings: Current research confirms pre-pregnancy and early life as unique periods of sensitivity during which seemingly small experiences have the potential to confer enduring effects. Recent findings point to a peptide component of cow's milk known as beta-casomorphin-7 (BCM7) as being a possible factor in the increased prevalence of autism. An analogous peptide is released from wheat-derived gluten, and studies have shown that a gluten-free/casein-free (GF/CF) diet can be beneficial in a significant proportion of autistic individuals. Schizophrenia patients also benefit from a GF/CF diet, indicating a similarity with autism.

Conclusion: Regardless of its relation to autism, the milk an infant receives helps set foundational systems that will produce lifelong effects. Further research should track a large, randomized sample of women from pre-pregnancy until the child is 5 years old to assess if there is a correlation between an autism diagnosis and any encounters in pre-pregnancy, pregnancy and/or early life. Special attention should be given to the milk a child receives, particularly whether it is breast milk or formula milk. Further research is also warranted in the effects of milk on adult health and implications for pre-pregnancy. Combining autism research with research on schizophrenia and other similar disorders may reveal insights about factors that contribute to both conditions.

Background

Autism is no longer a rare disorder. Since Leo Kanner's initial description of autism in 1943, the prevalence of autism and autism spectrum disorders (ASD) has steadily increased from 1 in 10,000 in 1970 to 66 in 10,000 in 2002 and recently to 1% of the population in 2012 (Stanković *et al.* 2012). This drastic increase raises important questions, and there are a number of theories that attempt to explain the autism epidemic. First, it has been proposed that autism is better recognized now than it was 40 years ago. It has also been put forth that the diagnostic criteria has changed over time and broadened to include children who previously may have been diagnosed with varying levels of mental retardation (MR) (Lenoir *et al.* 2009) or other neurological disorders. Whether it is autism, Asperger's, pervasive developmental disorder (PDD) or MR, the fact remains that there is something causing disturbances in the neuronal development of a significant number of children.

The cause of ASD is still said to be unknown, although recent research is providing significant direction. In 1949, Kanner concluded autism was caused by *refrigerator parents*. This was based on his observations of the autistic childrens' parents as being cold, unfeeling, and overly analytical. Kanner assumed that frigid parenting styles had turned children inward and directly caused the disorder. However, this idea has since been rejected as research into genetic predisposition and environmental influences have been linked to autism risk. Among environmental factors, milk consumption may place parents in a pivotal role to substantially decrease the risk of having an autistic child.

Findings: Pre-pregnancy, Pregnancy, and Early life

The long-term health of a newborn baby is influenced well before birth and even before conception. Pre-pregnancy maternal health has been shown to affect the risk of a range of later complications. Most recently, the use of periconceptual prenatal vitamins, specifically taking 800 mg of folic acid even BEFORE conception, was associated with a reduced risk of autism (Schmidt *et al.* 2011). Compared to mothers of typically developing children, mothers of children with autism were less likely to report having taken prenatal vitamins during the first 3 months before pregnancy or the first month of pregnancy. Sufficient iron intake prior to conception has also been linked to a decreased risk, reflecting the requirement of 300 mg or more of iron reserves during gestation (Viteri and Berger 2005). Women of reproductive age are especially at risk for developing iron deficiencies, which could progress to anemia. In the United States, 5% of non-pregnant women, 17% of pregnant women, and 33% of pregnant women of low socioeconomic status are anemic. Long-term weekly supplementation with iron and folic acid for ALL women of reproductive age could be significantly beneficial in the prevention of autism as well as other disorders.

Once pregnancy is confirmed, it is not too late to increase the chance of delivering a healthy baby. This can be achieved by avoiding stress. Independent of other biomedical risk factors, enhanced levels of depression and anxiety symptoms during pregnancy contribute to adverse obstetric, fetal, and neonatal outcomes (Alder *et al.* 2007). An animal study found that when pregnant mice were exposed to stress, their male babies presented with changes in the expression and DNA methylation status of the stress-related genes corticotrophin-releasing factor (CRF) and glucocorticoid receptor (GR) (Bale *et al.* 2010). Early pregnancy is a period of vulnerability and the sex specificity of effects from maternal stress may provide insight into predominantly male disorders such as autism, which affects four times as many males as females (Stanković *et al.* 2012).

Gastrointestinal (GI) problems are very common among autistic children. A study of 51 children with ASD and 40 typically developing children ages 3-15 found that 63% of the children with ASD had moderate or severe chronic diarrhea and/or constipation as compared with only 2% of the controls (Adams *et al.* 2011). Similar GI research found abnormal intestinal permeability test (IPT) values among autistic children. An investigation of IPT levels and the leaky gut hypothesis in patients with autism and their first degree relatives found that 36.7% of autistic children, along with 21.2% of their relatives, showed increased IPT values in comparison with only 4.8% of typically developing controls (de Magistris *et al.* 2010). This suggests a contribution of hereditary factors for GI complications in autism.

Milk: A1 vs. A2

All newborn mammals are raised on mother's milk, but the components of the milk vary greatly between species. For all species, mother's milk is one of the newborn's first encounters with the outside environment. From this perspective, it's easy to see how the gut is a doorway into the body, especially during development. It's fairly safe to say that any autism-related problems associated with milk will be because of a difference in the components present in cow's milk (or cow's milk-based formula) that is not found in human milk or because of a difference in the balance of these components. Human milk is much higher in lactose but much lower in calcium, sodium, potassium, and proteins than cow's milk (Shah 2000). The protein level in human milk begins around 1.6% with the initial postpartum milk (colostrum) and subsequently drops to about 0.9%. In comparison, the protein level of cow's milk is roughly 3-4% depending on the breed and other factors. Also, 80% of the protein in cow's milk is from casein proteins, whereas the major proteins in human milk are whey proteins. These components are not just providing a short term source of nourishment for the baby – they are establishing the foundation of future growth and development for all levels of functioning.

In his 2007 book titled *Devil in the Milk: Illness, Health, and the Politics of A1 and A2 Milk*, Keith Woodford provides a comprehensive analysis of milk. Woodford's research focuses on the major casein of milk, beta-casein, of which there are two primary types: A1 and A2.

All human beta-casein is of the A2 type, whereas cow beta-casein can be of the A1 or A2 type (Brantl and Teschemacher 1994). The beta-casein protein is 209 amino acids long, and the difference between the A1 and A2 types is that 1 of those 209 amino acids is not the same. Position 67 of A2 beta-casein contains the amino acid proline, whereas the same position in the A1 beta-casein contains the amino acid histidine (Bradley *et al.* 1998). This change from A2 milk to A1 milk is the result of a mutation that most likely happened 8,000 years ago when the proline was replaced by histidine. This may seem to be a small, insignificant change, but it has a huge and very significant effect when it's time to digest the milk.

When A1 milk is digested, it produces a small protein fragment of 7 amino acids called beta-casomorphin-7 (BCM7) (Naito 1972). However, the proline-histidine switch affects the digestion of beta-casein: The bonds formed by proline with other amino acids are more resistant to hydrolysis and are especially stronger than the bonds histidine shares with other amino acids. Therefore, during digestion, A1 beta-casein is easily cleaved at the weak histidine bond at position 67, while A2 beta-casein is not as readily cleaved because of its proline. Thus, A1 milk releases a lot of BCM7, while A2 milk releases only a little.

BCM7 is a powerful opioid. In healthy adults, it should be difficult for BCM7 to pass into the bloodstream, but for those with leaky gut syndrome and other GI complications, large molecules such as BCM7 may pass into the bloodstream and possibly through the blood-brain barrier (Cade *et al.* 2000). Early life is a period of developmental vulnerability during which the release of a powerful opioid has the potential to confer permanent effects. A number of studies have linked opioid substances and their receptors to autism (Panksepp and Sahley 1987; Modahl *et al.* 1992).

Our lab recently reported the discovery of a new action of Mu opiate receptor activation that promotes inflammation. This action involves inhibition of cellular uptake of the amino acid cysteine by a specific transporter known as Excitatory Amino Acid Transporter 3 (EAAT3) (Deth *et al.* 2008). EAAT3 is located in neurons as well as in the epithelial cells of the intestine and in the white blood cells of the immune system. BCM7 activates the Mu opiate receptor, which inhibits EAAT3 and decreases cysteine uptake, leading to a decrease in synthesis of the antioxidant glutathione, causing a state of oxidative stress.

Oxidative Stress

The body's ability to regulate oxidation (the loss of an electron) is a highly evolved, critical ability of all cells, and brain cells are unable to grow and function properly when antioxidant levels are abnormally low, a condition known as oxidative stress. Antioxidant capacity is dependent on the developmental stage and is lowest in pre-term infants compared with full-term newborns and highest in adults (Turcot et al. 2009). The low antioxidant capacity in early life renders infants particularly vulnerable to complications induced by an oxidative environment. Neonatal oxidative stress can initiate permanent modifications in cell development and can lead to cell death. Glutathione (GSH) is the biggest contributor to maintaining the intracellular balance between the reduction and oxidation (redox) environment of the cell (Turcot et al. 2009). In autistic individuals, cysteine and GSH levels are abnormally low, indicating an oxidative state (Jameset al. 2004; Deth et al. 2008; Frustaci et al. 2012).

Discussion: "Breast is best"

The World Health Organization (WHO) recommends exclusive breastfeeding for the first 6 months, at which point complementary feeding may begin in conjunction with breastfeeding to continue until the infant is at least 2 years old (World Health Organization 2008). A recent case study by Al-Farsi et al. in 2012 found that deviations from this recommendation increased the risk of autism. This increased risk was especially prominent in cases with delayed onset of breastfeeding, non-intake of colostrum, and bottle feeding. These findings highlight the value of colostrum in the initial breast milk and the benefits associated with exact adherence to the WHO recommendations.

Breastfeeding could also reduce the risk of other diseases. Breastfed infants have lower blood pressure later in life than those fed with infant formulas (Turcot et al. 2009). Breastfed babies are less likely to get inflammatory bowel diseases such as Crohn's disease and ulcerative colitis (Clement et al. 2004). This might be because of the protective maternal antibodies in colostrum, which further highlights the importance of immediate breastfeeding. Similar to the recent increase in autism diagnosis, the prevalence of Crohn's disease and ulcerative colitis has also greatly increased in the past 50 years (Gearry *et al.* 2006).

Besides providing possible decreased health risks, breastfeeding could additionally provide a slight cognitive advantage. A longitudinal study by Andres *et al.* in 2012 found that breastfed infants scored higher than formula-fed infants on the Mental Developmental Index, Psychomotor Development Index, and the Preschool Language Scale during the first year. This study also compared the development of infants fed milk-based formula (MF) versus soy protein-based formula (SF) and concluded there were no significant developmental differences between the MF and SF groups. This suggests the advantages of breastfeeding are exclusive and may not be replicated through *only* the elimination of A1 cow's milk from the diet. It is clear that breastfeeding provides extraordinary benefits to an infant.

Eliminating A1 casein from the diet

For children already diagnosed with ASD, eliminating A1 from the diet could be beneficial. Along with GI problems, autistic individuals can show signs of excessive systemic opioid activity as evidenced by peptides found in their urine and cerebrospinal fluid (Millward *et al.* 2008). Therefore, a GF/CF diet could reduce those symptoms of autism caused by these peptides (Hjiej *et al.* 2008). Autistic children placed on a GF/CF diet have significantly lower levels of IPT compared with autistic children on unrestricted diets (de Magistris *et al.* 2010).

Autism and Schizophrenia

Much can be learned from the similarities between disorders. Pre-pregnancy, pregnancy, and early life events have also been associated with the development of schizophrenia (Bale *et al.* 2010). Autism and schizophrenia are both chronic disorders of unknown etiology, and each affects approximately 1% of the population. Both autism and schizophrenia are diagnosed in a disproportionate number of males versus females. Autism affects four times as many males as females, while the onset of schizophrenia occurs during adolescence when major sex differences in the brain occur (Bale *et al.* 2010). As in autism, schizophrenic patients also have high concentrations of opiate peptides found in their urine. A study in 2000 by Cade *et al.* found that 85% of autistic and schizophrenic patients had significantly enhanced IgG antibodies to casein and gluten. Furthermore, levels of GSH are lower in both autism and schizophrenia (Vojdani *et al.* 2008; Do *et al.* 2009), suggesting that sufferers from both disorders could benefit from a GF/CF diet (Woodford 2007).

Perhaps autism and schizophrenia are different manifestations of the same underlying metabolic abnormality. If this is the case, researchers investigating the causes of autism would benefit from the expertise of those researching schizophrenia and *vice versa*. Such collaboration would be beneficial in possibly finding more effective treatments for either one or both of these disorders.

Conclusion

The GI tract of a newborn is a doorway into the developing body and brain. Breastfed babies may have an advantage over bottle-fed babies by the assurance of receiving A2 milk and the associated possibility of preventing oxidative stress that could lead to an autism spectrum disorder. Further research should track large, randomized samples of women from pre-pregnancy until the child is 5 years old to assess if there is a correlation between an autism diagnosis and any encounters in pre-pregnancy, pregnancy, and/or early life. Special attention should be paid to the milk a child receives as to whether it is breast milk or formula milk. For mothers who are unable to breastfeed, availability of formula made from A2 milk could be pivotal in reducing the prevalence of autism. Further research is warranted into the effects of milk on adult health and the implications for pre-pregnancy. Combining autism research with research into schizophrenia and other similar disorders should be encouraged. Regardless of its relation to autism, it is clear that the milk an infant receives helps set foundational systems that will produce lifelong effects.

References

Adams J, Johansen L, Powell L, *et al*. Gastrointestinal flora and gastrointestinal status in children with autism comparisons to typical children and correlation with autism severity. *BMC Gastoenterology*. 2011;11:22.

Alder J, Fink N, Bitzer J, *et al*. Depression and anxiety during pregnancy: A risk factor for obstetric, fetal and neonatal outcome? A critical review of the literature. *Journal of Maternal, Fetal, and Neonatal Medicine*. 2007;20(3):189-209.

Al-Farsi Y, Al-Sharbati M, Waly M, *et al*. Effect of suboptimal breast-feeding on occurrence of autism: A case control study. *Nutrition* 2012;28(7-8):e27-e32.

Andres A, Cleves M, Bellando J, *et al*. Developmental Status of 1-year-old infants fed breast milk, cow's milk formula, or soy formula. *Pediatrics* 2012;129:1134-1140.

Bale TL, Baram TZ, Brown AS, *et al*. Early Life Programming and Neurodevelopmental Disorders. *Society of Biological Psychiatry* 2010;68:314-319.

Bradley DG, Loftus RT, Cunningham P. Genetics and domestic cattle origins. *Evolutionary Anthropology* 1998:79-86.

Brantl V, Teschemacher L. Beta casomorphins and related peptides. *VCH Weinheim, Germany* 1994:207-219.

Cade R, Privette M, Fregly M, *et al*. Autism and schizophrenia: intestinal disorders. *Nutritional Neuroscience* 2000;3:57-72.

Cummins AG, and Thompson FM. Effect of breast milk and weaning on epithelial growth of the small intestine in humans. *Gut* 2002;51:748-754.

de Magistris L, Familiari V, Pascotto A, *et al*. Alterations of the Intestinal Barrier in Patients With Autism Spectrum Disorders and in Their First-degree Relatives. *Gastroenterology* 2010;00: 1-7.

Deth R, Muratore C, Benzecry J, *et al*. How environmental and genetic factors combine to cause autism: a redox/methylation hypothesis. *NeuroToxicology*. 2008;29:190-201.

Dietert RR, Dewitt JC, Germolec DR, *et al*. Breaking Patterns of Environmentally Influenced Disease for Health Risk Reduction: Immune Perspectives. *Environmental Health Perspectives* 2010;118:1091-1099.

Do K, Cabungcal J, Frank A, *et al*. Redox dysregulation, neurodevelopment, and schizophrenia. *Current Opinion in Neurobiology* 2009;19(2):220-230.

Frustaci A, Neri M, Cesario A, *et al*. Oxidative stress-related biomarkers in autism: Systematic review and meta analyses. *Free Radical Biology and Medicine* 2012;52(10):2128-2141.

Gearry RB, Richardson A, Frampton CM, *et al*. High incidence of Crohn's disease in Canterbury, New Zealand: results of an epidemiologic study. *Inflammatory Bowel Disease* 2006;12(10):936-943.

Hjiej H, Doyen C, Couprie C, *et al*. Substitutive and dietetic approaches in childhood autistic disorder: interests and limits. *Encephale* 2008;34(5):496-503.

James J, Cutler P, Melnyk S, *et al*. Metabolic biomarkers of increased oxidative stress and impaired methylation capacity in children with autism. *American Journal of Clinical Nutrition* 2004;80:1611–7.

Kanner, L. Problems of nosology and psychodynamics in early childhood autism. *American Journal of Orthopsychiatry* 1949;19:416–426.

Lenoir P, Bodier C, Desombre H, *et al.* Prevalence of pervasive developmental disorders. A review. *Encephale* 2009;35(1):36-42.

Millward C, Ferriter M, Calver S, *et al.* Gluten- and casein-free diets for autistic spectrum disorder. *Cochrane Database System Review.* 2008;(2):CD003498.

Modahl C, Fein D, Waterhouse L, *et al.* Does oxytocin mediate social deficits in autism? *Journal of Autism and Developmental Disorders* 1992;22(3):449-51.

Naito H, Kawakami A, and Imamura T. In vitro formation of phosphopeptide with calcium-binding property in the small intestinal tract of the rat fed on casein. *Agriculture and Biological Chemistry* 1972;36:409-415.

Panksepp J, Sahley TL. Possible brain opioid involvement in disrupted social intent and language development of autism. *Neurobiological issues in autism.* Plenum Press; New York: 1987

Rescigno M, and Di Sabatino A. Dendritic cells in intestinal homeostasis and disease. *The Journal of Clinical Investigation* 2009;119:2441-2450.

Schmidt RJ, Hansen RL, Hartiala J, *et al.* Prenatal vitamins, one-carbon metabolism gene variants, and risk for autism. *Epidemiology* 2011;22(4):476-85.

Shah N. Effects of milk-derived bioactives: an overview. *British Journal of Nutrition* 2000;84, Supplement 1:S3-S10.

Stanković M, Lakić A, and Ilić N. Autism and Autistic Spectrum Disorders in the Context of New DSM-V Classification, and Clinical and Epidemiological Data. *Srp Arh Celok Lek* 2012;140(3-4):236-243.

Turcot V, Rouleau T, Tsopmo A, *et al.* Long-term impact of an antioxidant-deficient neonatal diet on lipid and glucose metabolism. *Free Radical Biology and Medicine* 2009;47:275-282.

Viteri FE, and Berger J. Importance of Pre-Pregnancy and Pregnancy Iron Status: Can Long-Term Weekly Preventive Iron and Folic Acid Supplementation Achieve Desirable and Safe Status? *Nutrition Reviews* 2005, 63: S65–S76.

Vojdani A, Mumper E, Granpeesheh D, *et al.* Low natural killer cell and cytotoxic activity in autism: The role of glutathione, IL-2 and IL-15. *Journal of Neuroimmunology* 2008;205(1-2):148-154.

Woodford, Keith. Devil in the Milk: Illness, Health, and the Politics of A1 and A2 Milk. *Chelsea Green Publishing* 2007. White River Junction, VT.

World Health Organization. Indicators for assessing infant and young child feeding practices. Geneva: World Health Organization; 2008.

CHAPTER THIRTEEN

IS IT EVER TOO LATE? USING A BIOMEDICAL APPROACH AND DIETARY INTERVENTION TO TREAT CHILDREN AND ADULTS WITH AUTISM

By Pamela Ferro, RN, ASN; Raman Prasad, MS; and Carol Wester, RN, MSN, PMHCNS, BC

> *The role of a clinician is different than that of an administrator in that you cannot "require" that someone feel and function better; you must care, nurture, nurse, support, and heal them into doing so. You must go above and beyond. You must be creative and do whatever it takes.* - Carol Wester, RN, MSN, PMHCNS, BC

Introduction

In October 2009, at a conference banquet hall of 250 people, a white-haired mom stood with tears in her eyes and held up a T-shirt, size large, with dozens of holes bitten through the chest. Projected on the screen in the front of the room was a photo of her son Paul, a handsome-looking 34-year-old who lives in a group home. Paul, who suffers from symptoms of autism, had spent nearly all his life banging his head against the wall hard enough to damage the hair follicles. Unable to communicate, Paul used yelling, banging, and biting his shirt in an attempt to escape his physical pain and express his discomfort.

The theme of the conference, "How Intestinal Health Impacts Brain and Behavior," reflected our clinical experiences and results. As a dramatic illustration of the theme, one of us (Ferro) reported at the podium that Paul's destructive behaviors had recently stopped after the group home staff implemented dietary changes with support from our nursing practice. Paul's new diet and his body's reaction to the food clearly played a role in his improvement. Over a two-month period after beginning the diet, Paul's behavior changed from erratic to predictable. After so many years of helplessly witnessing her son's pain, the stress that Paul's mother had endured suddenly lifted.

Attendees at nearly every table in the hall could tell a comparable story. A child whose speech acquisition and growth had stopped, leaving him with a failure to thrive (FTT) diagnosis, was now excelling in elementary school. A girl who had been diagnosed with autism started making eye contact and smiling at her parents. A toddler who had stopped walking and talking and had begun losing weight was back to normal. An elementary school boy with Crohn's disease was in remission and had tapered off of heavy medication. All of these stories provided direct evidence of the intricate relationship between gut health, the brain, and behavior.

The shortcomings of the standard mental health model

As nurses with extensive backgrounds in psychiatric and mental health nursing, we (Ferro and Wester) did not always recognize the gut-brain connection. This was not necessarily surprising, given the relatively narrow focus of baccalaureate and graduate nursing programs on nursing, clinical therapy, psychopharmacology, and theories of care for individuals and groups. For each of us, a mixture of personal and professional experiences led us to confront the limits of standard mental health treatment and begin to develop a different, more comprehensive model of practice.

In my case (Wester), I remember standing in my backyard as a young girl, listening to screaming from the state psychiatric hospital across the river. Although most people didn't want to think about state hospitals, much less hear people screaming, I wanted to learn about what the institution's residents experienced and how I could help them. Following completion of two nursing degrees, I, therefore, spent a number of years working first in psychiatric hospitals and then with developmentally disabled adults at one of Massachusetts' state schools. These institutions, now defunct, housed individuals with some of the most complex and challenging medical and behavioral problems: people with mental disabilities, Down syndrome, or autism (often undiagnosed). When the schools shut down in the mid-1990s, I went to work at a local community health agency, where I met Pam.

I (Ferro) was a dedicated professional from a family of nurses. I worked in maternity, cardiac, and intensive care hospital settings for a number of years before transferring to community mental health. I enjoyed a happy marriage, and we had one child. Our household's day-to-day joys and struggles were no different from those of any young family. However, our life changed after our second son was born.

Isaiah was born in 1991 as a typical, bright-eyed, happy, strapping baby who progressed easily through his first year, but by age two, Isaiah had regressed, turning into a child who was as much absent as present. Isaiah's regression began after a sequence of events that started with exposure to chickenpox at a party. When I took him in for a routine doctor's visit that same week, the practice decided to vaccinate him with DTP (diphtheria, tetanus, and pertussis vaccine) and OVP (oral live virus polio vaccine) despite the varicella exposure. When I questioned the nurse about the wisdom of administering the vaccines to Isaiah under the circumstances, she gestured with a careless sweep of her hand, saying, "Ah, it'll be fine!" The following week, however, Isaiah broke out with a severe case of the chickenpox, and his regression began. He lost language and eye contact, and his digestion began to alternate between constipation and diarrhea. He also developed food and seasonal allergies. Often in pain from these conditions, Isaiah cried and screamed. The doctors diagnosed Isaiah with regressive autism, lymphoid hyperplasia, and what would come to be known as autistic enterocolitis. Although I knew about autism and had worked professionally with patients suffering from autism, the challenges of caring for Isaiah were overwhelming.

Previously, I had always looked forward to my extended family's annual Christmas party, but even that became stressful after Isaiah's regression. The people and noise would confuse Isaiah, overloading his senses. He would cry and throw tantrums, and I would end up spending my time comforting him rather than being with the family.

When the two of us met, Carol was traveling between multiple community mental health agency sites, and I was the nurse in charge of one of the sites. The umbrella agency managed hundreds of patients with major issues including schizophrenia, bipolar disorder, major depressive disorder, and substance abuse. All were further complicated by poverty and medical illnesses such as heart disease, diabetes, and chronic respiratory diseases.

Many residents of the state school where I (Wester) used to work now lived in the community, usually at group homes. These patients began visiting the clinic to receive psychiatric care. Typically, I prescribed medications to help these individuals control anxiety, aggression, unstable moods, poor sleep, or poor appetites. Gradually, these adults with mental disabilities began to make up most of my caseload.

The agency expected us to see four to five patients per hour. In our experience, 12 to 15 minutes per patient was not nearly enough. To help the individuals with mental disabilities who increasingly relied on us, we began to ignore the clock. We took time to find out as much as we could about each patient and to recommend appropriate medical care. However, the visits were challenging because our patients often were nonverbal and couldn't speak for themselves. When individuals can't report how they feel or what's going on, it becomes necessary to "intuit" or fill in the blanks.

We increasingly came to realize that the standard community mental health model—with its 12-15-minute time slots, emphasis on talk therapy, and reliance on generic psychological testing—did not fit our patient population. We began searching for an agency that would offer the flexibility to accommodate our unique patients. When this search was unsuccessful, we worked with a forward-thinking executive at the Massachusetts Department of Developmental Services (formerly the Department of Mental Retardation) to set up our own practice to meet the needs of adults with pressing psychiatric needs. The practice, which was incorporated in 1996, emphasized appropriate, respectful, and resourceful biopsychosocial care without the tight time constraints of the community mental health model.

Developing a more comprehensive treatment model
Our practice initially provided habilitative, psychopharmacology-based, advanced practice nursing services to adults in a low-key and nonthreatening environment. We welcomed adults with

Table 1. Examples of medical problems and sensory issues that may influence behavior

Type of trigger	Examples
Medical	– Infection (e.g., urinary, respiratory, fungal, sinus, strep) – Drug-drug interaction – Idiosyncratic drug reaction – Pain (e.g., dental, migraine, endometriosis, sinus) – Irritable bowel disease (IBD), irritable bowel syndrome (IBS), celiac disease, food allergies – Gastroesophageal reflux (GERD) – Thyroid irregularities (hyperthyroidism, hypothyroidism) – Diabetes
Sensory: Physical environment	– Fluorescent lighting – Mold – Off-gassing of new carpets, drapes, furniture – Spraying of insecticides, herbicides, or fungicides – Building/room temperature (too hot or too cold)
Sensory: Auditory	– Loud, agitating music (e.g., on van rides) – Disruptive, noisy meal routines (e.g., overcrowded tables, talking and/or grabbing, loud television, staff talking on cell phones)
Sensory: Food	– Food texture, sight, smell (prompting avoidance, gagging, or vomiting) – Caffeinated beverages or cigarettes
Sensory: Other	– Clothing and shoes (e.g., ill-fitting, uncomfortable, or constrictive; seasonal changes; fabric type) – Changes in routine (e.g., staff changes, roommate changes, family events, transportation-related changes)

developmental disabilities who suffered from complex and difficult-to-address behavioral and psychiatric problems. We scheduled initial appointments for a minimum of 2 hours and subsequent appointments for 30-60 minutes. In addition to giving patients a thorough psychiatric assessment, we also carefully evaluated them for medication responses and side effects. We reviewed behavioral data, studied consultations and reports from other care providers, and considered recommendations.

Over time, it became clear that patients who visited us for psychiatric and psychopharmacologic treatment often had underlying medical or sensory issues (see Table 1). For example, we frequently found that medical problems such as urinary tract infections, respiratory infections, constipation, dental problems, and other issues involving pain could be the source of agitation, aggression, or sleeplessness. In some patients, we discovered undiagnosed diabetes as well as thyroid irregularities. Sensory problems also could masquerade as psychiatric problems (such as agitation, self-injury, aggression, isolation, anxiety, screaming, and other reactions) and could sometimes be directly traced to an inappropriate or overstimulating environment. We learned that even minor disruptions to schedules and routines (such as the change of a seat on a van, a different relief staff for an overnight shift, or a detour from an established route) could cause agitation and aggression in routine-oriented patients with developmental disabilities. In one instance, a patient became agitated when his parents changed their visiting schedule. We did not believe that the appropriate treatment for disappointment or unhappiness was antipsychotic medication.

The *Diagnostic and Statistical Manual of Mental Disorders* of the American Psychiatric Association (DSM-IV-TR) points out that problems should only be diagnosed and treated as psychiatric problems after other potential causes have been ruled out. Psychiatric-like symptoms often can be red herrings (see Figure 1). We, therefore, began to put considerable effort into seeking out information and problem-solving regarding our clients' underlying medical, sensory, and interpersonal issues. In addition to correcting these issues, where possible, this approach included supporting the person with what they needed to be comfortable, such as headphones, a different type of clothing, a different method of communication, lab tests, referrals to medical providers or specialists, or a different seat on the van.

Figure 1. Psychiatric symptoms as possible red herrings for medical problems or environmental and sensory issues

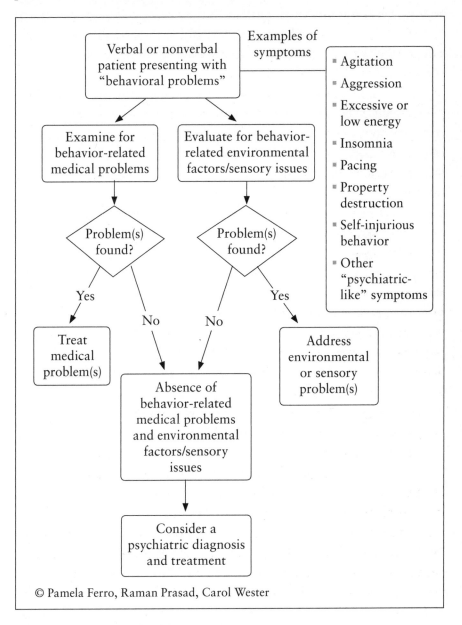

© Pamela Ferro, Raman Prasad, Carol Wester

Learning about gut health

As our practice developed, I (Ferro) continued to struggle at home with Isaiah's constant suffering, crying, physical discomfort, and poor health. Medical textbooks and doctors described autism as a genetically caused, unchangeable disease of the brain with no effective treatment options. There was no Internet information available at that time, and few support groups existed. Parents, however, including many of us in the medical profession, could not stand idly by as our children suffered. I began talking to other mothers and visited my local health food store often to learn about alternative treatments.

In 1998, we attended a conference at which two nurses (Maureen McDonnell, RN, and Jayne Barese, RN) explained the connection between bowel function and health. The talk highlighted the impact of toxins (ranging from environmental chemicals and pesticides to antibiotics and junk foods), noting that they could deplete essential gut bacteria, compromise the immune system, and jeopardize overall health. To repair an injured gut, the two speakers emphasized the use of a gluten-free/casein-free (GF/CF) diet, along with digestive enzymes, probiotics, nutrient supplementation, and fatty acids. Although we had heard of the GF/CF diet, until the conference we had not understood its rationale. The information shared by the two speakers seemed relevant both to Isaiah, who was then 6 years old, and to our adult patients with ostensible psychiatric challenges. Many of our clients had major issues with constipation or diarrhea. Could the problematic behaviors we saw so often (self-injury, acting out, agitation, irritation) be bowel-based?

To learn more, we arranged a two-day consultation with Maureen McDonnell and Jayne Barese, poring over theoretical material and talking about people's response to the interventions they had presented. From these two nurses, we learned how to comprehensively assess biomedical problems. For example, when taking a child's medical history, we began to also look at the *mother's* medical history, including occupational exposures, antibiotic use, and diet during pregnancy and labor. In addition, we learned how to relate behaviors to underlying causes. For example, toe walking is usually seen in children with constipation, chicken-bumps on the back or upper arms may suggest fatty acid problems, and extreme anxiety and obsessive-compulsive disorder (OCD) behaviors can be due to *Candida* or bacterial pathogens. We learned to identify dozens of symptoms and behaviors, ranging from reflux to fecal smearing, and how they relate to gastrointestinal (GI) dysfunction. Finally, we learned about laboratory tests that can help detect underlying medical issues that are related to GI issues. These include the CBC (complete blood count), the methylmalonic acid test for vitamin B12 deficiency, celiac screening, diagnostics for vitamin and nutrient levels, and comprehensive digestive stool analysis.

The Specific Carbohydrate Diet™

Armed with new information about the gut-brain connection, I (Ferro) started Isaiah on the GF/CF diet as well as selected supplements. Encouragingly, Isaiah's attention and behavior initially improved. However, these outward signs of behavioral progress stopped within months. Isaiah's tantrums and outbursts returned, and diarrhea and constipation still afflicted him, along with stomach pain, gas, and bloating. Nonetheless, I realized that the diet was doing some good and that going off the diet would lead to worsening behavior.

At work, we began to expand our practice beyond adults, seeing a handful of children with autism to teach their parents about the GF/CF diet. In 2003, when Isaiah was 12, one of these parents told me about another diet, the Specific Carbohydrate Diet™ (SCD™). This parent urged me to read a book titled *Breaking the Vicious Cycle*, by Elaine Gottschall. Initially, I was not interested. I already was teaching people about the GF/CF diet and was busy working and caring for Isaiah. When I finally read the book, I knew immediately that the SCD was an important key to understanding the effects of diet on autism.

Originally published under the title *Food and the Gut Reaction*, *Breaking the Vicious Cycle* was written for sufferers of Crohn's disease, ulcerative colitis, and celiac disease. The book focuses on digestion and what is going on in the intestines of people with these diseases. Specifically, the book explains that when the intestinal mucosa is damaged, the enzymes that are needed to break down complex carbohydrates are either not present or are separated from the carbohydrate molecules by a mucus layer. As a result, the carbohydrates cannot be broken down and absorbed by the intestine. Instead, the undigested carbohydrates remain in the intestine and fuel bacterial overgrowth. In turn, these bacteria produce harmful metabolic byproducts. If the intestinal cells do not heal and complex carbohydrates continue to be ingested, a vicious cycle may develop involving further injury to the small intestinal mucosa, more bacterial overgrowth, an increase in harmful metabolic byproducts, diarrhea or constipation, and potentially abnormal brain function and behavior.

As a method to heal the intestines, *Breaking the Vicious Cycle* describes the Specific Carbohydrate Diet™, which eliminates most complex carbohydrates, including those in rice and soy. In addition, the SCD™ avoids all processed foods and added sugars. For people with Crohn's disease, ulcerative colitis, and celiac disease, the SCD™ allows dairy products such as ghee, butter, low-lactose hard cheeses, yogurt fermented for at least 24 hours to break down all of the lactose, and dry-curd cottage cheese (another dairy product with almost no lactose). However, because children with autism typically cannot tolerate casein (the protein in milk), our practice advocates implementing the SCD™ minus all dairy products except ghee, which contains neither lactose nor casein.

After reading the book, I found Elaine Gottschall's phone number and spoke to her. Elaine had just started to hear about people using the SCD™ for autism. When she began to read some of the research on autism and GI problems, the relevance of the SCD™ for autism made sense. Intrigued by the possibilities, she agreed to visit our area. The then-82-year-old Elaine possessed the vigor of someone much younger. She simply told me, "I'll drive down. I'll take a friend with me. It's only a few hours from the Toronto area." And that's what she did. Over 50 people came to hear Elaine explain her ideas and share her experience via numerous case histories.

Elaine's visit was both hopeful and illuminating. Although we knew that children with autism did not tolerate gluten and casein and that most improved to some extent on a GF/CF diet, we also had observed that after a few months, the vast majority of children on a GF/CF diet peaked or even declined. When they stopped improving, we typically assumed that we had failed to eliminate all hidden sources of gluten or casein. Elaine's visit prompted us to step back, look at the bigger picture, and recognize that everything we ingest (including both food and medicine) influences the composition of the gut bacteria. Elaine's visit shifted our thinking, allowing us to understand that foods other than gluten and casein also have an impact on the gut, including the sugars added to GF/CF products and other complex-carbohydrate-rich foods such as rice and potatoes.

In November 2003, two months after Elaine's visit, we joined Maureen McDonnell, Jayne Barese, and nutritional supplement expert Ilene Buchholz, RN, to plan the May 2004 conference of the network formerly known as Defeat Autism Now! or DAN! Our goal was to develop a nurses' curriculum for the network. We proposed including the SCD™ as the main diet in the curriculum. Although Maureen had had years of experience with the GF/CF diet, it was apparent to all of us that the SCD™ had great potential to help children with autism. We could not ignore the science or the improvements we were beginning to witness. As a result, the SCD™ went into the nurses' curriculum, helping plant the idea of the SCD™ firmly in the autism community.

What the science says

In recent years, prominent medical journals have published a number of findings that illuminate the gut-brain connection first described to us by Maureen McDonnell and Jayne Barese. The relationship between diet, the gut flora, brain chemistry, and behavior is apparent in these studies.

1. A study involving a group of autistic children with GI problems found that complex carbohydrates (disaccharides and polysaccharides) were not fully digested and fed pathogenic gut bacteria.[1]
2. Studies that have analyzed stool and urine samples from children suffering from autism consistently find abnormal gut bacteria.[2-8] In studies that compare the gut flora of autistic children with that of siblings and non-related healthy children, the flora of the children with autism differs dramatically. Depending on the focus of the study, researchers have also found high levels of pathogenic clostridia[6-7] as well as *Desulfovibrio*[8] species of bacteria in children with autism.
3. A high percentage of children with autism have been found to have a "leaky gut," supporting the theory that harmful molecules may be entering the bloodstream, possibly causing opioid reactions.[9]
4. Even in healthy subjects, the intestinal flora communicate with the central nervous system through the gut-brain axis to alter brain chemistry and, therefore, behavior.[10] Research is beginning to intensify to elucidate the connection between intestinal flora and behavior.[11-12]

5. Dietary modifications change the composition of human gut flora, and these changes may start occurring within 24 hours.[13] Manipulating the diet of mice has been shown to alter the intestinal microflora as well as memory and learning.[14]

Although no one has determined what initiates the disruption of intestinal flora in people with autism, it is becoming clearer that autism involves many metabolic processes. More importantly, given our current understanding, the gut provides a window to improve metabolism, behavior, and, ultimately, quality of life.

Implementing the Specific Carbohydrate Diet™ with children

I (Ferro) started Isaiah on the SCD™ even before Elaine Gottschall's visit. Isaiah had suffered from digestive issues from ages 2 to 12, but within one week of starting the SCD™ his alternating diarrhea and constipation had cleared up. One week! Over the next two months, Isaiah's other symptoms lessened as his gut healed, and he became calmer and happier. The year before starting the SCD™, Isaiah had missed 50 days of school due to illness, mostly abdominal pain. He frequently cried, performed obsessive-compulsive routines and rituals, became distracted, and could not sit still. When he did make it to school, he spent all of his time with an individual teacher so as not to distract the class. During Isaiah's first year on the SCD™ (his 6th grade year), he was able to stay in class for the full day with some supports. That Christmas, after ten years of staying away, Isaiah actually enjoyed going to the family holiday party.

After seeing that substantial individual improvements of this type were not uncommon, I began helping other parents to implement the SCD™, starting with the children I had previously assisted with the GF/CF diet. Regardless of their baseline condition, these children showed dramatic improvements. The progress was not always linear, since setbacks in the 3rd and 6th months were typical, but the focus of the SCD™ on bowel function inevitably led to positive behavioral changes. Nonsocial children began making eye contact, hyperactive children calmed down, delayed children became more verbal, and overly thin children gained weight. Several mothers tried the diet for themselves and experienced clearing of brain fog that they hadn't even realized existed.

When I examined the charts of families I had previously followed on the GF/CF diet, I observed that most children initially improved when bread and dairy products were removed from the diet. In many cases, however, these products were quickly replaced with rice, potato, and soy, all of which contain complex carbohydrates that the children could not adequately digest. In the two cases where the children continued to improve on a GF/CF diet alone, the parents had replaced gluten and casein with meats, fruits, vegetables, and no junk, effectively following the SCD™.

As I began to help one family after another, word of mouth spread. I kept in touch with Elaine, calling her for advice on especially difficult cases until she passed away in the fall of 2005. By 2006, my active patients numbered over 200, with many more on the waiting list. I began to ask mothers experienced with SCD™ to mentor parents who were new to the diet. One mother, whose son and several nephews followed the diet, started a business for freshly baked SCD™ goods. To keep up with demand, she had to install commercial ovens and hire an employee.

One family of recent immigrants made an appointment for their 13-year-old nonverbal daughter. Because English was the family's second language, making it difficult to talk meaningfully about specific foods, I visited their house to teach them the diet. Together we went through the kitchen, shelf by shelf. Three months later, the girl spoke her first words.

Working with the adult population

Meanwhile, I (Wester) continued to see adult clients with conditions including autism, mental retardation of unknown etiology, Down syndrome, and attention-deficit/hyperactivity disorder (ADHD). Many of these adults had bowel and immune problems. As I gained experience with biomedical approaches and the SCD™, I began to treat these adult patients differently. Although I always had spent a lot of time trying to figure out the source of my clients' problems, my main treatment as a board certified clinical nurse specialist consisted of prescribing medication. Pam's experiences with kids taught us how to treat adults. When families or agencies were willing to try new approaches, I began recommending dietary changes for adult patients.

Jack, a 50-year-old former state school resident with autism, mental retardation, and significant speech issues, illustrates some of the successes that we experienced. For years, Jack had struggled with aggressive and self-injurious behavior. Psychiatrists and behavior control medications failed to help him. Both the staff and residents of his group home labeled Jack as "dangerous." During van rides Jack would unbuckle his seat belt and attack the driver with his fists or try to open the door and jump out of the moving van. The group home staffed Jack 2:1— two staff devoted their attention to Jack at all times. Jack experienced a poor quality of life, and his family lived with the constant anxiety of waiting to hear whether someone (Jack or the staff) had gotten hurt.

Jack also had a history of constipation. For this reason, even before our practice learned about the SCD™, I suggested that Jack try the GF/CF diet. However, the staff at Jack's home inconsistently or inaccurately implemented the diet, and the experiment ended in failure. A year later, with new staff in place and the family on board with dietary interventions, we tried again, introducing Jack to the SCD™. Within weeks of seriously implementing the diet, Jack began moving his bowels regularly and eating and sleeping well. His mood and behavior improved dramatically: the agitation, aggression, and self-injury stopped.

At present, years later, Jack is easily staffed by one person, participates in small groups without issue, and rides in the van safely. He laughs and smiles regularly and goes out to eat with staff. They all know the eating plan well, as do the local restaurants. Despite Jack's limited language skills, occasionally he will name or request a food that is not on his eating program. Staff will merely ask him "Can you have that?" and he will slyly smile and say "Nooooo..." Together, they will figure out something appealing that he can have.

Jack continues to take his previous medication as well as probiotics and fish oil. The combination of diet, medication, supplements, family involvement, and staff diligence has changed the landscape of Jack's life. None of the current staff can remember him being restrained. Former staff members who have not seen Jack in years cannot believe he is the same person.

It has become clear to me that developmental disabilities involve the entire body. The SCD™ has made all the difference for Jack and other adults who have what I sometimes call an "autistic-like metabolism." Moreover, the dietary changes suggested by the SCD™ are effective for almost everyone. The diet typically results in less agitation, an increased sense of calmness, better sleep, improved bowel function, and more interaction in those who have language. When group home staff witness these results, they are usually willing to sustain the dietary changes.

When I worked at the state school, the school had a special behavioral unit where patients walked around with swollen faces, bloody lips, and black eyes from punching and hitting themselves. One man, now deceased, would bite huge chunks of flesh out of his shoulders and arms. In retrospect, it is clear that many of these behaviors had to do with the individuals' inability to get any relief from GI and other types of pain. The people who ended up on that unit were like the children who suffer from autism. They could not tolerate the noise, the bad food, the overstimulation, and everything else going on in their environment. Although the professional staff spent considerable time trying different treatments and interventions, they lacked the knowledge to address the underlying problems. Those patients would be treated very differently now, given our knowledge of the gut-brain connection. Given my long history of working with mentally disabled adults, many of whom led difficult lives, it is gratifying to now be able to sometimes facilitate dramatic improvements for people long considered to have static, unchanging disorders.

Moving forward

At our nursing practice, our protocol relies on spending quality time with patients, taking thorough histories, and doing detective work when needed. Over time, we have expanded the nature of the histories to gather more indicators of bowel health. Specialized diets, supplements, vitamins, probiotics, and antifungals play a prominent role in treatment of both children and, when possible, adults. Our goals are to take a person out of physical pain and improve quality of life.

As scientists gain a better understanding of the gut-brain connection, we find that more medical practitioners and organizations are interested in our work. To channel this interest, in 2002, I (Ferro) founded the Gottschall Autism Center, a nonprofit organization that seeks to provide educational opportunities for parents and meaningful work opportunities for adults with autism. In the fall of 2009, we also held the conference referred to at the beginning of this chapter ("When the Belly is the Beast: How Intestinal Health Impacts Brain and Behavior"), followed by a second conference in the spring of 2011. Notably, many staff members employed by local group homes voluntarily attended the second conference after hearing about successes with adult patients such as Paul and Jack. As our own understanding of the gut-brain connection continues to evolve, we hope that this enhanced understanding will allow us to continue to provide a higher quality of life to children and adults with autism.

We want to emphasize that *it is never too late to use biomedical approaches and therapeutic diets to treat people with autism.* In our practice, we have seen substantial improvement in both children and adults, both initially and over time. We focus on steadily improving digestive function, which then leads to improved behavior. Our approach varies, depending on a person's age and the resources available. We set high goals for developing toddlers and young children because we recognize that successful treatment at an early age may significantly alter the course of that child's life. With treatment, the younger children move toward more typical patterns of age-appropriate development. In many cases, children with no language rapidly develop rudimentary language skills, which progress as additional growth and learning take place. All of the younger children we have treated have shown dramatic improvement in bowel function, awareness, alertness, social relatedness, behavioral control, eye contact, mood, attention, sleep, appetite, and weight.

With adults, we have seen biomedical treatments result in quality-of-life improvements, although not as dramatically as with the children. We have never helped a nonverbal adult acquire language, but we have witnessed significant increases in signing, gesturing, eye contact, social smiling, and playfulness with other people. We also observe improvement in mood and behavioral control, decreases in psychomotor agitation, and relief from overwhelming anxiety. Self-injury, skin picking, and property destruction often diminish or stop completely. These adults also participate in social activities (including horseback riding) more frequently and successfully. An adult individual may become able to enjoy recreational activities available in the community, go into a store, attend a concert, or take an art class.

With regard to medication, with children our goal is to avoid having them on lifelong drugs. We avoid mood stabilization and sleep medications, including antidepressants. However, we will use medication for emergencies or short-term relief of intolerable symptoms. Medication should not be a standalone therapy, however, and with appropriate biomedical support is usually not necessary in young children. With adults, we have not been able to remove them from the medications that they have been taking for years, often decades. However, we have not had to increase medication, and in several cases, we have been able to lower dosages or find alternatives with fewer side effects.

The type and degree of change possible depend on many factors, including the person's age, the nature of the autism spectrum disorder, the resources available, the skill and persistence of the treating clinicians, the diligence of family and caretakers, and the motivation of the affected individuals themselves. However, there is always realistic hope for improvement. One must try and then try some more. Everyone can always do better: it is NEVER too late.

References

1. Williams BL, Hornig M, Buie T, Bauman ML, Cho Paik M, Wick I, Bennett A, Jabado O, Hirschberg DL, Lipkin WI. Impaired carbohydrate digestion and transport and mucosal dysbiosis in the intestines of children with autism and gastrointestinal disturbances. *PLoS ONE*. 2011 Sep;6(9):e24585.
2. Finegold SM, Molitoris D, Song Y, Liu C, Vaisanen ML, Bolte E, McTeague M, Sandler R, Wexler H, Marlowe EM, Collins MD, Lawson PA, Summanen P, Baysallar M, Tomzynski TJ, Read E, Johnson E, Rolfe R, Nasir P, Shah H, Haake DA, Manning P, Kaul A. Gastrointestinal microflora studies in late-onset autism. *Clin Infect Dis*. 2002 Sep;35(Suppl 1):S6-S16.
3. Clarke F, Hill RJ, Silva MMDA. Gut bacterial and fermentation profiles are altered in children with autism. *J Gastroen Hepatol*. 2010;25:116-9.
4. Finegold SM, Dowd SE, Gontcharova V, Liu C, Henley KE, Wolcott RD, Youn E, Summanen PH, Granpeesheh D, Dixon D, Liu M, Molitoris DR, Green JA 3rd. Pyrosequencing study of fecal microflora of autistic and control children. *Anaerobe*. 2010 Aug;16(4):444-53.
5. Yap IK, Angley M, Veselkov KA, Holmes E, Lindon JC, Nicholson JK. Urinary metabolic phenotyping differentiates children with autism from their unaffected siblings and age-matched controls. *J Proteome Res*. 2010 Jun;9(6):2996-3004.

6. Parracho HM, Bingham MO, Gibson GR, McCartney AL. Differences between the gut microflora of children with autistic spectrum disorders and that of healthy children. *J Med Microbiol.* 2005 Oct;54(Pt 10):987-91.

7. Song Y, Liu C, Finegold SM. Real-time PCR quantitation of clostridia in feces of autistic children. *Appl Environ Microbiol.* 2004 Nov;70(11):6459-65.

8. Finegold SM. *Desulfovibrio* species are potentially important in regressive autism. *Med Hypotheses.* 2011 Aug;77(2):270-4.

9. de Magistris L, Familiari V, Pascotto A, Sapone A, Frolli A, Iardino P, Carteni M, De Rosa M, Francavilla R, Riegler G, Militerni R, Bravaccio C. Alterations of the intestinal barrier in patients with autism spectrum disorders and in their first-degree relatives. *J Pediatr Gastroenterol Nutr.* 2010 Oct;51(4):418-24.

10. Heijtz RD, Wang S, Anuar F, Qian Y, Björkholm B, Samuelsson A, Hibberd ML, Forssberg H, Pettersson S. Normal gut microbiota modulates brain development and behavior. *Proc Natl Acad Sci U S A.* 2011 Feb;108(7):3047-52.

11. Neufeld KM, Kang N, Bienenstock J, Foster JA. Reduced anxiety-like behavior and central neurochemical change in germ-free mice. *Neurogastroenterol Motil.* 2011 Mar;23(3):255-64, e119.

12. Forsythe P, Sudo N, Dinan T, Taylor VH, Bienenstock J. Mood and gut feelings. *Brain Behav Immun.* 2010 Jan;24(1):9-16.

13. Turnbaugh PJ, Ridaura VK, Faith JJ, Rey FE, Knight R, Gordon JI. The effect of diet on the human gut microbiome: a metagenomic analysis in humanized gnotobiotic mice. *Sci Transl Med.* 2009 Nov;1(6):6ra14.

14. Li W, Dowd SE, Scurlock B, Acosta-Martinez V, Lyte M. Memory and learning behavior in mice is temporally associated with diet-induced alterations in gut bacteria. *Physiol Behav.* 2009 Mar;96(4-5):557-67.

CHAPTER FOURTEEN

DIAGNOSING AND TREATING INFLAMMATORY BOWEL DISEASE IN THE GENOMIC ERA

Stephen Walker, PhD

Inflammatory bowel disease (IBD) refers to a group of intestinal disorders that exhibit overlapping symptoms and a highly variable disease trajectory from individual to individual. Early diagnosis and effective treatment are clinical imperatives to assure the most positive outcomes for individuals with IBD. This chapter provides a brief overview of some current tools in place for IBD classification and diagnosis. In addition to presenting some of the standard diagnostic criteria, the bulk of the chapter is focused on a discussion of the newer molecular approaches and technologies that are being used to clarify issues such as susceptibility, heterogeneity, and heritability within and between IBD subtypes, features that make definitive diagnosis challenging. Within the chapter, a potential IBD variant that occurs in autism spectrum disorder (ASD) children is discussed and used as an example of how some of the newer research strategies may be useful for the characterization and classification of IBD and IBD subtypes at the molecular level. These detailed characterizations, in turn, will support more personalized treatment approaches.

Inflammatory bowel disease

The term *inflammatory bowel disease* refers to a genetically, immunologically, and histopathologically heterogeneous group of conditions classified as Crohn's disease (CD), ulcerative colitis (UC), and indeterminate colitis (IC)[1] or inflammatory bowel disease unclassified (IBDU).[2] IBD develops during childhood and adolescence in up to 25% of patients[3] and, although it is relatively common in modern Westernized industrial societies – current prevalence of IBD in developed countries is estimated to be 2-3/1000[4] – there is no consensus as to the underlying etiology. One prevailing model is that the intestinal microbiome drives an unmitigated immune and inflammatory response in a genetically susceptible host.[5-7] The key difference between those with and without IBD, then, is the ability of the latter to maintain the normal state of the intestinal immune system, i.e., immune tolerance.[5]

Within the gut there are a variety of cell types, whose activities are orchestrated in a highly regulated fashion, that are responsible for maintaining *immunologic tolerance.* Immune tolerance (sometimes referred to as "controlled physiologic inflammation") is the normal state of the intestinal immune system.[5] There is a balance within the gut to maintain this tolerance and at the same time maintain the capacity to mount an immune and inflammatory response within the mucosa in response to the diverse *insults* (i.e., exposures deemed by the immune system to be foreign) encountered there. Individuals susceptible to IBD tend towards a state of uncontrolled chronic or relapsing inflammation, with a failure/inability to downregulate the inflammation that resulted from the initial insult. The specific molecular events that underlie this loss of control have not been completely characterized; however, defects in innate and adaptive immune pathways have been identified.[8] When the ability to regulate the immune response has been compromised or lost, a disease phenotype emerges. The extent and duration of the IBD phenotype is highly variable from person to person, rendering accurate diagnosis and effective treatment as constantly evolving paradigms. This highlights the need for individualized diagnostic and therapeutic approaches designed to identify and treat the condition before serious tissue damage occurs.

Classification and diagnosis

"Past: the era of description. Present: the era of explanation. Future: the era of prediction." (Sands, 2007)

Diagnosing IBD in the clinic is based upon the evaluation of a variety of information that includes the current symptom presentation together with patient history, histology findings following endoscopy/colonoscopy procedures, and clinical test results.[10] In order to guide treatment, patients must be assessed to determine IBD phenotype, disease distribution, disease activity and severity, and, whenever possible, drug responsiveness.[1, 9] Due to overlapping symptoms in IBD, extensive heterogeneity, and clinical test results that display less than 100% sensitivity and specificity, definitive diagnosis is not always possible.[1, 11] Therefore, although there would likely be general diagnostic agreement among gastroenterologists in cases that represent *classic* disease presentations: "classic" Crohn's disease (e.g., with features such as perianal disease or small intestinal stricturing patholgy[2]) or "classic" UC (e.g., with a finding of rectal involvement and continuous and confluent colonic involvement with clear demarcation of inflammation[1]), there are a significant number of cases where, even after all of the available information has been evaluated, the specific IBD diagnosis is still uncertain. It is for this reason, and because the diseases themselves exhibit such broad heterogeneity, that existing diagnostic and classification tools are insufficient.

What new tools are available to characterize IBD?

IBD manifests clinically and subclinically in a variety of ways, and it is becoming more widely accepted that Crohn's disease and ulcerative colitis, as well as indeterminate colitis, are actually groups of disorders with a spectrum of underlying mechanisms resulting in similar clinical manifestations.[9] A key strategy, therefore, in the latest efforts to characterize these IBD subtypes is to use molecular techniques such as (1) genome-wide association studies (GWAS) and single nucleotide polymorphism (SNP) analyses to identify high-risk genotypes; (2) gene expression analysis in gastrointestinal biopsy tissue to gain insights into the different biological mechanisms and pathways that underlie IBD phenotypes; and (3) peripheral biomarker identification to provide a rapid and easy access diagnostic and treatment response assessment tool. Each of these approaches has the potential to provide significant new information for the diagnosis and treatment of IBD.

Using genome-wide association to study complex disease

Genomics, the study of an individual's particular DNA sequence, is rapidly becoming an area of significant interest in terms of understanding complex diseases like IBD. This is important to the field of clinical diagnostics because within the genome lies fundamental information that can be used to identify individuals at risk for disease as well as those who would likely respond to a particular therapeutic agent used to treat the condition.

Unlike DNA sequencing that can be used to "read" every nucleotide in a person's entire genome (3-4 billion nucleotide pairs), genome-wide association studies take more of a shotgun approach and measure single nucleotide polymorphisms (differences) in thousands to hundreds of thousands of locations in the genome, in hundreds or sometimes thousands of individuals. These SNP results are then used to identify genotypic markers that confer disease susceptibility within individuals and populations. Although the resulting associations and risk assessments, determined on the basis of sophisticated statistical analyses of the comprehensive SNP data, can provide useful information, the field is still very early in development, and the results must be interpreted with caution. There are three key reasons for this: (1) many of the identified SNPs that are found within individuals who have the disease but not in control individuals who don't have the disease are not located within genes *known to be associated with the disease*; (2) even when a SNP occurs in a gene known to have functional relevance to the disease, the SNPs are often not associated with any known biological function themselves; and (3) the genotypic associations, while compelling, do not take into account environmental risk factors that are often equally important in predicting who does and does not develop a disease phenotype.

The use of GWAS data to assess disease risk in populations and in individuals is becoming more commonplace, including in the field of gastroenterology. For example, a public company, 23andMe, has performed SNP analyses on thousands of individuals in a number of different complex disease categories (e.g., Parkinson's, IBD, type 2 diabetes) as well as healthy controls and provides risk assessment, based on SNP results, for a number of diseases that include Crohn's disease and ulcerative colitis.[12] When one submits a DNA sample (via a saliva sample) to the company, it will genotype the DNA at approximately one million SNP locations. The individual's SNP data can then be compared to the large database at the 23andMe portal to gauge relative risk for developing a number of diseases. For example, the Crohn's disease "risk" panel consists of a dozen SNPs that are each significantly more prevalent in individuals with CD than those without CD. Based on an individual's SNP profile in relation to those 12 markers, a person can assess their relative risk of CD at each of those 12 markers. Again, it is important to keep in mind that these risk calculations are based on statistical associations to population-wide genotype data and are not typically, at this point in time at least, supported by compelling clinical data.

Functional genomics studies

Another important genomic-based tool being used to characterize and distinguish between IBD subtypes is referred to as *functional genomics (transcriptomics)* or gene expression analysis. In these studies, rather than DNA, one is measuring mRNA levels and comparing those levels between different groups of samples (IBD versus control, CD versus UC, etc.) as a means to distinguish the groups and to learn something about the biology that underlies a particular phenotype. Detailed molecular information, gleaned from clinical specimens derived from patients with gastrointestinal (GI) symptoms, will provide the potential to add new and important diagnostic tools to those that already exist for IBD. The analysis of differential gene expression in relevant ileocolonic tissue from this group of affected individuals is leading to a better understanding of the molecular processes involved, including pathways that have been significantly impacted, and will provide a more detailed understanding of the biology that underlies IBD and especially IBD subtypes.

Several published studies describe the use of gene expression profiling of gastrointestinal biopsy tissue to distinguish between IBD (Crohn's disease and ulcerative colitis) and non-IBD samples.[13-16] In each study, significant gene expression differences were identified between IBD and non-IBD samples, as well as between samples derived from different IBD conditions; however, no universal and reproducible diagnostic panel of differentially expressed transcripts has resulted from these efforts. Moreover, relatively few studies have applied gene expression profiling to complex disease tissue like intestinal mucosa, reflecting the unique challenges inherent to this type of analysis.[17] In one recent study, this type of approach was used to identify a biomarker panel that could be used as a means to distinguish IBD (Crohn's disease and ulcerative colitis) from non-IBD (in this case irritable bowel syndrome – IBS). The study further identified a subset of transcripts, consisting of seven genes, whose differential expression was useful in distinguishing the two main IBD classes, Crohn's disease and ulcerative colitis (UC), with a high degree of sensitivity and specificity.[17, 18] These data have not yet been reproduced in a separate study population, but they point to the potential for this type of approach.

Overall, gene expression profiling in intestinal mucosal tissue has shown promise in differentiating disease and non-disease tissue as well as for distinguishing between different disease phenotypes. The inherent problems in this type of approach are at least threefold: (1) the limited availability of relevant tissue specimens; (2) the limited reproducibility of results from different studies (probably largely due to non-overlapping experimental design from study to study); and (3) extreme heterogeneity across IBD cases. As with GWAS, functional genomic studies can provide another layer of important information in IBD characterization, but should be viewed with a critical eye.

Combining genotypic and gene expression data increases power to detect causal associations

Variation in gene expression is an important mechanism underlying susceptibility to complex disease. The simultaneous genome-wide assay of gene expression (functional genomics) and genetic variation (SNP analysis via GWAS) *within the same sample* allows the mapping of the genetic factors that underlie individual differences in quantitative levels of expression (expression QTL – eQTL). The availability of systematically generated eQTL information could provide immediate insight into a biological basis for disease associations identified through genome-wide association studies and can help to identify networks of genes involved in disease pathogenesis.[19] Combining genomic and transcriptomic data offers the potential to uncover disease-predisposing variants. Such an approach has already proven useful in identifying genetic associations in other complex diseases. For example, in multiple sclerosis this practice has identified IL7R polymorphisms,[20] an association confirmed in two large cohorts.[21, 22] There has been a growing interest in assessing the contribution of single nucleotide polymorphisms (SNPs) and copy number variants (CNVs) to the genetic variation influencing gene expression. Projects such as GENEVAR illustrate the success of such analyses.[23]

Surrogate markers in peripheral blood

Peripheral blood gene expression is being used extensively to identify surrogate markers for disease, and, relevant to this chapter, specifically for discrimination and classification of IBD subtypes.[24-26] This approach is based on the premise that peripheral blood, as it interacts with the tissues and cells of the body, may manifest gene expression changes in response to or because of the disease tissue they encounter.[26] The popularity of this approach is due to the fact that it fulfills a need for minimally invasive, yet informative, ways to monitor disease presence, activity, and efficacy of therapy.

In order for a biomarker to be broadly useful, it needs to correlate with the phenotype *and* be relatively easy to measure in the target population. While ileocolonic tissue gene expression data will likely provide important clues to the biology underlying the inflammation seen in IBD, the invasive nature of procurement limits the utility of mucosal biopsies as a practical tissue source for routine diagnostic testing. Whole blood, on the other hand, is a readily accessible and viable alternative. There are numerous reported successes using whole blood gene expression profiling for differentiating subtypes in a wide range of clinical conditions: neuropsychiatric conditions,[27] cancer,[28] and even differentiating autism spectrum disorder (ASD) children. In one recent study, gene expression profiles from peripheral blood were used to identify differences in children with autism and autism spectrum disorders compared with general population controls.[29] The authors were able to detect significant gene expression differences between (a) autism and controls; (b) early-onset autism and controls; (c) autism with regression and controls; and (d) early-onset autism compared to autism with regression. They concluded that their "data strongly support the idea that transcriptional profiling of cells in peripheral blood could be particularly promising for providing mechanistic insights and surrogate markers in autism."

Profiling of peripheral blood gene expression in IBD patients has demonstrated that this strategy can be used to differentiate between CD and UC,[24] UC from CD and non-inflammatory diarrhea,[26] and UC and CD from non-IBD colitis.[25] In each of these studies, the differential expression levels of specific sets of transcripts provided the discriminative power of the approach. In one case, the authors reported that UC and

CD cases could be distinguished by five genes with 100% specificity and sensitivity.[25] They further reported a correlation between several differentially expressed transcripts (DETs) in blood and differential expression of those same transcripts in inflamed colonic tissue. They postulate that combining peripheral blood gene expression results with differential gene expression results from inflamed tissue from the same patients may provide a more reliable biomarker.

IBD in autism spectrum disorder – a novel subtype?

It is clear that the latest genetic and functional genomic approaches are allowing research teams to make significant headway in the identification of specific disease phenotypes, which is relevant to disease risk assessment and even in predicting a patient's response to therapeutics. These same approaches are now being applied to an IBD-like condition that has yet to be characterized at a molecular level.

An IBD variant has been reported in the literature and describes the histopathological, immunohistochemical, and cytokine profiles in GI-symptomatic autism spectrum disorder (ASD[GI]) children.[30, 31] Typical endoscopic findings include lymphonodular hyperplasia (LNH) in the terminal ileum. A retrospective review of ileocolonic histopathology obtained from 143 consecutive ASD[GI] children undergoing routine diagnostic ileocolonoscopy reported ileocolitis in 69% of the children.[32] The presence of ileocolitis imparts significance to the finding of exaggerated LNH in these children as LNH is a well established comorbid occurrence in a variety of inflammatory and autoimmune disorders of the GI tract.

A number of recent studies have reported an increased frequency of GI symptoms in ASD children compared with typically developing children and those with other developmental delays.[33-36] Prospective, systematic studies suggest that as many as 70% of autistic children suffer from chronic GI symptoms.[33, 37, 38] These symptoms include diarrhea, constipation, abdominal distension, failure to thrive, weight loss, and abdominal pain. In addition, many children suffer episodes of extreme irritability, aggression, and self-injury that appear to be related to abdominal pain since these symptoms improve with treatment of the underlying GI inflammation. Since ASDs are diagnosed clinically via neurodevelopmental and neurocognitive criteria, it is tempting to speculate about the temporal relationship between chronic GI inflammation – especially in very young children – and neurodevelopmental problems. At a minimum, there appear to be specific behavioral associations with chronic GI symptoms.

Currently, it is unclear if GI symptoms and intestinal mucosal inflammatory changes seen in children with ASD represent a variant of IBD versus non-specific colitis or "normal" mucosal cellular composition. It is possible that a thorough molecular characterization of inflamed tissue from ASD[GI] cases will provide additional evidence of a disease process that, while similar in many respects to recognized types of IBD, is distinct.

Summary

"The real challenge for the future is to develop a tailored (i.e. pharmacogenomic) approach to prevention of the initiation and perpetuation of the inflammatory cascade before tissue injury occurs." (Baumgart & Carding, 2007)

The goal of this chapter was to provide a brief overview of current ways in which state-of-the-art genetic and genomic approaches are being used for the diagnosis, characterization, and treatment of complex disease, specifically IBD. Genetics, including GWAS and SNP analyses, are being used to provide a measure of risk assessment and to begin to stratify disease sub-phenotypes. Functional genomics, specifically gene expression analysis in bowel biopsy tissue, is being used both as a tool to distinguish between IBDs and also to provide a more detailed understanding of the specific biological pathways involved in the different disease presentations. Surrogate biomarker profiling in peripheral blood holds promise for stratifying disease sub-phenotypes, but, more importantly, provides a readily accessible avenue for diagnostic and prognostic testing. Moreover, if differential gene expression in blood can be shown to correlate directly with gene expression changes in inflamed bowel tissue from the same individual, it may be possible one day to circumvent the need for more invasive procedures like colonoscopy by performing a blood test for definitive diagnosis instead.

The complementary molecular approaches discussed here are being used in an overall effort to make diagnosis and treatment of IBD easier, more precise, less invasive, and more effective. Understanding who is at risk *before* they actually present with symptoms would provide the benefit of being able to initiate preventative care. Being able to predict which medications and therapeutics would be most effective in an individual patient would provide the benefit of having to spend less time and resources on trial-and-error approaches. Having simpler diagnostic tools, like a blood-based test that is both highly sensitive and highly specific, would likewise save time and resources. Taken together, these tools that enable a "personalized medicine" approach have the potential to revolutionize the way medicine is practiced.

References

1. Vucelic B. Inflammatory bowel diseases: controversies in the use of diagnostic procedures. (2009) *Dig Dis*. 27(3): 269-277.
2. Martland GT and Shepherd NA. Indeterminate colitis: definition, diagnosis, implications and a plea for nosological sanity. (2007) *Histopathology*. 50: 83-96.
3. Levine A, Griffiths A, Markowitz J, Wilson DC, Turner D, et al. Pediatric modification of the Montreal classification for inflammatory bowel disease: the Paris classification. (2011) *Inflamm Bowel Dis*. 17(6):1314-1321.
4. de Mesquita MB, Civitelli F, Levine A. Epidemiology, genes and inflammatory bowel diseases in childhood. (2008) *Dig Liver Dis*. 40(1):3-11
5. Sands BE. Inflammatory bowel disease: past, present, and future. (2007) *J Gastroenterol*. 42(1): 16-25.
6. Iebba V, Aloi M, Civitelli F, Cucchiara S. Gut microbiota and pediatric disease. (2011) *Dig Dis*. 29(6):531-539.
7. Cryan JF and Dinan TG. Mind-altering microorganisms: the impact of the gut microbiota on brain and behaviour. (2012) *Nat Rev Neurosci*. 13(10):701-712.
8. Rutgeerts P, Vermeire S, Van Assche G. Biological therapies for inflammatory bowel diseases. (2009) *Gastroenterology*. 136(4): 1182-1197.
9. Targan SR and Karp LC. Inflammatory bowel disease diagnosis, evaluation and classification: state-of-the art approach. (2007) *Curr Opin Gastroenterol*. 23(4): 390-394.
10. Sands BE. From symptom to diagnosis: clinical distinctions among various forms of intestinal inflammation. (2007) *Gastroenterology*. 126(6): 1518-1532.
11. Bousvaros A, Antonioli DA, Colletti RB, Dubinsky MC, Glickman JN, et al. Differentiating ulcerative colitis from Crohn disease in children and young adults: report of a working group of the North American Society for Pediatric Gastroenterology, Hepatology, and Nutrition and the Crohn's and Colitis Foundation of America. (2007) *J Pediatr Gastroenterol Nutr*. 44(5): 653-674.
12. Crohn's Disease Genetic Risk - 23andMe. (n.d.). Retrieved from https://www.23andme.com/health/Crohns-Disease/ Last accessed January 18, 2013.
13. Wu F, Dassopoulos T, Cope L, Maitra A, Brant SR. Genome-wide gene expression differences in Crohn's disease and ulcerative colitis from endoscopic pinch biopsies: insights into distinctive pathogenesis. (2007) *Inflamm Bowel Dis*. 13(7): 807-821.

14. Galamb O, Sipos F, Dinya E, Spisak S, Tulassay Z, et al. mRNA expression, functional profiling and multivariate classification of colon biopsy specimen by cDNA overall glass microarray. (2006) *World J Gastroenterol.* 12(43): 6998-7006.

15. Costello CM, Mah N, Häsler R, Rosenstiel P, Waetzig GH, et al. Dissection of the inflammatory bowel disease transcriptome using genome-wide cDNA microarrays. (2005) *PLoS Med.* 2(8): e199.

16. Lawrance IC, Fiocchi C, Chakravarti S. Ulcerative colitis and Crohn's disease: distinctive gene expression profiles and novel susceptibility candidate genes. (2001) *Hum Mol Genet.* 10(5): 445-456.

17. von Stein P. Inflammatory bowel disease classification through multigene analysis: fact or fiction? (2009) *Expert Rev Mol Diagn.* 9(1): 7-10.

18. von Stein P, Lofberg R, Kuznetsov NV, Gielen AW, Persson JO, et al. Multigene analysis can discriminate between ulcerative colitis, Crohn's disease, and irritable bowel syndrome. (2008) *Gastroenterology.* 134(7): 1869-1881; quiz 2153-1864.

19. Cookson W, Liang L, Abecasis G, Moffatt M, Lathrop M. Mapping complex disease traits with global gene expression. (2009) *Nat Rev Genet.* 10:184-194.

20. Booth DR, Arthur AT, Teutsch SM, Bye C, Rubio J, et al. The Southern MS Genetics Consortium. Gene expression and genotyping studies implicate the interleukin 7 receptor in the pathogenesis of primary progressive multiple sclerosis. (2005) *J Mol Med.* 83:822-830.

21. Zhang Z, Duvefelt K, Svensson F, Masterman T, Jonasdottir G, et al. Two genes encoding immune-regulatory molecules (LAG3 and IL7R) confer susceptibility to multiple sclerosis. (2005) *Genes Immun.* 6:145-152.

22. Gregory SG, Schmidt S, Seth P, Oksenberg JR, Hart J, et al. Interleukin 7 receptor alpha chain (IL7R) shows allelic and functional association with multiple sclerosis. (2007) *Nat Genet.* 39:1083-1091.

23. Stranger BE. Nica AC, Forrest MS, Dimas A, Bird CP, et al. Population genomics of human gene expression. (2007) *Nat Genet.* 39:1217-1224.

24. Burczynski ME, Peterson RL, Twine NC, Zuberek KA, Brodeur BJ, et al. Molecular classification of Crohn's disease and ulcerative colitis patients using transcriptional profiles in peripheral blood mononuclear cells. (2006) *J Mol Diagn.* 8(1): 51-61.

25. Sipos F, Galamb O, Wichmann B, Krenács T, Tóth K, et al. Peripheral blood based discrimination of ulcerative colitis and Crohn's disease from non-IBD colitis by genome-wide gene expression profiling. (2011) *Dis Markers.* 30(1): 1-17.

26. Burakoff R, Hande S, Ma J, Banks PA, Friedman S, et al. Differential regulation of peripheral leukocyte genes in patients with active Crohn's disease and Crohn's disease in remission. (2010) *J Clin Gastroenterol.* 44(2): 120-126.

27. Glatt SJ, Everall IP, Kremen WS, Corbeil J, Sásik R, et al. Comparative gene expression analysis of blood and brain provides concurrent validation of SELENBP1 up-regulation in schizophrenia. (2005) *Proc Natl Acad Sci U S A.* 102(43):15533-15538.

28. Laversin SA, Phatak VM, Powe DG, Li G, Miles AK, et al. Identification of novel breast cancer-associated transcripts by uniGene database mining and gene expression analysis in normal and malignant cells. (2013) *Genes Chromosomes Cancer.* 52(3):316-329.

29. Gregg JP, Lit L, Baron CA, Hertz-Picciotto I, Walker W, et al. Gene expression changes in children with autism. (2008) *Genomics.* 91(1):22-29.

30. Wakefield AJ, Ashwood P, Limb K, Anthony A. The significance of ileo-colonic lymphoid nodular hyperplasia in children with autistic spectrum disorder. (2005) *Eur J Gastroenterol Hepatol.* 17:827-836.

31. Ashwood P and Wakefield AJ. Immune activation of peripheral blood and mucosal CD3+ lymphocyte cytokine profiles in children with autism and gastrointestinal symptoms. (2006) *J Neuroimmunol.* 173:126-134.

32. Krigsman A, Boris M, Goldblatt A, Stott C. Clinical presentation and histologic findings at ileocolonoscopy in children with autistic spectrum disorder and chronic gastrointestinal symptoms. (2010) *Autism Insights.* 1: 1–11.

33. Valicenti-McDermott M, McVicar K, Rapin I, Wershil BK, Cohen H, et al. Frequency of gastrointestinal symptoms in children with autistic spectrum disorders and association with family history of autoimmune disease. (2006) *Dev Behav Ped.* 27:128-136.

34. Ming X, Brimacombe M, Chaaban J, Zimmerman-Bier B, Wagner GC. Autism spectrum disorders: concurrent clinical disorders. (2008) *J Child Neurology.* 23:6-13.

35. Buie T, Campbell DB, Fuchs GJ 3rd, Furuta GT, Levy J, et al. Evaluation, diagnosis, and treatment of gastrointestinal disorders in individuals with ASDs: a consensus report. (2010) *Pediatrics.* 125 Suppl 1: S1-18.

36. Bauman ML. Medical comorbidities in autism: challenges to diagnosis and treatment. (2010) *Neurotherapeutics.* 7(3): 320-327.

37. Horvath K and Perman JA. Autistic disorder and gastrointestinal disease. (2002) *Current Opinion in Ped.* 14:583–587.

38. Levy SE. Relationship of dietary intake to gastrointestinal symptoms in children with autistic spectrum disorders. (2007) *Biol Psychiatry.* 61:492-497

39. Baumgart DC and Carding SR. Inflammatory bowel disease: cause and immunbiology. (2007) *Gastroenterology.* 369:1627-1640.

CHAPTER FIFTEEN

FOOD ALLERGY AND THE GUT-BRAIN AXIS

By Andrew Wakefield, MB, BS

Category	Presenting condition
Gastrointestinal	
IgE-mediated	IgE-mediated food allergy
Non-IgE-mediated	Non-IgE-mediated food allergy Celiac disease Gastroesophageal reflux disease
Conditions of overlapping IgE and non-IgE mediated allergy	Eosinophilic esophagitis Eosinophilic gastritis Eosinophilic enterocolitis
Skin	
IgE-mediated	Extrinsic eczema (often associated with IgE-mediated food allergy)
Non-IgE-mediated	Intrinsic eczema
Respiratory	
IgE-mediated	Allergic conjunctivitis Allergic rhinitis Atopic asthma
Non-IgE mediated	Non-allergic rhinitis Non-atopic asthma Recurrent or chronic rhinosinusitis† Recurrent otitis media Adenoid hypertrophy

The issue of food allergy and its role in ASD will be discussed in some detail for three reasons: First, food allergy is common in children and becoming increasingly so. Second, from the clinical perspective, food allergy seems particularly prevalent in children with ASD. Third, it provides a prototypic mechanism for a link between the gut and the brain.

Some of the strongest evidence for a plausible disease mechanism (pathogenesis) in ASD is emerging from studies that have focused not on the brain but on the intestine. Among the more consistent and compelling discoveries is that of GI pathology in some affected children with an associated chronic immune system activation and inflammation—a process that may be driven, in part, by some form of food allergy. Recognition of the contribution of food protein antigens— molecules that activate an immune response—to this inflammatory cycle in the form of food allergy are receiving growing attention. So is the possibility that an aberrant immune reaction to food, set up in the gut, can have immune and inflammatory knock-on (secondary or incidental) effects in the brain. Such a mechanism has been identified in celiac disease, and it is not a stretch for ASD by any means.

Adverse reactions to food, recognized from at least the time of Hippocrates over two millenia ago, come in many guises. Food-allergic disorders are common and are becoming more so, affecting in the region of 8% of children under three years old and up to 35% based upon parental reporting.[1] Nontoxic reactions may be immunologic reactions (allergic) or non-immunologic (e.g., food intolerances due to digestive enzyme deficiencies). Both immunologic and non-immunologic mechanisms may coexist. In turn, allergic reactions to ingested foods may be mediated through different axes of the immune system. Accordingly, they manifest differently and require different diagnostic approaches and treatment.

The stage for food allergy may be set during the earliest encounters between the infant's intestine and the food they eat. It has even been observed that, occasionally, initial sensitization to food proteins may occur in the fetus, presumably via the mother's diet.[2]

Alternatively, the sterile, immunologically naïve intestine of the newborn is bombarded with foreign proteins and other potential allergens from the moment of delivery. The optimal outcome of this encounter is the development of immunological tolerance—a state of non-overreactivity—to beneficial bacteria and foodstuffs. The evolution of this ecological optimization is limited by the immaturity of certain aspects of newborn intestinal physiology, including low output of sterilizing stomach acid, low digestive enzyme activities, and immune system immaturity, e.g., low levels of the antibody (IgA) that protects mucosal surfaces of the body such as the intestinal lining. The net effect of this immaturity is that the earlier the introduction of solid foods the greater the likelihood of allergic reactions to these foods.[3] In addition, it is possible that immune perturbation from infection or vaccination may provoke allergy to previously innocuous foods.

It is not surprising that food allergies come in a variety of forms, given the complexity of the immune system and the extraordinary range of foreign substances to which the intestinal lining is exposed. Food allergic reactions mediated by IgE antibodies are those with which the public is most familiar. This is the immediate or anaphylactic type that is seen with, for example, peanut allergy. Symptoms caused by immediate GI hypersensitivity typically develop within two hours of consuming the offending food and often much sooner. They include nausea, colicky abdominal pain, vomiting and/or diarrhea. These may be accompanied by skin reactions such as urticaria[4] (hives) and asthma. Repeated exposure leads to a degree of reduced sensitivity and less obvious clinical reactions, such as failure to thrive (poor appetite and weight gain) and intermittent abdominal pain.

A second category is non-IgE-mediated or delayed-type food allergy, frequently due to dietary protein intolerance. This condition may present early in life and is associated with irritability, protracted vomiting and diarrhea, and consequent dehydration. Symptoms usually occur 4 to 72 hours after food ingestion. Because of the delay in the onset of symptoms, it may be difficult to link them to food. Re-exposure to the offending food(s)—commonly cow's milk or soy protein formulas in younger children and eggs, wheat, rice, oat, peanuts, chicken, turkey, and fish in older children—may lead to diarrhea (sometimes bloody), abdominal distention, and failure to thrive. Celiac disease, an immunologic intolerance to wheat gliadin (a protein present in wheat), is a specific disorder within the subset of non-IgE-mediated disorders. The third category involves mixed IgE- and non-IgE-mediated food allergies.

Non-IgE-mediated food allergy includes conditions in which inflammation of the intestinal lining is associated with swelling of the lymph glands (lymphoid nodular hyperplasia [LNH]). Under the microscope, biopsies frequently show infiltration of the mucosa by immune cells called eosinophils (allergy cells).[5] These findings (LNH[6] and an eosinophilic inflammation) have been reported in children with autism as part of their GI disease.

Eosinophilic esophagitis, gastritis, and gastroenteritis are examples of this form of food allergy. Clinically, allergic esophagitis presents most commonly from infancy through to adolescence and is associated with reflux, intermittent vomiting, food refusal, abdominal pain, irritability, and sleep disturbance. These symptoms do not typically respond to conventional reflux medication such as acid-blocking drugs.

In the latter two categories—IgE and non-IgE-mediated food allergies—GI symptoms such as diarrhea, abdominal pain, and failure to thrive usually predominate. However, food-allergic GI reactions may be accompanied by symptoms ranging from arthritis to asthma, migraine, cluster headaches, eczema, fatigue, heartburn, and behavioral disturbances—particularly in children. Alternatively, the GI disease may be "occult" or clinically silent and surprisingly, perhaps, the non-GI symptoms such as behavioral issues may be the *only* manifestations of intestinal food allergy.

The diagnosis of food allergy
As in all clinical encounters, in the diagnosis of food allergy, the patient's history and physical examination findings are paramount. The history should ascertain the nature of the symptoms, the identity and amount of the suspect food(s), the time to reaction from ingestion, whether the same reaction occurs with repeated exposure to that food, and when the last reaction occurred. Allergic shiners, coarse hair, and dry skin with or without eczema may be present. The physical examination should include anthropomorphic measures such as height and weight and a thorough general examination. Attention to signs of abdominal disease is an obvious requirement, whereas eliciting signs of neurological and behavioral deficits, although not as obvious, may be equally important.

Beyond the history and examination, the differential diagnosis of food allergy generally follows one of two paths. If an IgE-mediated allergy is suspected, it can usually be confirmed by skin tests. Testing involves subcutaneous injection with small quantities of glycerinated extracts of common food allergens and measurement of any consequent skin reaction.[8] An alternative, the RAST (radioallergosorbent test) is a blood test performed in the laboratory that looks for IgE antibodies against specific foods.

Skin prick tests are negative in non-IgE-mediated food allergy, and, until recently, specific testing had been relatively unhelpful in the identification of foods responsible for non-IgE-mediated reactions. On its own, testing for the presence of alternative types of antibodies such as IgG (immunoglobulin G) to foods is not helpful for predicting a non-IgE-mediated food allergy. More recently, commercial laboratory testing has become available for food-related antibodies in the blood that form complexes with molecules called complement molecules that are also present in the blood. It is these complexes that are thought to promote the allergic inflammation and tissue damage.[9] Food-related immune complexes can be detected against a range of common foods using a sample of the patient's blood. It has been suggested that testing in this way can help the physician or nutritionist determine what foods should form part of any trial of dietary exclusion; however, further formal scientific study of the merits of this particular testing is required. Clinical testing for non-IgE-mediated food allergy has also progressed with the development of patch testing, the application of suspect foods to the skin in a series of Finn Chambers[10] which allow the measurement of any positive reaction following prolonged exposure.

If a non-IgE-mediated food allergy is suspected, upper and lower GI endoscopy and biopsy are necessary and may confirm the diagnosis by finding eosinophilic inflammation of the intestinal mucosa and/or a lymphocytic infiltrate in the lining epithelial cells.

Thereafter, the real test of whether a particular food(s) is responsible for the patient's symptoms is an allergy elimination diet followed by rechallenge with the suspect food(s). Ideally, this is done in circumstances where neither the patient nor the doctor is aware of when the food is eliminated or reintroduced. Resolution of symptoms following removal and their subsequent provocation upon re-exposure provides the definitive diagnosis.

The natural history of non-IgE-mediated food allergy is that it resolves over time.[11] The interval to recovery is highly variable; for example, some children grow out of a milk allergy in a matter of months while others may take 8 to 10 years.

Food allergy and neurological disease

In building the scientific argument for a link between the gut and the brain—and specifically abnormal immune reactions to ingested food and autism symptoms—a good starting point is a review of the evidence for gut-immune-brain interactions as a more general concept. Specifically in the context of a non-IgE-mediated food allergy, the best-studied example of the neurological knock-on effects of intestinal disease is untreated celiac disease. Celiac disease is an immune-mediated (allergic) disorder triggered by ingestion of wheat gliadin and related proteins in genetically susceptible individuals. This susceptibility is encoded in immune response genes designated DR3-DQ2 (present in 90%–95% of celiac sufferers) and DQ8 (present in 5%–10% of celiac sufferers). However, hereditary factors alone do not explain the development of celiac disease, and infectious triggers have been proposed. In the continued presence of gluten, the disease is self-perpetuating; if untreated, it can lead to severe complications such as lymphoma.

In addition to the characteristic intestinal changes, including small intestinal mucosal flattening, inflammation, and malabsorption, celiac disease is associated with various extraintestinal manifestations. These include neurological complications such as neuropathy, nerve inflammation (neuritis), ataxia (lack of muscle coordination), seizures, and behavioral changes. Celiac disease is a classical example of a disease in which a primary intestinal food allergy can lead to secondary brain injury.

It is important for families affected by ASD to recognize that neurological complications arising in the setting of gluten sensitivity may occur in the absence of GI symptoms, with the only sign of this cryptic gluten sensitivity being ataxia, dementia, seizures, or affective symptoms such as depression. In the setting of ASD, this may include behavioral symptoms that, given their prominence, mask any less obvious GI issues. Cryptic gluten sensitivity includes the situation where the patient suffers no overt GI symptoms but has antibodies against wheat gliadin and experiences extraintestinal symptoms that are often neurological in nature. For example, Dr. Marios Hadjivassiliou and colleagues from Leeds in the UK investigated patients with neurological disease of unknown cause for the presence of antigliadin antibodies.[12] Antibody levels in the blood were compared with those in patients with a specific neurological diagnosis such as stroke, multiple sclerosis (MS), and Parkinson's disease (PD).

Positive titers for antigliadin antibodies—as evidence of an immune response to gluten—were present in 30 of 53 (57%) patients with neurological disease of unknown cause compared with much lower proportions of the stroke/MS/PD group (5%), and healthy blood donors (12%). Interestingly, despite these patients having no GI symptoms, duodenal biopsies in 26 out of 30 antigliadin antibody-positive patients revealed mucosal pathology, including celiac disease in 9 and non-specific duodenal inflammation in 10. Clearly, gluten sensitivity is common in patients with neurological disease of unknown cause and may be present without overt GI symptoms. Moreover, this gluten sensitivity may be causally related to the neurological disease.[13]

In pursuing this association further, Hadjivassiliou and colleagues focused upon patients suffering from ataxia, the commonest neurological manifestation of celiac disease. Notably, ataxia is reported frequently by parents of children with regressive autism, being particularly prominent during the regressive phase.[14] In some individuals with a genetic susceptibility to celiac disease and serological evidence of gluten sensitivity (antigliadin antibodies), gluten ataxia is the sole manifestation of their disease.

The authors identified 28 patients with ataxia and antigliadin antibodies. Brain scans showed that 6 patients had evidence of cerebellar atrophy—shrinkage due to loss of nerve cells. Necropsies performed on 2 patients who died showed inflammation in the cerebellum and damage to the spinal cord. These observations led the authors to the conclusion that gluten ataxia occurs as a result of immunological damage to these areas of the brain. Of note, despite no GI symptoms, 16 of the 28 patients had GI pathology consistent with celiac disease with the presence of an alternative inflammatory disease in another 2.

In a larger study, Hadjivassiliou identified a high prevalence of gluten sensitivity among 41% of a group of 132 patients with ataxia of unknown cause. In those with a genetically-based ataxia and in healthy blood donors, the prevalence was low. GI symptoms were present in only a small minority (13%) of those with gluten ataxia. The authors concluded that gluten ataxia is the single most common cause of ataxia of unknown origin and urged that newly-presenting patients with this condition get antigliadin antibody testing.[15]

So how might antibodies that develop against gluten in the intestinal lining cause problems in the brain? Hadjivassiliou's theory was that antibodies made against wheat proteins travel in the bloodstream to the brain where they cross-react, possibly through a lookalike process of molecular mimicry, with brain proteins of a structure similar to those of wheat proteins. They suggested that in a similar manner to celiac disease, an autoimmune reaction occurs in the brain, particularly the cerebellum—the part that is principally responsible for controlling balance and coordination.

When the authors put serum (the antibody-containing part of the blood) from patients with gluten ataxia onto slices of human cerebellum in the laboratory, a strong antibody reaction was detected in specific cells unique to the cerebellum—Purkinje cells—for 12 of the 13 patients tested. Commercial antigliadin antibody also stained human Purkinje cells in a similar manner. Purkinje cells, named after the Czech anatomist Jan Evangelista Purkyně, are like lights at a busy intersection; these cells effectively control the flow of information from the cerebellum.

Broadly, the study confirmed two things: first, patients with gluten ataxia have antibodies against cerebellar Purkinje cells; second, antigliadin antibodies cross-react with Purkinje cell-associated antigens.[16] The findings raise the subsidiary question: does binding of these antibodies to the Purkinjie cells impair their health and function? One study that might advance the argument for a pathologic role of these antigliadin antibodies in causing ataxia would be to isolate them and inject them into an experimental laboratory animal to see if they reproduced the symptoms and brain damage described by Hadjivassiliou and colleagues.

Their observations also raise the tantalizing possibility that there may be target molecules in the brain that bind antigliadin antibodies as a precursor to immune damage. Alaedini et al. from Cornell University identified one of these molecular targets as Synapsin I, one of a family of brain proteins involved in regulating neurotransmitter release at synapses. Theoretically, therefore, antigliadin antibodies might upset brain function by interfering with neurotransmission.[17]

And anti-Synapsin 1 antibodies are not the only players. In fact, the major target of autoimmunity across the whole spectrum of gluten sensitivity is an enzyme called tissue transglutaminase (transglutaminase type II). Hadjivassiliou and colleagues described the binding of antibodies against this enzyme in the cerebellum and brain stem as well as in the intestine of patients with gluten ataxia. This binding was similar to that seen in patients with celiac disease, supporting the proposition that gluten ataxia, in common with celiac disease, is an immune-mediated disorder that starts with food allergy.[18]

From a clinical perspective, the deal-breaker for a gut-immune-brain interaction in the neurologic manifestations of celiac disease is whether removal of gluten from the diet, which is known to cause celiac antibodies to fall and eventually disappear from the blood, leads to an improvement in the clinical symptoms of gluten ataxia. Hadjivassiliou's team put this to the test in a study of 43 patients with gluten ataxia. All were offered a strict gluten-free diet and monitored every six months. All patients underwent a battery of tests to assess their ataxia at baseline and after one year on the diet. Twenty-six patients (treatment group) adhered to the gluten-free diet and had evidence of elimination of antigliadin antibodies by one year. Fourteen patients refused the diet and were allocated to the untreated control group. Three patients had persistently raised antigliadin antibodies despite adherence to the diet and were therefore excluded from the analysis. After one year, there was a significant improvement in all of the ataxia tests in the treatment group compared with the control group. They observed that gluten ataxia responded to a strict gluten-free diet even in the absence of obvious intestinal disease. Crucially, they had identified a neurological disease that was treatable by diet. This made the correct diagnosis of gluten sensitivity in patients presenting with ataxia, a vital step in their potential for recovery.[19]

Celiac disease and affective symptoms
Beyond ataxia, celiac disease is associated with a range of psychological

and behavioral problems. Reports on adult celiac sufferers indicate that between 30–69% have depressive symptoms,[20] and 42% have depressive disorders.[21] Of the few studies that have focused upon young people with celiac disease, disorders of sleep and the ability to relax have been described in adolescents,[22] and the frequency of behavioral disorders and depressive problems was higher in children with untreated celiac disease when compared with those on a gluten-free diet and those without celiac disease.[23]

Where celiac disease is clinically silent due to a lack of GI symptoms, a careful history often reveals that, in many such cases, there is low intensity comorbid illness associated with decreased well-being, which in children includes behavioral disturbances with a tendency to depression, irritability, and impaired school performance.[24] Fabiani et al. described an increase in weight and height velocity, appetite, mood amelioration and an improvement in physical and school performance in adolescents whose celiac disease was apparently asymptomatic at diagnosis once they began following a gluten-free diet.[25]

From Finland, Pynönnen et al. reported that celiac patients had a significantly higher lifetime prevalence of a major depressive disorder (31% versus 7%) and disruptive behavior disorder (28% versus 3%) than non-celiac controls.[26] These differences were evident for the celiac group before a gluten-free diet but not after, suggesting that diet may reduce affective symptoms. The authors recommend that patients presenting with affective disorders and behavioral disturbances should be screened for gluten sensitivities.

Celiac disease and autism

The first report of autism occurring in association with celiac disease dates from 1971.[27] Barcia and colleagues subsequently reported an increased incidence of biopsy-confirmed celiac disease in their patients with pervasive developmental disorder (PDD) at a frequency that was three and a half fold higher than in the developmentally normal population.

Advancing the argument for a similar gut-immune-brain axis in autism would be supported by reports in which autism or autistic symptoms have occurred in some children with celiac disease and for these symptoms to have abated with a gluten-free diet. It is not necessary that all children with celiac disease have symptoms of ASD or that the bowel pathology found in many children with ASD overlaps with celiac disease. Proof of principle requires only that in well-described cases of celiac disease where autism symptoms are present that such symptoms resolve following the removal of gluten.

For example, Genuis et al. provided a detailed description of a five-year-old boy with regressive autism and chronic GI symptoms who not only had very high celiac disease antibody titers but also evidence of malabsorption with nutritional and vitamin deficiencies. A gluten-free diet led rapidly to relief of his GI symptoms and improvement in his behavior and cognitive function. Two and a half years later he no longer had autism and his mother described him as "...doing incredibly well and [he] is so very happy."[28]

The bowel and behavior beyond celiac disease

The link between food allergy and behavioral disturbances goes beyond celiac disease; a link between certain foods and aberrant behavior has long been recognized, although support from well-designed scientific studies has only come more recently. In 1947, Randolf reviewed "the fatigue syndrome" of allergic origin as a common cause of irritability and abnormalities of behavior in children.[29] He described how this syndrome usually results from chronic food allergy involving sensitivity to more than one food, while "sensitivity to wheat and corn is encountered most frequently."[30]

He divided the affected children into two groups: first, the chronically tired, sluggish, and depressed child, and second, the hyperkinetic and hyperexcited child. Randolf commented: "Both are inclined to be irritable and fretful in their behavior and to be maladjusted in both the home and school. Their schoolwork suffers because of a characteristic difficulty in concentration and impairment of memory."[31]

Although food allergy is more commonly associated with a history of one or more GI symptoms, Randolf recognized that behavioral symptoms may be the sole allergic manifestation exhibited by a child. He also recognized the need to prioritize the allergy symptoms over the behavioral, stating: "When dealing with allergic children, the significance of psychic and emotional factors in the genesis of irritability and behavior problems may be judged to best advantage after the allergic reactions are brought under control."[32] Put another way, he is saying that we should exclude a medical disorder before assuming that the problem is all in the mind.

By 1979, it was recognized that states of excessive excitability and fatigue associated with food allergy in children could be part of a continuous process operating in two stages, rather than operating as two distinct sets of responses occurring in different children. This was characterized by a "high" or tension (hyperkinetic) stage followed by a "low" or fatigue stage, usually in that order but sometimes reversed. This phenomenon became known as the allergic tension-fatigue syndrome.[33]

The observation that food intolerances, likely of an allergic origin, could be linked not only to behavioral changes in children but also to infectious environmental triggers had been reported some years earlier. In 1956, Daynes presented his findings of "Naughtiness, depression, and fits due to wheat sensitivity" to the Royal Society of Medicine in London.[34] He made the following observations:

Typically a child between 1 and 5 years becomes naughty and difficult a few days after the onset of an acute infectious illness . . . such as measles or gastroenteritis. He is irritable, negativistic, and spiteful, sleep is disturbed and he wakes up in the night and often screams; his appetite is poor, he fails to gain weight, his abdomen is often distended and the stools may become bulky, pale and offensive. This condition, if left untreated, usually rights itself after a month or two, but it may last for much longer in which case slight petit mal attacks may develop in addition to worsening of the other symptoms. I have been placing these children on a gluten-free diet at the earliest opportunity and the symptoms respond dramatically, usually within two or three days. They relapse if a premature return to a normal diet is made. Study of over 40 cases has led me to formulate a syndrome – pre-coeliac syndrome.

Here we have an early report of an infection such as measles triggering likely food allergy. In addition, Daynes also described the first informal observation of clinical improvement following an exclusion diet followed by return of symptoms upon re-exposure, a wheat-withdrawal-rechallenge effect.

Some aspects of the relationship between food allergy and behavioral problems remain controversial. In order to make the case, the early observational studies required support from both controlled clinical trials and mechanistic science to underpin a plausible biological basis for interactions between food and behavior. This evidence has been provided by studies such as that by Egger et al., who examined 76 "overactive" children treated with a diet that was very low in substances capable of eliciting an immune response (oligoantigenic).[35] They reported:

> *Sixty-two [children] improved, and a normal range of behaviour was achieved in 21 of these. Other symptoms, such as headaches, abdominal pain, and fits, also often improved. Twenty-eight of the children who improved completed a double-blind, crossover, placebo-controlled trial in which foods thought to provoke symptoms were reintroduced. Symptoms returned or were exacerbated much more often when patients were on active material than on placebo. Forty-eight foods were incriminated. Artificial colorants and preservatives were the commonest provoking substances, but no child was sensitive to these alone.*

Sleep disturbances are a recurring theme in parental reports of food-related behavioral disturbances. Not only are they a prominent feature in children with food allergy and the incipient decline of children into autism, but also improvement in sleep is often the first sign of improvement reported by parents when the child with ASD starts the gluten- and casein-free diet. To confirm that sleeplessness in infants can be related to an undiagnosed allergy to cow's milk proteins, Kahn et al. studied 71 infants including 20 with chronic insomnia, and 31 who suffered skin or digestive symptoms attributed to cow's milk intolerance, 13 of whom also had insomnia. Control infants consisted of 20 with no history of sleep disturbance or milk allergy. Laboratory tests revealed allergic reactions to milk in all the infants in the first two groups. The sleep of the infants with insomnia normalized after cow's milk was eliminated from the diet. Insomnia reappeared when the infants in the first group were rechallenged with milk. The findings confirmed that food allergy is an important cause of sleep disturbance in infants.[36]

Laboratory studies have since provided some insights into possible mechanisms for this gut-brain interaction. For example, in 2003 Basso et al.[37] administered the egg protein ovalbumin to previously sensitized laboratory mice. Mice allergic to ovalbumin had higher levels of anxiety, activation of emotionality-related brain areas, and aversion to the ovalbumin-containing solution. Either administration of antibodies that neutralized IgE antibody or the induction of immune tolerance to ovalbumin prevented both the food aversion and the brain activation. These important findings established a direct relationship between brain function and food allergy, creating, as the authors described, "a solid ground for understanding the [cause] of psychological disorders in allergic patients."

Mast cells and the gut-brain axis

A key player, not only in food allergy but emerging also in the link between ASD's environmental cause(s) and its devastating effect, is the mast cell. Mast cells are present in most tissues characteristically surrounding blood vessels and nerves and are especially prominent near the boundaries between the outside world and the tissues, such as the skin, lungs, and digestive tract. The *Mastzellen*, or mast cell, was first described by Nobel Laureate Paul Ehrlich, a scientist born in 1854 in the German kingdom of Prussia. His doctoral thesis, awarded from the University of Leipzig in 1878, described mast cells on the basis of their unique staining characteristics in tissues and the large granules that they contain. They were so named from the German *Mast* (food) in the belief that these granules provided nourishment for surrounding tissues. Now more appropriately considered to be part of the immune system, their relationship to food has emerged in the alternative guise of mediators of food allergic responses – ironically, their granules potentially toxic rather than nourishing.

Mast cells are one of the body's early warning systems – a system that can sometimes be difficult to shut down or override – causing more harm than good. Their profound and far-reaching effects are due, in part, to their tendency to "explode" on exposure to allergens, releasing their granules (degranulation) of highly reactive proinflammatory chemicals. With time, the complex role of these cells as an integral part of the immune/inflammatory response has emerged. In fact, so important is this role that animals lacking mast cells cannot develop inflammation.

Recognition of the importance of mast cells in ASD has come from Dr. Theoharis Theoharides and his team from Tufts University School of Medicine in Boston. His interest started not with autism but with a spectrum of rare disorders associated with excessive mast cell activity, collectively termed mastocytosis. Mastocytosis is associated with both food intolerances and disturbances in cognition and behavior. This evident gut-brain connection and the emerging parallels with autism led him to examine the prevalence of ASD in children with a diagnosis of mastocytosis. In a landmark observation, ASD turned out to be 10 times higher in those with mastocytosis compared with the current prevalence of around 1 in 100 children for ASD![38]

The Tufts University group is pursuing the theory that mast cells, principally those situated at the body's natural barriers such as the bowel-blood barrier and the blood- brain barrier, cause these barriers to leak when the mast cells become overly activated by, for example, food allergens. This, they propose, leads to the ingress of proinflammatory molecules into the brain and neuroinflammation.

Mastocytosis involves proliferation and activation of mast cells, which, in the skin, is evident clinically as a rash – urticaria pigmentosa (UP). Theoharides et al. reported a highly relevant clinical example of possible mast cell triggering in the setting of ASD. The authors described one child with UP, diagnosed at 1 year, whose UP worsened following routine immunization at 3 years. His exaggerated skin reaction was associated with concurrent developmental regression leading to a diagnosis of PDD-NOS.[39]

Dr. Theoharides and his team have contributed greatly to our understanding not only of the potential role of these cells in ASD but also how their excessive activation and harmful effects might be prevented with pharmacologically active foodstuffs. They are currently investigating whether inflammation in the brain can be reduced with naturally occurring flavonoids such as quercetin and luteolin, which act to stabilize mast cells and inhibit their release of inflammatory mediators.[40] It remains to be seen what beneficial effects these compounds might have in ASD.

Food allergy and ADHD

By 1998, elimination diets of low immunogenicity (low allergic potential) had been examined in at least seven controlled studies[41] and had demonstrated either significant improvement compared with a placebo of full-diet[42] or deterioration when rechallenge with offending foods was undertaken after a trial of diet.[43] Based upon these studies, Arnold suggested that the profile of a probable responder is a middle- or upper-class preschooler with atopy—a predisposition to allergic disease—and prominent irritability and sleep disturbance, with physical as well as behavioral symptoms.[44] Again, across the spectrum of associated behavioral abnormalities, sleep disturbance has emerged as one of the most prominent and consistent hallmarks of food allergy.

By 2010 from a Dutch team headed by Dr. Buitelaar in Nijmegen, robust data from a randomized controlled study had confirmed the efficacy of a restricted elimination diet in improving symptoms of ADHD. The diet group, which was allowed only certain foods,[45] was compared with an unrestricted diet control group. After 9 weeks, eleven of 15 (73%) in the diet group showed a decrease by 50% or more on parent rating scales compared with none of 12 (0%) in the control group. Similarly, with teacher ratings, 7 of 10 (70%) in the diet group showed improvement compared with none of 7 controls.[46]

And by 2011, Buitelaar and colleagues had completed and reported a two-phase study consisting of food removal and a randomized double-blind food rechallenge. The study was substantially larger than their earlier one, involving 50 children in each of the diet and control groups. Not only was there a highly significant improvement of behaviors on diet but there was a similarly significant relapse rate once the restriction diet was stopped.[47]

The authors concluded by "supporting the implementation of a dietary intervention in the standard of care for all children with ADHD."[48] While the study did not examine the role of non-IgE-mediated food allergy in this relationship, it means that the debate over whether food affects behavior is effectively a done deal.

Does food allergy play a role in autism?

The science of celiac disease has helped to establish a gut-immune-brain axis. The immunologic and inflammatory mechanisms that have been elucidated for such an axis are by no means exclusive—inflammatory cytokines may have a direct effect on mood and behavior, independent of autoimmunity, for example. What the research has established, nonetheless, is a plausible and coherent chain of potential cause and effect. Similarly, in order to establish a role for food allergy in autism symptoms, a number of links in the chain of causation need to be forged. Studies that would help include:

1. the demonstration of abnormal immune (e.g., antibody) responses to specific foods
2. an inflammatory reaction associated with this immune response
3. a cellular or biochemical neurological response to these immune/inflammatory events
4. modulation of the foregoing effects by an elimination diet and/or pharmaceutical control of the associated immune/inflammatory process

Inspired initially by anecdotal parental observations that various food intolerances influenced autism symptoms in their children, some interesting clinical observations have been reported. In 1995, Lucarelli et al. found high levels of antibodies to a variety of milk proteins[49] in patients with autism compared with developmentally normal subjects.[50] The authors then examined the effect of an exclusion diet free of cow's milk and other foods that gave a positive skin test (IgE-mediated allergy) in 36 patients. They reported a marked improvement in behavioral symptoms after a period of eight weeks on the elimination diet.

Beyond IgE-mediated food allergy, more substantial evidence has emerged of a role for non-IgE-mediated food allergy in autism in support of the popular and growing awareness that reactions to common foods like dairy and wheat can have neurological and behavioral knock-on effects.

In a logical progression that has paralleled the work of Hadjivassiliou and others in celiac disease, Vojdani et al. pursued the possibility that autism is associated with antibodies that develop against food proteins that then recognize and react with similar proteins in human neural tissues, leading to changes in brain development and behavior. This proposed model moved the autism-immune association from food allergy alone to food-induced autoimmunity—a situation in which a "confused" immune system mounts a damaging response against its host. As preliminary evidence for this "horror autotoxicus"[51] Vojdani et al. demonstrated, for the first time, that in some children with autism and predisposing immune response genes, the dietary peptides (molecule consisting of two or more amino acids) gliadin and casein bound to enzymes on the host cell surface. These children produced antibodies against gliadin, casein, and the cell's own molecules, resulting in an autoimmune reaction.[52]

They subsequently compared this food-induced autoimmune reaction in patients with autism with that seen in patients with established autoimmune disease ("mixed connective tissue disease"). In both groups, antigliadin antibodies were present and cross-reacted with human cell surface proteins—on this occasion, peptidase enzymes. The authors proposed that these autoantibodies might cause membrane enzyme dysfunction and immune dysregulation affecting the nervous system.[53] Vojdani et al. also showed that some children with autism have antibodies against a milk protein (butyrophilin); these antibodies cross-reacted with certain important brain proteins such as myelin basic protein (MBP)—a constituent of the insulation that surrounds nerves—suggesting a mechanism by which, in autism, milk antigens may contribute to autoimmune responses to nerve tissues.[54]

From molecules to inflammation

An autoimmune *reaction*, for example, the binding of antibodies that are cross-reactive with foods and host antigens, does not on its own constitute an autoimmune *disease*. It is also necessary to have inflammatory pathology and/or disturbance of cell function arising as a consequence of this immunologic interaction. On a potentially convergent track to Vojdani and colleagues, Ashwood et al.[55] reported the novel observation of marked disturbances in immune cell (lymphocyte) numbers and function in the intestines of children with autistic regression and GI symptoms. Lymphocytes isolated from the intestinal lining of such children exhibited a striking increase in the level of the potent proinflammatory molecule tumor necrosis factor-alpha (TNF-α) and a decrease in the level of interleukin-10 (IL-10), a counter-regulatory cytokine that acts to downgrade the immune response and limit inflammation. The findings of microscopic inflammation and a marked proinflammatory immune cell activation in the intestinal mucosa are reminiscent of other inflammatory bowel diseases and put the gut front and center stage in some forms of ASD.

Independently, Dr. Harumi Jyonouchi, an immunologist from the University of Medicine & Dentistry of New Jersey, and her colleagues reported an association between immune reactivity to common dietary proteins and excessive proinflammatory cytokine production in a subset of ASD children when their blood lymphocytes were exposed to endotoxin, a component of bacteria that is highly prevalent in the gut, is better known for causing fever during infections, and is a major stimulant of innate (natural) immunity in the gut mucosa.[56]

Jyonouchi and her colleagues then sought to resolve whether such abnormal immune responses were just part of these children's innate immune constitution or whether they were the result of chronic GI disease secondary to allergic reactivity to food.[57] To do so, they studied cytokine responses of immune cells from the blood that were exposed to bacterial endotoxin. Responses in children with ASD, with and without GI symptoms, including those on unrestricted and elimination diets, were compared with neurotypical children with non-IgE-mediated food allergy on similar diets and healthy children.

The first observation was that, regardless of dietary interventions, endotoxin-exposed immune cells from the blood of children with ASD and those with non-IgE-mediated food allergy produced higher levels of TNF-α than did healthy children. In support of the original findings of Ashwood et al., ASD children with GI symptoms on an unrestricted diet produced more of the proinflammatory cytokine IL-12 and less anti-inflammatory IL-10 than other groups. Those children with ASD, GI symptoms, and an unrestricted diet had the most marked immune imbalance.

Overall, their findings indicated intrinsic defects of innate immune responses in ASD children with GI symptoms, supporting the probability of a gut-immune-brain axis operating in these children to produce the manifestations of autism.[58] An interesting observation that set the ASD children apart from more common forms of non-IgE-mediated food allergy is their apparent failure to generate IL-10—the anti-inflammatory cytokine—in an effort to limit the inflammatory response. This observation clearly requires further study.

In order to determine which common foods might be driving the inflammatory responses in ASD children with GI symptoms, the authors measured cytokine production in response to whole cow's milk protein (CMP) and its major components[59] as well as to gliadin and soy. Exposed to milk proteins, ASD children with GI symptoms produced more proinflammatory cytokines than did control subjects. They also produced more TNF-α with gliadin. Even in those ASD children with no GI symptoms, cow's milk protein stimulated lymphocytes to produce more proinflammatory cytokines than did control subjects. The findings provided clear evidence of a link between food allergy and GI symptoms in children with ASD.[60]

As the evidence continues to mount for a gut-immune-brain interaction in some children with ASD—perhaps a majority of the current epidemic wave—a   pathogenic mechanism is consolidating around food allergy, intestinal inflammation, autoimmune responses in neural tissue, and symptomatic disease. As with celiac disease, the proof of the pudding is in *not* eating; do diets that exclude potentially allergenic foods lead to resolution of the behavioral symptoms of ASD?

Selective food exclusion in the treatment of autism

For autism, the mainstay of dietary intervention has been the gluten- and casein-free diet. In 2010, the results of two randomized controlled clinical trials were available that confirmed the benefit of this approach in ameliorating the behavioral symptoms of autism.

Anne-Marie Knivsberg and her colleagues in Norway performed a single-blind, controlled study to evaluate the effect of a gluten- and casein-free diet for children with autism. Twenty children with autism were randomly assigned to either the diet or the control group and underwent developmental and behavioral testing. The experimental period was one year, after which observations and tests were repeated. A significant reduction in autistic behaviors was found for participants in the diet group but not for those in the control group.[61]

Replication is a key to scientific validation; in the recent study titled "The ScanBrit Randomised Controlled Study of Gluten- and Casein-free Dietary Intervention for Children With Autism Spectrum Disorders," Whiteley et al. undertook a 2-stage, 24-month controlled trial in which 72 Danish children aged four to ten years were randomly assigned to either diet or non-diet groups.[62] At Stage One, all children were tested at baseline, 8, and 12 months with respect to any behavioral changes. After 12 months, 17 children in the non-diet group were switched to the diet, and 18 already on the diet were asked to continue. Inter- and intra-group comparison of symptoms revealed evidence of sustained clinical improvements for those children on the diet. This effect eventually plateaued at a higher level of functioning.

The authors concluded that ". . .the data provided evidence of sustained clinical improvements in groups receiving the dietary intervention compared to controls. . . dietary intervention may possibly affect developmental outcome for ASD children."[63]

For autism, by 2010, the threads of a compelling pathological axis of gut-immune-brain interaction in ASD were coming together. Key aspects of the gut-immune-brain axis in ASD were consistent in many respects with the prototypic model of celiac disease. Jyonouchi and colleagues were to add a further piece to the jigsaw by linking the beneficial clinical and immunological responses to dietary intervention in a preliminary study. In their patients with ASD, the elimination diet helped to resolve GI symptoms and autistic behaviors while, at the same time, normalizing cytokine responses in these patients' immune cells. The authors concluded that "Dysregulated production of inflammatory and counter-regulatory cytokines may be associated with non-IgE-mediated adverse reaction to common dietary proteins in some ASD children, indicating therapeutic significance of dietary interventions. . . ."[64]

Jyonouchi and her colleagues had succeeded in linking non-IgE-mediated food allergy, GI symptoms, and elevated inflammatory cytokine production in a substantial number of ASD children in response to clinically suspect foods like cow's milk protein, soy, and gliadin. They had also linked normalization of these parameters to dietary intervention, at least in preliminary studies.[65] But many questions remain unanswered. For example, in children with cow's milk protein-associated non-IgE-mediated food allergy, dietary exclusion leads to sustained improvement in GI symptoms. In contrast, for some children with ASD and this same allergy, GI symptoms recur despite a strict exclusion diet. Jyonouchi et al. found that after having started the appropriate diet, these children's immune reactivity to milk and wheat proteins declined over three months but rebounded by six months, despite their having continued with the diet.[66] This was not seen in food allergic children who did not have ASD. While GI symptoms also improved initially, they returned in these children with ASD. On the other hand, behavioral symptoms including irritability, hyperactivity, and lethargy improved on diet and did not relapse. There is something different about the ASD group that distinguishes their response from more typical non-IgE-mediated food allergy; Jyonouchi believes that they have a continued problem with innate immunity that might lead them to react to a succession of foods—not just those initially eliminated from the diet. I believe that this effect may be linked to their apparent difficulty in producing adequate counter-regulatory or anti-inflammatory cytokines like IL-10 that restore and maintain immune tolerance in the intestine. Whatever the basis of this anomaly, it requires continued vigilance and reassessment of these children, based at the very least on the status of their GI symptoms, in order to manage their continuing dietary issues and intestinal disease.

Conclusion

By 2010, there was good evidence of immunological intolerances to common foodstuffs in a significant proportion of patients with ASD. It was also evident that these intolerances may be mediated through a variety of immunologic and inflammatory mechanisms and may directly or indirectly impact behavior.

References

1. Rona RJ, Kiel T, Summers C, et al. The prevalence of food allergy: a meta-analysis *J Allergy Clin Immunol*. 2007;120:638-46.
2. Ward CM, Geng L, Jyonouchi H. Fetal sensitization to cow's milk protein and wheat: cow's milk protein and wheat-specific TNF-alpha production by umbilical cord blood cells and subsequent decline of TNF-alpha production by peripheral blood mononuclear cells following dietary intervention. *Pediatr Allergy Immunol*. 2007;18:276-80.

3. Fergusson DM, Horwood LJ, Shannon FT. Early solid feeding and recurrent eczema: a 10-year longitudinal study. *Pediatrics*. 1990;86;541-6.
    A prospective study of over 1200 infants demonstrated a direct relationship between the number of solid foods introduced into the diet by 4 months of age and the subsequent development of atopic dermatitis, with a 3-fold increase in recurrent eczema at 10 years of age in infants who had received 4 or more different solid foods before 4 months of age.
    Halken S. Prevention of allergic disease in childhood: clinical and epidemiological aspects of primary and secondary allergy prevention. *Pediatr Allergy Immunol*. 2004;15 Suppl 16:4-5, 9-32.

4. Urticaria refers to a raised, itchy area of skin that is usually a sign of an allergic reaction.

5. An eosinophil is a type of white blood cell involved in allergic and other immune responses that releases histamine and other potentially toxic molecules when activated. The name comes from the characteristic intense red staining seen under the microscope when the dye eosin is used.

6. Wakefield AJ, Ashwood P, Limb K, et al. The significance of ileo-colonic lymphoid nodular hyperplasia in children with autistic spectrum disorder. *Eur J Gastroenterol Hepatol*. 2005;17:827-36.
    Krigsman A, Boris M, Goldblatt A, et al. Clinical presentation and histologic findings at ileocolonoscopy in children with autistic spectrum disorder and chronic gastrointestinal symptoms. *Autism Insights*. 2010;2:1-11.

7. Chen B, Girgis S, El-Matary W. Childhood autism and eosinophilic colitis. *Digestion*. 2010;81:127-9.
    Wakefield AJ, Anthony A, Murch SH, et al. Enterocolitis in children with developmental disorders. *Am J Gastroenterol*. 2000;95:2285-95.

8. Food allergens eliciting a wheal (a raised mark on the skin) that is at least 3 mm greater than the saline control injection are considered positive. See: Sampson HA. Food allergy. Part 2: diagnosis and management. *J Allergy Clin Immunol*. 1999;103:981-9.

9. See www.foodallergytest.com for additional explanation.

10 http://www.truetest.com/PhysicianPDF/HCP23_FinnCh%20details.pdf

11. Wood RA. The natural history of food allergy. *Pediatrics*. 2003;111:1631-7.

12. Hadjivassiliou M, Gibson A, Davies-Jones GA, et al. Does cryptic gluten sensitivity play a part in neurological illness? *Lancet*. 1996;347:369-71.

13. Ibid.

14. Wakefield AJ, Stott C, Limb K. Gastrointestinal co-morbidity, autistic regression and measles-containing vaccines: positive re-challenge and biological gradient effects. *Medical Veritas*. 2006;3:796-802.

15. Hadjivassiliou M, Grünewald R, Sharrack B, et al. Gluten ataxia in perspective: epidemiology, genetic susceptibility and clinical characteristics. *Brain*. 2003;126:685-91.

16. Hadjivassiliou M, Boscolo S, Davies–Jones GA, et al. The humoral response in the pathogenesis of gluten ataxia. *Neurology*. 2002;58:1221-6.

17. Alaedini A, Okamoto H, Briani C, et al. Immune cross-reactivity in celiac disease: anti-gliadin antibodies bind to neuronal synapsin I. *J Immunol*. 2007;178;6590-5.

18. Hadjivassiliou M, Maki M, Sanders DS, et al. Autoantibody targeting of brain and intestinal transglutaminase in gluten ataxia. *Neurology*. 2006;66:373–7.

19. Hadjivassiliou M, Davies-Jones GA, Sanders DS, et al. Dietary treatment of gluten ataxia. *J Neurol Neurosurg Psychiatry*. 2003;74:1221-4.

20. Goldberg D. A psychiatric study of patients with diseases of the small intestine. *Gut.* 1970;11:459-65.
Ciacci C, Iavarone A, Mazzacca G, et al. Depressive symptoms in adult coeliac disease. *Scand J Gastroenterol.* 1998;33:247-50.
Addolorato G, Capristo E, Ghittoni G, et al. Anxiety but not depression decreases in coeliac patients after one-year gluten-free diet: a longitudinal study. *Scand J Gastroenterol.* 2001;36:502-6.

21. Carta MG, Hardoy MC, Boi MF, et al. Association between panic disorder, major depressive disorder, and celiac disease: a possible role for thyroid autoimmunity. *J Psychosom Res.* 2002;53:789-93.

22. Ljungman G, Myrdal U. Compliance in teenagers with celiac disease: a Swedish follow-up study. *Acta Paediatr.* 1993;82:235-8.

23. Hernanz A, Polanco I. Plasma precursor amino acids of central nervous system monoamines in children with celiac disease. *Gut.* 1991;32:1478-81.

24. Fasano A, Catassi C. Current approaches to diagnosis and treatment of celiac disease: an evolving spectrum. *Gastroenterology.* 2001; 120: 636-51.

25. Fabiani E, Taccari LM, Ratsch IM, et al. Compliance with gluten-free diet in adolescents with screening-detected celiac disease: a 5-year follow-up study. *J Pediatr.* 2000; 136: 841-3.

26. Pynnönen PA, Isometsä ET, Verkasalo MA, et al. Gluten-free diet may alleviate depressive and behavioural symptoms in adolescents with coeliac disease: a prospective follow-up case-series study. *BMC Psychiatry.* 2005;5:14.

27. Goodwin MS, Cowen MA, Goodwin TC. Malabsorption and cerebral dysfunction: a multivariate and comparative study of autistic children. *J Autism Child Schizophr.* 1971;1:48-62.

28. Genuis SJ, Bouchard TP. Autism presenting as celiac disease. *J Child Neurol.* 2010;25: 114-9.

29. Randolph TG. Allergy as a causative factor of fatigue, irritability, and behavior problems of children. *J Pediatr.* 1947;31:560-72.

30. Ibid.

31. Ibid.

32. Ibid.

33. Mayron LW. Allergy, learning, and behavior problems. *J Learn Disabil.* 1979;12:32-42.

34. Atkins FM. Food allergy and behavior: definitions, mechanisms, and a review of the evidence. *Nutr Rev.* 1986;44(Suppl):104–12.

35. Controlled trial of oligoantigenic treatment in the hyperkinetic syndrome. Egger, J., Stolla, A., & McEwen, LM. *Lancet*, 1985;325:540-5.

36. Kahn A, Rebuffat E, Blum D, et al. Difficulty in initiating and maintaining sleep associated with cow's milk allergy in infants. *Sleep.* 1987;10:116-21.

37. Basso AS, Pinto FAC, Russo M, et al. Neural correlates of IgE-mediated food allergy. *J Neuroimmunol.* 2003;140:69-77.

38. Theoharides TC. Autism spectrum disorders and mastocytosis. *Int J Immunopathol Pharmacol.* 2009;22:859-65.

39. Theoharides TC, Angelidou A, Alysandratos KD, et al. Mast cell activation and autism. *Biochim Biophys Acta.* 2010 Dec 28. [Epub ahead of print]

40. Asadi S, Zang B, Weng Z, et al. Luteolin and thiosalicylate inhibit HgCl2 and thimerosal-induced VEGF release from human mast cells. *Int J Immunopathol Pharmacol.* 2010;23:1015-20.

41. Breakey J. The role of diet and behaviour in childhood. *J Paediatr Child Health.* 1997;33:190-4.

42. Kaplan BJ, McNicol J, Conte RA, et al. Dietary replacement in preschool-aged hyperactive boys. *Pediatrics.* 1989;83:7-17.

43. Egger J, Carter CM, Graham PJ, et al. Controlled trial of oligoantigenic treatment in the hyperkinetic syndrome. *Lancet.* 1985;1:540-5.
   Pollock I, Warner JO. Effect of artificial food colors on childhood behavior. *Arch Dis Child.* 1990;65:74-7.
   Carter CM, Urbanowicz M, Hemsley R, et al. Effects of a few food diet in attention deficit disorder. *Arch Dis Child.* 1993;69:564-8.
   Rowe KS, Rowe KJ. Synthetic food coloring and behavior: a dose-response effect in a double-blind, placebo-controlled, repeated-measures study. *J Pediatr.* 1994;125(5 Pt 1):691-8.
   Boris M, Mandel FS. Foods and additives are common causes of the attention deficit hyperactive disorder in children. *Ann Allergy.* 1994;72:462-8.
   Schmidt MH, Mocks P, Lay B, et al. Does oligoantigenic diet influence hyperactive/conduct-disordered children—a controlled trial? *Eur Child Adolesc Psychiatry.* 1997;6:88-95.

44. Arnold LE. Treatment alternatives for attention deficit hyperactivity disorder. *NIH Consensus Development Conference on Diagnosis and Treatment of Attention Deficit Hyperactivity Disorder.* November 16–18, 1998. National Institutes of Health, Bethesda, MD.

45. Rice, turkey, lamb, vegetables, fruits, margarine, vegetable oil, tea, pear juice, and water.

46. Pelsser LMJ, Frankena K, Toorman J, et al. A randomized controlled trial into the effects of food on ADHD. *Eur Child Adolesc Psychiatry.* 2009;18:12-19.

47. Pelsser LM, Frankema K, Toorman J, et al. Effects of a restricted elimination diet on the behaviour of children with attention-deficit hyperactivity disorder (INCA study): a randomized controlled trial. *Lancet.* 2011;377:495-503.

48. Ibid.

49. IgA antibodies to casein, α-lactalbumin and β-lactogloduin and IgG and IgG to casein.

50. Lucarelli S, Frediani T, Zingoni AM, et al. Food allergy and infantile autism. *Panminerva Med.* 1995;37:137-41.

51. Horror autotoxicus, literally meaning the horror of self-toxicity, was a term coined by the great German bacteriologist and immunologist Paul Ehrlich (1854-1915) to describe the body's innate aversion to immunological self-destruction. However, the immune system can upon occasion attack itself and does so in autoimmune disorders.

52. Infections, toxic chemicals, and dietary peptides binding to lymphocyte receptors and tissue enzymes are major instigators of autoimmunity in autism. See: Vojdani A, Pangborn JB, Vojdani E, et al. Infections, toxic chemicals and dietary peptides binding to lymphocyte receptors and tissue enzymes are major instigators of autoimmunity in autism. *Int J Immunopathol Pharmacol.* 2003;16:189-99.

53. Vojdani A, Bazargan M, Vojdani E, et al. Heat shock protein and gliadin peptide promote development of peptidase antibodies in children with autism and patients with autoimmune disease. *Clin Diagn Lab Immunol.* 2004;3:515–24.

54. Vojdani A, Campbell B, Anyanwub E, et al. Antibodies to neuron-specific antigens in children with autism: possible cross reaction with encephalitogenic proteins from milk, *Chlamydia pneumonia* and *Streptococcus* group A. *J Neuroimmunol.* 2002;129:168-77.

55. Ashwood P, Anthony A, Pellicer AA, et al. Intestinal lymphocyte populations in children with regressive autism: evidence for extensive mucosal immunopathology. *J Clin Immunol.* 2003;23:504-17.
Wakefield AJ, Puleston J, Montgomery SM, et al. Entero-colonic encephalopathy, autism and opioid receptor ligands. *Aliment Pharmacol Ther.* 2002;16:663-74.
Ashwood P, Anthony A, Torrente F, et al. Spontaneous mucosal lymphocyte cytokine profiles in children with regressive autism and gastrointestinal symptoms: mucosal immune activation and reduced counter regulatory interleukin-10. *J Clin Immunol.* 2004:24:664-73.

56. Jyonouchi H, Sun S, Itokazu N. Innate immunity associated with inflammatory responses and cytokine reduction against common dietary proteins in patients with autism spectrum disorder. *Neuropsychobiology.* 2002;46:76–84.

57. Jyonouchi H, Geng L, Ruby A, et al. Dysregulated innate immune responses in young children with autism spectrum disorders: their relationship to gastrointestinal symptoms and dietary intervention. *Neuropsychobiology.* 2005;51:77–85.

58. Jyonouchi H, Geng L, Ruby A, et al. Evaluation of an association between gastrointestinal symptoms and cytokine production against common dietary proteins in children with autism spectrum disorders. *J Pediatr.* 2005;146:605-10.

59. Casein, β-Lactoglobulin, and α-Lactalbumin.

60. Jyonouchi H, Geng L, Ruby A, et al. Dysregulated innate immune responses in young children with autism spectrum disorders: their relationship to gastrointestinal symptoms and dietary intervention. *Neuropsychobiology.* 2005;51:77–85.

61. Knivsberg AM, Reichelt KL, Høien T, et al. A randomised, controlled study of dietary intervention in autistic syndromes. *Nutr Neurosci.* 2002;5:251-61.

62. Whiteley P, Haracopos D, Knivsberg AM, et al. The ScanBrit randomised, controlled, single-blind study of a gluten- and casein-free dietary intervention for children with autism spectrum disorders. *Nutr Neurosci.* 2010;13:87-100.

63. Ibid.

64. Jyonounchi H, Geng L, Cushing-Ruby A, et al. Mechanisms of non-IgE mediated adverse reaction to common dietary proteins (DPs) in children with autism spectrum disorders (ASD). *J Allergy Clin Immunol.* 2004;113:S208.

65. Jyonouchi H, Sun S, Itokazu N. Innate immunity associated with inflammatory responses and cytokine production against common dietary proteins in patients with autism spectrum disorder. *Neuropsychobiology.* 2002;46:76-84.

66. Jyonuchi H, Geng L, Ruby A, et al. Suboptimal responses to dietary intervention in children with autism spectrum disorder and non-IgE-mediated food allergy. In *Autism Research Advances*, Zhao LB (Ed). (pp. 169-184). Hauppauge, NY: Nova Science Publishers, Inc., 2007.

BIOGRAPHIES

Thomas Borody, MD, PhD, FRACP, FACP, FACG, AGAF, is the founder and medical director of the Centre of Digestive Diseases in Sydney, Australia. He has published over 220 scientific papers and was a clinical fellow in gastroenterology at the Mayo Clinic in Rochester, MN. www.cdd.com.au

***

James Jeffrey Bradstreet, MD, MD(H), FAAFP, is widely published on the various aspects of autism- related biology and comorbidities. He is an adjunct professor of pediatrics at Southwest College of Naturopathic Medicine in Tempe, Arizona, and is licensed in Georgia, Florida, California, and Arizona. www.drbradstreet.org.

***

Geri Brewster, RD, MPH, CDN, is a certified dietitian-nutritionist with a Master of Public Health, who practices in NY. She has advanced areas of study in functional medicine and biomedical therapies. Geri speaks nationally on pediatric special needs, children's health, and nutritional needs. www.geribrewster.com

***

Jordana Campbell, BSc, serves as Research Officer at the Centre for Digestive Diseases in Sydney, Australia. www.cdd.com.au

***

Judy Chinitz, MS, MS, is in private practice at New Star Nutritional Consulting (www.newstarnutrition.com). With Dr. Sidney Baker, Judy cofounded Medigenesis, an Internet-based interactive medical database (www.medigenesis.com). In 2007, Judy published a book on the *Specific Carbohydrate Diet, We Band of Mothers: Autism, My Son and The Specific Carbohydrate Diet.*

***

Richard Deth, PhD, is a Professor of Pharmacology at Northeastern University, where he has maintained a research laboratory since 1976. Currently his lab is focused on understanding the relationship between antioxidant status and methylation reactions, including its role in autism and other neurological disorders.

***

Krystal D. Dubé graduated from Northeastern University with a degree in behavioral neuroscience. She combines her knowledge of the brain with applied behavior analysis strategies for a comprehensive approach to meaningful growth. Krystal currently works as a social educator and behavior therapist at Skills for Living in Norwell, MA.

***

Pamela J. Ferro, RN, ASN, is the cofounder of Hopewell Associates, Inc., and founder of the Gottschall Autism Center. Pam is widely recognized as being an authority on the Specific Carbohydrate DietTM as used in autism. Pam was also one of the original nursing collaborators who developed the DAN! (Defeat Autism Now!) Nurses' Curriculum.

***

Sydney Finegold, MD, is a globally respected microbiologist with more than 50 years of research in intestinal microorganisms. He is chief of the Anaerobic Bacteria

Laboratory at UCLA. He was honored with the Lifetime Achievement Award for his exhaustive work in the field of research at the Veterans Administration in West Los Angeles.

***

Martha R. Herbert, PhD, MD, is a pediatric neurologist and neuroscientist at Massachusetts General Hospital, Harvard Medical School, and the Harvard-MIT-HST-Martinos Center for Biomedical Imaging. Her TRANSCEND Research Program uses advanced brain imaging techniques and biomarkers to look at the relationship of metabolism, perfusion, and brain function, and at brain change with treatment.

***

John H. Hicks II, MD, is the cofounder and medical director of Elementals Living, which is located in Delavan, WI. For over 30 years, Dr. Hicks has dedicated himself to the art and science of integrated holistic medicine. www.elementalsliving.com

***

Nathaniel Hodgson is a doctoral student at Northeastern University.

***

Arthur Krigsman, MD, is a pediatrician and board certified pediatric gastroenterologist who has evaluated and treated over 1700 children suffering from autism and a variety of GI problems. He maintains offices in NYC and Austin, is actively involved in clinical research, and has presented his findings in peer-reviewed journals, scientific meetings, and at a congressional hearing. www.autismgi.com

***

Nancy Mullan, MD, is an author, lecturer, and clinician best known for her natural approach to treatment and recovery from ASD. Practicing for 30 years, she currently practices nutritional medicine and psychiatry in Burbank, California, treating children on the autism spectrum and adults with hormonal, gastroenterologic, neurologic, and/or metabolic dysfunction. www.nancymullanmd.com

***

Raman Prasad, MS, has successfully followed the Specific Carbohydrate Diet™ for more than 15 years. In 1998, he founded the online recipe database www.scdrecipe.com. Raman is the author of the non-fiction memoir *Colitis & Me: A Story of Recovery* and the two SCD™ cookbooks *Recipes for the Specific Carbohydrate Diet* and *Adventures in the Family Kitchen*.

***

Daniel A. Rossignol, MD, FAAFP, has had, in the last seven years, 23 publications and 3 book chapters concerning autism and related conditions. Dr. Rossignol is a Fellow of the American Academy of Family Physicians (FAAFP) and is president of the Medical Academy of Pediatric Special Needs (MAPS), which provides education and long-term support for practitioners.

***

Malav Trivedi is a doctoral student at Northeastern University.

***

Biographies

Lauren Underwood, PhD, received her doctorate in biology from Tulane University and was awarded an NIH Post-Doctoral Fellowship. She works for NASA, Office of the Chief Technologist. Dr. Underwood co-authored several chapters in the book *Understanding Autism for Dummies* and has served as the scientific consultant for *Autism Science Digest*.

***

Michael Wagnitz is employed as a chemist in the toxicology section of a public health laboratory. Michael has spent the last 12 years doing whatever is possible to address the underlying medical problems of children diagnosed with autism spectrum disorders.

***

Andrew Wakefield, MB, BS, is an academic gastroenterologist. He received his medical degree from St. Mary's Hospital Medical School (part of the University of London) in 1981. Dr. Wakefield is the author of *Callous Disregard* and *Waging War on the Autistic Child*. He has published over 140 original scientific articles, book chapters, and invited scientific commentaries.

***

Stephen Walker, PhD, has been a member of the FDA-sponsored International Microarray Quality Control (MAQC) consortium since its inception in 2005. He is currently an associate professor at the Wake Forest Institute for Regenerative Medicine. He is on the graduate faculty and serves as faculty in the neuroscience and medical genetics programs.

***

Carol Wester, RN, MSN, PMHCNS, BC, is the cofounder of Hopewell Associates, Inc., and is a board certified clinical nurse specialist in psychiatric and mental health nursing, who has worked with adults with developmental and intellectual disabilities for over 30 years. Carol was one of the original collaborators who developed the DAN! (Defeat Autism Now!) Nurses' Curriculum.

***

Amy Yasko, PhD, AMD, FAAIM, was a consultant to the medical, pharmaceutical, and research communities for almost 20 years with an expertise in biochemistry, molecular biology, and biotechnology. She holds doctorates in microbiology, immunology, infectious diseases, naturopathy, and natural health.